MEDICINE IN LITERATURE

ENGLISH AND HUMANITIES SERIES

ADVISORY EDITOR: Lee A. Jacobus
University of Connecticut, Storrs

Adolescence in Literature
Thomas West Gregory

Business in Literature
Charles A. Burden, Elke Burden, Lynn Ganim, and Sterling Eisiminger

Fifty Contemporary Poets: The Creative Process
Alberta T. Turner

Medicine in Literature
Joseph Ceccio

Sharing Literature with Children: A Thematic Anthology
Francelia Butler

Short Stories from Around the World
Lee A. Jacobus

Sports in Literature
Henry B. Chapin

Writing in the Margin: From Annotation to Critical Essay
Ronald Primeau

MEDICINE IN LITERATURE

JOSEPH CECCIO
Wright State University

LONGMAN
New York and London

PN
6071
.M38
M4

*For my wife, Cathy,
and my mother, Tina*

MEDICINE IN LITERATURE

Longman Inc., New York

Associated companies, branches, and representatives throughout the world.

Copyright © 1978 by Longman Inc.

Developmental Editor: Gordon T. R. Anderson
Manuscript and Editorial Supervisor: Nicole Benevento
Design: Pencils Portfolio, Inc.
Manufacturing and Production Supervisor: Louis Gaber
Composing: The Book Press
Printing and Binding: The Book Press

Library of Congress Cataloging in Publication Data
Ceccio, Joseph F.
    Medicine in literature.
    (English and humanities series)
    Bibliography:
    1.   Medicine—Literary collections. I. Title.
II. Series.
PN6071.M38C4   808.8′031   77–18308
ISBN 0–582–28051–6

Manufactured in the United States of America

Acknowledgments

"On the Examination Table" by Vassar Miller. Reprinted from *If I Could Sleep Deeply Enough*, poems by Vassar Miller. By permission of Liveright Publishing Corporation. Copyright © 1968, 1972, 1973, 1974 by Vassar Miller.

"The Consultation" by Richard Selzer. From *Rituals of Surgery* by Richard Selzer. Copyright © 1974 by Richard Selzer. By permission of Harper & Row, Publishers.

"Diabetes" by James Dickey. "Diabetes" from *The Eye-Beaters, Blood, Victory, Madness, Buckhead and Mercy* by James Dickey. Copyright © 1968, 1969, 1970 by James Dickey. Reprinted by permission of Doubleday & Company, Inc.

"The Use of Force" by Wiliam Carlos Williams. William Carlos Williams, *The Farmers' Daughters*. Copyright 1938 by William Carlos Williams. Reprinted by permission of New Directions Publishing Corporation.

"A Country Doctor" by Franz Kafka. Reprinted by permission of Schocken Books Inc. from *The Penal Colony* by Franz Kafka. Copyright 1948 by Schocken Books Inc. Copyright renewed © 1975 By Schocken Books Inc.

"The Hospital" by Robert Lowell. Reprinted with the permission of Farrar, Straus & Giroux, Inc. from *Notebook 1967–68* by Robert Lowell, copyright © 1967, 1968, 1969 by Robert Lowell.

"Unknown Girl in the Maternity Ward" by Anne Sexton. From *To Bedlam and Part Way Back*, by Anne Sexton. Copyright © 1960 by Anne Sexton. Reprinted by permission of Houghton Mifflin Company.

"The Surgeon at 2 A.M." by Sylvia Plath. From *Crossing the Water* by Sylvia Plath. Copyright © 1962 by Ted Hughes. By permission of Harper & Row, Publishers.

"The Horse Dealer's Daughter" by D. H. Lawrence. From *The Complete Short Stories of D. H. Lawrence*, Volume II. Copyright 1922 by Thomas B. Seltzer, Inc., 1950 by Frieda Lawrence. Reprinted by permission of The Viking Press.

"Doctor's Wife" by Joyce Carol Oates. Reprinted by permission of Louisiana State University from *Anonymous Sins and Other Poems* by Joyce Carol Oates, copyright © 1969.

"The Dentist's Wife" by William Melvin Kelley. Reprinted by permission of William Morris Agency, Inc. Copyright © 1958 by William Melvin Kelley.

"Doctor, I can't . . . I won't have a child" by A. J. Cronin. Copyright 1935, 1937, 1938, 1939, 1943, 1946, 1948, 1949, 1950, 1951, 1952 by A. J. Cronin. From *Adventures in Two Worlds* by A. J. Cronin, by permission of Little, Brown and Co.

Contents

Introduction

The course that I teach at Wright State University called Medicine in Literature forms the basis for this thematic book. My dual background as a college teacher of writing and literature and as a former surgical technician at military hospitals in Texas and Kansas has enabled me to develop this course and the resulting anthology, as well as to derive great satisfaction from exploring this fascinatingly interdisciplinary field.

In terms of enjoyment and enlightenment, this critical anthology offers much to a wide variety of readers. It can appeal to students of English composition who seek a context within which to write meaningful papers, to students of medicine and literature who need a solid textbook for a quarter or semester, as well as to general readers who just want to expand their horizons. The book is suitable as a basic text for thematic courses *both* in literature *and* in writing at two-year and four-year colleges. University premedical and medical students, and students in the allied health technologies, will be especially challenged by this intriguing collection of relevant readings.

Planned and written for the nonspecialist, *Medicine in Literature* progresses thematically and is divided into six parts; there is an overall balance among the genres of fiction, poetry, and drama. Not only are twentieth-century American authors and their works generally emphasized, but many writers who are also physicians or nurses are represented. Significant contributions come from women and members of minority groups. All selections are reasonably short, self-contained, and eminently readable. Each part of the book is preceded by an original introduction which places that part's selections in proper context and suggests several approaches for interpretation. And each part concludes with a set of classroom-tested topics for discussion and for writing.

This anthology is unique in that it includes more readings on the medicine-in-literature theme from American, British, and world literature than have ever appeared together before. Instructors of courses in Medicine in Literature—myself included—now have a single volume that reflects the great breadth and scope of the subject. And the selected bibliography at the book's end makes it easy for readers to follow up in more detail any one of the six major thematic areas.

The six parts of *Medicine in Literature*—on the individual themes of medicine and interpersonal relationships, medicine and humor, medicine and mental health, medicine and the scientific impulse, medicine and the nurse, and medicine and its limitations—possess an essential unity in at least two ways. First, the six parts reveal a general-specific-general movement. Second, the parts, when taken as a whole, give a rather comprehensive picture of the medicine-in-literature topic.

The opening part, "Medicine and Interpersonal Relationships," provides a general orientation for the reader. Here we are introduced to the patient-doctor relationship as expressed in literature as well as to three important subtopics: the medical examination, the medical institution, and the doctor's world. The central four parts then go on to explore key facets of our overall theme. The second part, "Medicine and Humor," shows that creative works dealing with medicine-in-literature themes do not always tell a sad, serious, or morbid story. While several selections in part 1 use humor primarily for comic relief, those in part 2 use humor as the major focus (contrast, for instance, "The Consultation" with *The Doctor in Spite of Himself*).

The third part, "Medicine and Mental Health," develops a theme already previewed by part 2's humorous tale, "The Haunted Quack." The fourth part, "Medicine and the Scientific Impulse," in turn treats the relationship between medical practice and medical science, a relationship that part 3's "Ward Six" previously touched upon. With the fifth part, "Medicine and the Nurse," we highlight allied health professionals, many of whom have appeared in earlier selections but who now take their turn at center stage. The last part, "Medicine and Its Limitations," probes the three broad themes of death, fate, and the limits of medicine. This return to a general orientation fulfills the promise of part 6. The final selection, "The Curse of Eve," lends itself to an illuminating analysis in which it is possible to trace throughout Doyle's short story the various resonances of this anthology's six major thematic areas.

In addition to this general-specific-general movement, my rationale for having these six linked parts springs from the fact that these are the major subject categories in which creative authors have done the most and the best work. The six parts, when taken together, paint a fairly comprehensive picture of the medicine-in-literature topic. Readers of the anthology will find a wealth of interesting material as they discover, throughout the six related parts, how and why the various thematic strands fit together. The journey through *Medicine in Literature* will be a pleasurable and a profitable one!

For her suggestions on form and content and for her assistance on several medical and technical matters, I wish to thank Cathy M. Ceccio, R.N. And I shall always be grateful to Professor Allan Holaday of the University of Illinois for his continuing guidance and sound advice on both literary and professional matters. Many thanks are also due to Longman senior editor, Gordon T. R. Anderson, and to advisory editor Lee A. Jacobus of the University of Connecticut, for taking time from their busy schedules to aid in the development of this textbook. Finally, I wish to acknowledge Wright State's Liberal Arts Research Committee for a grant that helped make *Medicine in Literature* a reality.

Part 1

Medicine and Interpersonal Relationships

This initial part introduces our central topic and simultaneously sets the stage for the five parts that successively develop it. The selections in this part illustrate three important themes: the medical examination, the medical institution or hospital, and the doctor's world. Here we are primarily interested in seeing how various interpersonal relationships grow, change, or become strained.

The first five selections show the authors' points of view about the medical examination and some of its consequences. Perhaps nothing is as personal—even sacred—to a patient as having the "knowing hand" of a physician touch, palpate, inspect, and percuss the parts of his or her body. This touching is essential in the doctor's role as "healer," but the very act of examining a patient can sometimes establish a relationship that demands too much from the doctor and very little from the patient. The use of touch is *the* significant concept in the examination: the patient lets down defenses and permits his or her body to be analyzed and viewed in the name of science and health. Yet the examination often provokes great feelings of alarm and inadequacy in the patient.

Vassar Miller's poem "On the Examination Table" is an especially moving statement. The poet-speaker, who herself is handicapped with cerebral palsy, describes her intense feelings of depersonalization during the physical examination. No doctor is mentioned in this poem, but the speaker's physical reactions to the examination indicate a strong sense of terror as her bodily integrity is diminished by what the poet perceives as a negative ritual of medical automaticity. The unspoken relationship between physician and patient seems cold, uncaring, and dehumanizing. Must it be this way?

Sociologists believe that rituals help organize our lives, give stability to our practices, defend our traditions. The ritual has always been important in medicine, too; hence, the creative literature dealing with medicine is abundantly filled with descriptions of different rituals. The physical examination is just such a ritual (surgery is another). As the doctor examines a patient to gather specific information upon which to base a diagnosis, the ritual of the examination frequently becomes a reassuring event for the patient—an event that many patients even seek out willingly. But what happens when the role of the patient is conferred upon a young woman most unwilling to accept the ritual of an examination? In "The Consultation," Richard Selzer, a contemporary American surgeon and short-story writer, recounts a strangely surprising examination ritual. Bored with technical exhibits at a medical convention, a surgeon arranges for a night's diversion with a prostitute. The level of the relationship soon turns from the personal to the professional after the doctor discovers a lump in the woman's right breast. A casual caress results in an expert examination; roles change as the man becomes the physician and the prostitute becomes the patient. *Tactus eruditus,* the knowing or wise touch of the doctor, assists Selzer's physician-lover in quickly reassuming his professional role.

Patients with chronic diseases often have acute difficulty in acknowledging their illnesses—a situation that is well portrayed in James Dickey's poem "Diabetes." Here the more important interpersonal relationship is not between the speaker and the young physician who makes the diagnosis, but between the speaker and the disease itself. Dickey shows how a man and his chronic disease coexist and even protect each other; ultimately, of course, they wage war and vie for supremacy over the beleaguered body. Perhaps Dickey's best revelation of the délicate relationship the man has with his disease comes in a scene that depicts one pocket holding an insulin syringe and the other laden with sugar. The diabetic needs insulin daily, for his body no longer produces the vital hormone that helps metabolize sugar; yet too much insulin can send a diabetic into a coma; so a quick source of carbohydrate ("sugar cubes to balance me in life") must be close at hand. Maintaining a diabetic's blood sugar "Level, level" can be a tricky business, and the fear of being an uncontrolled diabetic is constantly present in the poem.

Good doctors examine their patients quickly, deftly, with a minimum of discomfort, especially if their patients are children. A careful, thorough, and gentle touch aids in establishing rapport with the child and with the parents. In "The Use of Force," the famous physician-writer William Carlos Williams tells of a doctor's visit to a young patient's house. When he attempts to examine the little girl's throat, she is most uncooperative. The doctor grows angry and frustrated, but because he fears an epidemic of the dreaded diphtheria he must use force to examine the child. Dr. Williams masterfully portrays in this story the love-hate relationship that develops between the doctor, on the one hand, and the child and her parents, on the other.

The dreamlike, surrealistic ambience of Franz Kafka's "A Country Doctor" seems to keep the examination of a young boy with a serious hip wound on a symbolic level. Kafka takes us on a strange and frightful journey as he juxtaposes the natural, snowy world outside the sick boy's home and the closed atmosphere within the peasant sickroom. Because the relationships that unfold between the district physician and his patient's family are surrealistically stylized, in this case the ritual of the examination is less important than the ritual of healing. Only when the doctor is forcefully stripped of his clothes and status is he able to lie beside his patient and effect a "cure." We might profitably discuss how, specifically, Kafka's nightmarish tale—written as one long paragraph—is both similar to and yet different from the four selections that precede it.

The next three works are poems by twentieth-century American writers that deal with the medical institution or hospital and how it affects and is affected by interpersonal relationships. The irony of Robert Lowell's sonnet "The Hospital" is that the vague relationships hinted at in the poem are not really personal at all and that the obvious sources of information are false: for example, corpses look alive and living patients appear dead. Any suggestion of a caring human being would surely be welcome, but Lowell offers nothing except "tubes" and "jugs of dim blue doctored water."

The mother-child bond as first represented in Anne Sexton's "Unknown Girl in the Maternity Ward" holds great promise of fruition until the speaker tells the child: "But this is an institution bed. / You will not know me very long." The institution, that large and impersonal hospital with its "starch halls," seems to color the attitudes of "enamel" doctors and busy nurses. The hospital's coldness may even reflect the developing detachment between the girl and her new baby. Perhaps the young woman will give up her bastard child to but another institution in the near future.

Sylvia Plath's "The Surgeon at 2 A.M." specifies how at least one surgeon envisions himself at work in the middle of the night. The antiseptic atmosphere of the starkly hygienic hospital and operating room sets the tone for the relationship that the surgeon has with the patient, the patient's body, and the assistants with whom the surgeon works. The dehumanized hospital supports this godlike surgeon as he dissects, explores, even perfects the separate parts of the patient's body, which are compared to various aspects of nature, for instance, "I worm and hack in a purple wilderness" and "The blood is a sunset." In the end, we are forced to wonder if this doctor is capable of having any kind of a sensitive relationship with people where he is *not* like "the sun" in his "white coat" and where "Grey faces, shuttered by drugs" do *not* constantly follow him "like flowers."

The last four selections deal with the doctor's world. Aside from the relationship that the doctor forms with patients, the most significant associations in the doctor's world revolve around wife or husband, family, and friends. Traditionally, it has been hard for some physicians to believe they have a right to a personal life apart from their professional life. This theme informs much of D. H. Lawrence's "The Horse Dealer's Daughter," in which a young country surgeon rescues a poor girl from a suicide attempt, only to have her fall in love with him and he with her. The doctor becomes enmeshed in a swift but painful conversion to lover—a development that seems dramatically at odds with his previously measured and ordered life as the local physician.

In Joyce Carol Oates' poem "Doctor's Wife," we find an interesting if somewhat complex portrait of a doctor and his role as sketched by his angry wife. While she may well understand that her husband's married life must at many times give way to the demands of his profession, the doctor's wife seems to feel that her husband could and should control the level of his involvement with patients: "Your lips speak and never say 'Enough, enough—' "

The theme of the frustrated or unfulfilled wife continues as part of William Melvin Kelley's "The Dentist's Wife." Kelley, a contemporary black American author, writes with a subtly ironic twist; he focuses on a dentist's wife who is unhappy with her husband's Harlem practice. The wife, who once yearned for her husband's material success among white professionals, has now attained a heightened social consciousness and wonders if the dentist should not be doing "something good for our race." The dentist, for his part, wants to be rid of his wife. Kelley's perceptive handling of some thorny moral and sexual issues makes this story with its surprise ending well worth reading.

Finally, A. J. Cronin's pointed autobiographical sketch "Doctor, I can't . . . I won't have a child" illustrates the demands that patients who are also friends often make upon their physicians. A woman acquaintance asks Dr. Cronin for an abortion, but he refuses; she subsequently goes to a local abortionist, experiences complications, then desperately calls for Cronin's help. How he handles this intricate situation ethically but discreetly proves fascinating. This story, which like the Kelley piece raises the crucial topic of medical ethics, is clearly relevant for modern times despite changes in abortion laws during recent years.

VASSAR MILLER

On the Examination Table

My eyes, two birds
crazily threshing
in the trap of their sockets,

my tongue, dry leaf
ready to fall
to the pit of my throat,

my breath, fragile moth
caught in a cave-in
of my gullet's tight tunnel,

> my belly, overturned turtle,
> stripped from the shell
> of daily decorum,
>
> my body, dull dog,
> shies into terror's
> mythical monster.

RICHARD SELZER

The Consultation

He walked the center aisle of the convention hall, past stands of textbooks on *Surgical Anatomy, Complications of Surgery, Peripheral Vascular Diseases— Their Diagnosis and Treatment*. Other stalls gleamed with instruments—rows of proctoscopes, bronchoscopes, gastroscopes, rigid with potential, awaiting on one end a palpitating orifice, on the other a knowing eye. Here were forceps, clamps of the finest dentition. He tried one in his hand, listening to the impeccable click as the ratchets locked tight, tighter, tightest, a sound that had both frightened and comforted him all his professional life. There were scalpels of superior edge, their silver bellies as diverse as tropical fish, and retractors for holding open incisions, retractors of such cleverness as to match the ingenuity of a royal armorer.

Suddenly he was bored with it, the lectures, the instruments, the whole gadgetry of surgery, the rooms full of well-dressed men who all looked forty-five years old. . . . He would call her up.

She had a shockingly virtuous telephone voice which placed the brief arrangements over price in the grossest ill taste.

"Shall I pick you up at your hotel?"

"Fine."

"Oh, yes. Dinner first?"

"I'd love to. Where?"

"You choose it."

"What time?"

"Seven-thirty be all right?"

"Fine. Looking forward. . . ."

The illusion of romance was under way.

Gloria Snurkowski was the name he had been given to look up. He had laughed then at the idea of a Polish prostitute. Still, she had to be *something*.

He was reassured when he saw her an hour later in the lobby of the hotel, serpentine, icy, impeccably dehumanized. Except for one thing—a gesture. Now and then she would place the third and fourth fingers of her hand to the corner of her mouth and press them against the underlying teeth. It was a Polish peasant's move. He was certain that her grandmother had done it a thousand times in the middle of her wheat field. But that was the only thing she had overlooked. The rest was perfect.

In the morning he had awakened first. One eye was buried in the pillow but with the other he followed the tide of her breathing. She was lying on her side, part of her back resting against him. A golden stripe of sunshine appeared abruptly between two slats of the Venetian blind and lit up the mountain range of her shoulder. His eye skied down her neck, leaped off the ridge of her clavicle, and descended to the upper slope of the breast in a squinting shower of light. His vision paused for a moment at the foot of the slope, then moved on up the smooth ascent, slowly, gradually, passing through a small shaded declivity, then up again into the sunlight toward the nipple. He held it there until the strain of looking so far to the side made itself felt, then relaxed, and sped down the far side. Halfway down, his vision was jarred by a small rise. Automatically, he backed up the hill like a rewinding movie, then flicked the switch and let it go again. There, where the bump was on the trail, the skin was different, pitted by a shallow dimple. He raised his left arm to bring his hand around to the breast, and palmed it carefully. When she did not stir, he moved his fingers to the southern slope, sounding the depths as he went. He was moving over the rough spot now, his fingers growing exploratory, aggressive, deft. He picked up tissue between thumb and fingers, rotating it, fathoming. She moaned in discomfort, still asleep.

A cold white knowledge drifted into his mind like a snowfall, each flake of which was a bit of evidence. The lump was hard. It was discrete. It was irregular in shape. It was fixed to the overlying skin, fixed as well to the underlying muscle. It was immovable. It was tender. And his palpating fingers fled from her body like frightened fish in a pond. The suddenness of their departure was what fully awakened her.

He swung his feet to the floor and padded across the carpet to the bathroom, where he showered long and deliberately. He dried himself and went back to the bed, where he sat down and reached for his socks on the floor. She turned, and one of her hands reached around his waist, dipping.

"You're getting dressed?"

"Yes, I've got to be going."

With his back to her, he said, "I've got to talk to you."

"It's a hundred dollars."

"No, no, I don't mean that. I mean, that's O.K., a hundred dollars. Here." He reached for his wallet, counted out a fifty and five tens, and held it out to her.

She raised up on one elbow, watched this very carefully, and said, "Put it on the table." Then she sank back and watched him dress.

"You're buttoning your shirt wrong. You missed one."

He unbuttoned it and started again from the bottom. "There's something I've got to tell you," he began again.

"You're not sick, are you?" She was paying attention now.

"No, I'm not." ... A pause. "But you are."

"What do you mean?"

"Listen. I'm a doctor, as you know." His voice took on a deeper, more professional tone, but his armpits were wet. "I couldn't help but feel ..." Her open naïve mouth, her eyes wide and waiting ... "You've got a lump in your breast." He couldn't turn away from her.

Her face stayed vacant.

"A lump. I felt it. Right side."

She moved from her elbow to her back, settling onto the bed.

"Here." He picked up her hand as though it were a cup of coffee, and guided it to her breast. Holding the fingers, he led them toward the spot and pressed them down, moving them in a circular fashion. Her face changed slowly, tightened around enlarging eyes. Her lips were closed and dry.

"Do you feel it?"

She nodded slightly. "Yes."

"You've got to see a doctor. It must be taken care of."

"What is it?"

"I don't know." He shrugged and turned away. "Maybe it's nothing."

"It's something, isn't it?"

"I don't know. You can't tell until it's removed."

"You know."

"I don't know, I tell you."

"You're a doctor. You know. If it is, what do they do?"

He hadn't meant to go this far. "If it isn't, there's only a small scar. It won't show."

"And if it is? They will take off my breast." It was said as an announcement, flatly, without inflection. "I won't do it."

"You have to. It's important."

She covered her breasts with her arm, protectively, the palm of one hand gripping the opposite shoulder.

"Doctor." She was strange to him, formal, as though she had not just a few hours before felt him explode against her. "I can't do that."

"Look, I'm talking about your life, not your livelihood."

Their voices were low, surreptitious. They knew only words of one syllable. It was as though they kept them that way, afraid that if they raised them, spoke out loud, their sentences would crumble into meaningless noises.

"What is it? Tell me."

"I don't know."

"You ought to."
"But I don't."
"What should I . . . ?"
"It needs to come out."
"No!"
"Be sensible. It might be . . ."
"Cancer."

She had said it first. All along it had been a game, not unlike choosing sides by gripping a baseball bat to see who wins first choice. He had won; she had said it first. She reached for her slip and shyly lowered it over her head, then with small furtive movements she put her arms through the strap holes. There was about her the caved-in look of the victim. It made him vaguely nauseated. Not the strangeness of the word; certainly he knew it over and again in his daily work. Nor the translation of it into suffering. But rather what sickened him was the thought that he and the lump had been rivals, each feeding on her flesh, reaching within her, that they had been competing for her in a kind of race to have her before the other could use her all up, leaving none.

His fingers scuttled to the doorknob and locked around it like pincers. He turned to find her eyes fixed on his hand now palming the doorknob.

"Well, good-bye. Be sensible, now. You can only tell under the microscope. Anyway, it's a small price to pay in exchange for your life."

Her eyes never wavered from that doorknob, which was a hard lump in his hand. With sudden violence he twisted it as hard as he could and pulled as though to avulse it from the wood.

"Wait!" She walked to the table and picked up one of the ten-dollar bills. "Here. Thanks for the consultation." She was smiling just a little now.

He matched her smile, but his mouth was dry. "Sorry," he said softly then. "I don't make house calls."

JAMES DICKEY

Diabetes

I
Sugar

One night I thirsted like a prince
Then like a king
Then like an empire   like a world
On fire. I rose and flowed away and fell

Once more to sleep. In an hour I was back
In the kingdom   staggering, my belly going round with self-
Made night-water, wondering what
The hell. Months of having a tongue
Of flame convinced me: I had better not go
On this way. The doctor was young

And nice. He said, I must tell you,
My friend, that it is needles moderation
And exercise. You don't want to look forward
To gangrene and kidney

Failure   boils blindness infection skin trouble falling
Teeth coma and death.
                            O.K.
                                      In sleep my mouth went dry
With my answer   and in it burned the sands
Of time with new fury. Sleep could give me no water
But my own. Gangrene in white
Was in my wife's hand at breakfast
Heaped like a mountain. Moderation, moderation,
My friend, and exercise. Each time the barbell
                Rose   each time a foot fell
                Jogging, it counted itself
One death   two death   three death and resurrection
For a little while. Not bad! I always knew it would have to be
                                      somewhere around
                The house: the real
                Symbol of Time I could eat
And live with, coming true when I opened my mouth:
                True in the coffee and the child's birthday
                Cake   helping sickness be fire-
                tongued, sleepless and water-
                logged   but not bad, sweet sand
                Of time, my friend, an everyday—
                A livable death at last.

                            II
                      Under Buzzards

                                    [for Robert Penn Warren]

Heavy summer. Heavy. Companion, if we climb our mortal bodies
        High with great effort, we shall find ourselves
                Flying with the life

Of the birds of death. We have come up
Under buzzards   they face us

Slowly   slowly circling   and as we watch them they turn us
Around, and you and I spin
Slowly, slowly rounding
Out the hill. We are level
Exactly on this moment: exactly on the same bird-

plane with those deaths. They are the salvation of our sense
Of glorious movement. Brother, it is right for us to face
Them every which way, and come to ourselves and come
From every direction
There is. Whirl and stand fast!
Whence cometh death, O Lord?
On the downwind, riding fire,

Of Hogback Ridge.
                    But listen: what is dead here?
They are not falling but waiting   but waiting
Riding, and they may know
The rotten, nervous sweetness of my blood.
Somewhere riding the updraft
Of a far forest fire, they sensed the city sugar
The doctors found in time.
My eyes are green as lettuce with my diet,
My weight is down,
One pocket nailed with needles and injections, the other dragging
With sugar cubes to balance me in life
And hold my blood
Level, level. Tell me, black riders, does this do any good?
Tell me what I need to know about my time
In the world. O out of the fiery

Furnace of pine-woods, in the sap-smoke and crownfire of needles,
Say when I'll die. When will the sugar rise boiling
Against me, and my brain be sweetened
to death?
          In heavy summer, like this day.
All right! Physicians, witness! I will shoot my veins
Full of insulin. Let the needle burn
In. From your terrible heads
The flight-blood drains   and you are falling back
Back to the body-raising

Fire.
Heavy summer. Heavy. My blood is clear
For a time. Is it too clear? Heat waves are rising
Without birds. But something is gone from me,
Friend. This is too sensible. Really it is better
To know when to die   better for my blood
To stream with the death-wish of birds.
You know, I had just as soon crush
This doomed syringe
Between two mountain rocks, and bury this needle in needles

Of trees. Companion, open that beer.
How the body works   how hard it works
For its medical books is not
Everything: everything is how
Much glory is in it: heavy summer is right

For a long drink of beer. Red sugar of my eyeballs
Feels them turn blindly
In the fire   rising   turning   turning
Back to Hogback Ridge, and it is all
Delicious, brother: my body is turning   is flashing unbalanced
Sweetness everywhere, and I am calling my birds.

WILLIAM CARLOS WILLIAMS

The Use of Force

They were new patients to me, all I had was the name, Olson. Please come down as soon as you can, my daughter is very sick.

When I arrived I was met by the mother, a big startled-looking woman, very clean and apologetic who merely said, Is this the doctor? and let me in. In the back, she added. You must excuse us, doctor, we have her in the kitchen where it is warm. It is very damp here sometimes.

The child was fully dressed and sitting on her father's lap near the kitchen table. He tried to get up, but I motioned for him not to bother, took off my overcoat and started to look things over. I could see that they were all very nervous, eyeing me up and down distrustfully. As often, in such cases, they weren't telling me more than they had to, it was up to me to tell them; that's why they were spending three dollars on me.

The child was fairly eating me up with her cold, steady eyes, and no expression to her face whatever. She did not move and seemed, inwardly, quiet; an unusually attractive little thing, and as strong as a heifer in appearance. But her face was flushed, she was breathing rapidly, and I realized that she had a high fever. She had magnificent blonde hair, in profusion. One of those picture children often reproduced in advertising leaflets and the photogravure sections of the Sunday papers.

She's had a fever for three days, began the father and we don't know what it comes from. My wife has given her things, you know, like people do, but it don't do no good. And there's been a lot of sickness around. So we tho't you'd better look her over and tell us what is the matter.

As doctors often do I took a trial shot at it as a point of departure. Has she had a sore throat?

Both parents answered me together, No . . . No, she says her throat don't hurt her.

Does your throat hurt you? added the mother to the child. But the little girl's expression didn't change nor did she move her eyes from my face.

Have you looked?

I tried to, said the mother, but I couldn't see.

As it happens we had been having a number of cases of diphtheria in the school to which this child went during that month and we were all, quite apparently, thinking of that, though no one had as yet spoken of the thing.

Well, I said, suppose we take a look at the throat first. I smiled in my best professional manner and asking for the child's first name I said, come on, Mathilda, open your mouth and let's take a look at your throat.

Nothing doing.

Aw, come on, I coaxed, just open your mouth wide and let me take a look. Look, I said opening both hands wide, I haven't anything in my hands. Just open up and let me see.

Such a nice man, put in the mother. Look how kind he is to you. Come on, do what he tells you to. He won't hurt you.

At that I ground my teeth in disgust. If only they wouldn't use that word "hurt" I might be able to get somewhere. But I did not allow myself to be hurried or disturbed but speaking quietly and slowly I approached the child again.

As I moved my chair a little nearer suddenly with one catlike movement both her hands clawed instinctively for my eyes and she almost reached them too. In fact she knocked my glasses flying and they fell, though unbroken, several feet away from me on the kitchen floor.

Both the mother and father turned themselves inside out in embarrassment and apology. You bad girl, said the mother, taking her and shaking her by one arm. Look what you've done. The nice man . . .

For heaven's sake, I broke in. Don't call me a nice man to her. I'm here to look at her throat on the chance that she might have diphtheria and possibly die of it. But that's nothing to her. Look here, I said to the child, we're going to look at your throat. You're old enough to understand what I'm saying. Will you open it now by yourself or shall we have to open it for you?

Not a move. Even her expression hadn't changed. Her breaths however were coming faster and faster. Then the battle began. I had to do it. I had to have a throat culture for her own protection. But first I told the parents that it was entirely up to them. I explained the danger but said that I would not insist on a throat examination so long as they would take the responsibility.

If you don't do what the doctor says you'll have to go to the hospital, the mother admonished her severely.

Oh yeah? I had to smile to myself. After all, I had already fallen in love with the savage brat, the parents were contemptible to me. In the ensuing struggle they grew more and more abject, crushed, exhausted, while she surely rose to magnificent heights of insane fury of effort bred of her terror of me.

The father tried his best, and he was a big man but the fact that she was his daughter, his shame at her behavior and his dread of hurting her made him release her just at the critical moment several times when I had almost achieved success, till I wanted to kill him. But his dread also that she might have diphtheria made him tell me to go on, go on though he himself was almost fainting, while the mother moved back and forth behind us raising and lowering her hands in an agony of apprehension.

Put her in front of your lap, I ordered, and hold both her wrists.

But as soon as he did the child let out a scream. Don't, you're hurting me. Let go of my hands. Let them go I tell you. Then she shrieked terrifyingly, hysterically. Stop it! Stop it! You're killing me!

Do you think she can stand it, doctor! said the mother.

You get out, said the husband to his wife. Do you want her to die of diphtheria?

Come on now, hold her, I said.

Then I grasped the child's head with my left hand and tried to get the wooden tongue depressor between her teeth. She fought, with clenched teeth, desperately! But now I also had grown furious—at a child. I tried to hold myself down but I couldn't. I know how to expose a throat for inspection. And I did my best. When finally I got the wooden spatula behind the last teeth and just the point of it into the mouth cavity, she opened up for an instant but before I could see anything she came down again and gripping the wooden blade between her molars she reduced it to splinters before I could get it out again.

Aren't you ashamed, the mother yelled at her. Aren't you ashamed to act like that in front of the doctor?

Get me a smooth-handled spoon of some sort, I told the mother. We're going through with this. The child's mouth was already bleeding. Her tongue was cut and she was screaming in wild hysterical shrieks. Perhaps I should have desisted and come back in an hour or more. No doubt it would have been better. But I have seen at least two children lying dead in bed of neglect in such cases, and feeling that I must get a diagnosis now or never I went at it again. But the worst of it was that I too had got beyond reason. I could have torn the child apart in my own fury and enjoyed it. It was a pleasure to attack her. My face was burning with it.

The damned little brat must be protected against her own idiocy, one says to one's self at such times. Others must be protected against her. It is social necessity. And all these things are true. But a blind fury, a feeling of adult shame, bred of a longing for muscular release are the operatives. One goes on to the end.

In a final unreasoning assault I overpowered the child's neck and jaws. I forced the heavy silver spoon back of her teeth and down her throat till she gagged. And there it was—both tonsils covered with membrane. She had fought valiantly to keep me from knowing her secret. She had been hiding that sore throat for three days at least and lying to her parents in order to escape just such an outcome as this.

Now truly she *was* furious. She had been on the defensive before but now she attacked. Tried to get off the father's lap and fly at me while tears of defeat blinded her eyes.

FRANZ KAFKA

A Country Doctor

I was in great perplexity; I had to start on an urgent journey; a seriously ill patient was waiting for me in a village ten miles off; a thick blizzard of snow filled all the wide spaces between him and me; I had a gig, a light gig with big wheels, exactly right for our country roads; muffled in furs, my bag of instruments in my hand, I was in the courtyard all ready for the journey; but there was no horse to be had, no horse. My own horse had died in the night, worn out by the fatigues of this icy winter; my servant girl was now running round the village trying to borrow a horse; but it was hopeless, I knew it, and I stood there forlornly, with the snow gathering more and more thickly upon me, more and more unable to move. In the gateway the girl appeared, alone, and waved the lantern; of course, who would lend a horse at this time for such a journey? I strode through the courtyard once more; I could see no way out; in my confused distress I kicked at the dilapidated door of the yearlong uninhabited pigsty. It flew open and flapped to and fro on its hinges. A steam and smell as of horses came out from it. A dim stable lantern was swinging inside from a rope. A man, crouching on his hams in that low space, showed an open blue-eyed face. "Shall I yoke up?" he asked, crawling out on all fours. I did not know what to say and merely stooped down to see what else was in the sty. The servant girl was standing beside me. "You never know what you're going to find in your own house," she said, and we both laughed. "Hey there, Brother, hey there, Sister!" called the groom, and two horses, enormous creatures with powerful flanks, one after the other, their legs tucked close to their bodies, each well-shaped head lowered like a camel's, by sheer strength of buttocking squeezed out through the door hole which they filled entirely. But at once they were standing up, their legs long and their bodies steaming thickly. "Give him a hand," I said, and the willing girl hurried to help the groom with the harnessing. Yet hardly was she beside him when the groom clipped hold of her and pushed his face against hers. She screamed and fled back to me; on her cheek stood out in red the marks of two rows of teeth. "You brute," I yelled in fury, "do you want a whipping?" but in the same moment reflected that the man was a stranger; that I did not know where he came from, and that of his own free will he was helping me out when everyone else had failed me. As if he knew my thoughts he took no offense at my threat but, still busied with the horses, only turned round once towards me. "Get in," he said then, and indeed: everything was ready. A magnificent pair of horses, I observed, such as I had never sat behind, and I climbed in happily. "But I'll drive, you don't know the way," I said. "Of course," said he, "I'm not coming with you anyway, I'm staying with Rose." "No," shrieked Rose, fleeing into the house with a justified presentiment that her fate was inescapable; I heard the door chain rattle as she put it up; I heard the key turn in the lock; I could see, moreover, how she put out the lights in the entrance hall and in further flight all through the rooms to keep herself from being discovered. "You're coming with me," I said to the groom, "or I won't go, urgent as my journey is. I'm not thinking of paying for it by handing the girl over to you." "Gee up!" he said; clapped his hands; the gig whirled off like a log in a freshet; I could just hear the door of my house splitting and bursting as the groom charged at it and then I was deafened and blinded by a storming rush that steadily buffeted all my senses. But this only for a moment, since, as if my patient's farmyard had opened out just before my courtyard gate, I was already there; the horses had come quietly to a standstill; the blizzard had stopped; moonlight all around; my patient's parents hurried out of the house, his sister behind them; I was almost lifted out of the gig; from their confused ejaculations I gathered not a word; in the sickroom the air was almost unbreathable; the neglected stove was smoking; I wanted to push open a window; but first I had to look at my patient. Gaunt, without any fever, not cold, not warm, with vacant eyes, without a shirt, the youngster heaved himself up from under the feather bedding, threw his arms round my neck, and whispered in my ear: "Doctor, let me die." I glanced round the room; no one had heard it; the parents were leaning forward in silence waiting for my verdict; the sister had set a chair for my handbag; I opened the bag and hunted among my instruments; the boy kept clutching at me from his bed to remind me of his entreaty; I picked up a pair of tweezers, examined them in the candlelight and laid them down again. "Yes," I thought blasphemously, "in cases like this the gods are helpful, send the missing horse, add to it a second because of the urgency, and to crown everything bestow even a groom——" And only now did I remember Rose again; what was I to do, how could I rescue her, how could I pull her away from under that groom at ten miles' distance, with a team of horses I couldn't control. These horses, now, they had somehow slipped the reins loose, pushed the windows open from outside, I did not know how; each of them had stuck a head in at a window and, quite unmoved by the startled cries of the family, stood eyeing the patient. "Better go back at once," I thought, as if the horses were summoning me to the return journey, yet I permitted the patient's sister, who fancied that I was dazed by the heat, to take my fur coat from me. A glass of rum was poured out for me, the old man clapped me on the shoulder, a familiarity justified by this offer of his treasure. I shook my head; in the narrow confines of the old man's thoughts I felt ill; that was my only reason for refusing the drink. The mother stood by the bedside and cajoled me towards it; I yielded, and, while one of the horses whinnied loudly to the ceiling, laid my head to the boy's breast, which shivered under my wet beard. I confirmed what I already knew; the boy was quite sound, something a little wrong with his circulation, saturated with coffee by his solicitous mother, but sound and best turned out of bed with one shove. I am no world reformer and so I let him lie. I was the district doctor and did my duty to the uttermost, to the point where it became almost too much. I was badly paid and yet generous and helpful to the poor. I had still to see that Rose was all right, and then the boy might have his way and I wanted to die too. What was I doing there in that endless winter! My horse was dead, and not a single person in the village would lend me another. I had to get my team out of the pigsty; if they hadn't chanced to be horses I should have had to travel with swine. That was how it was. And I nodded to the family. They knew nothing about it, and, had they known, would not have believed it. To write prescriptions is easy, but to come to an understanding with people is hard. Well, this should be the end of my visit, I had once more been called out needlessly, I was used to that, the whole district made my life a torment with my night bell, but that I should have to sacrifice Rose this time as well, the pretty girl who had lived in my house for years almost without my noticing her—that sacrifice was too much to ask, and I had somehow to get it reasoned out in my head with the help of what craft I could muster, in order not to let fly at this family, which with the best will in the world could not restore Rose to me. But as I shut my bag and put an arm out for my fur coat, the family meanwhile standing together, the father sniffing at the glass of rum in his hand, the mother, apparently disappointed in me—why, what do people expect?—biting her lips with tears in her eyes, the sister fluttering a blood-soaked towel, I was somehow ready to admit conditionally that the boy might be ill after all. I went towards him, he welcomed me smiling as if I were bringing him the most nourishing invalid broth—ah, now both horses were whinnying together; the noise, I suppose, was ordained by heaven to assist my examination of the patient—and this time I discovered that the boy was indeed ill. In his right side, near the hip, was an open wound as big as the palm of my hand. Rose-red, in many variations of shade, dark in the hollows, lighter at the edges, softly granulated, with irregular clots of blood, open as a surface mine to the daylight. That was how it looked from a distance. But on a closer inspection there was another complication. I could not help a low whistle of surprise. Worms, as thick and as long as my little finger, themselves rose-red and blood-spotted as well, were wriggling from their fastness in the interior of the wound towards the light, with small white heads and many little legs. Poor boy, you were past helping. I had discovered your great wound; this blossom in your side was destroying you. The family was pleased; they saw me busying myself; the sister told the mother, the mother the father, the father told several guests who were coming in, through the moonlight at the open door, walking on tiptoe, keeping their balance with outstretched arms. "Will you save me?" whispered the boy with a sob, quite blinded by the life within his wound. That is what people are like in my district. Always expecting the impossible from the doctor. They have lost their ancient beliefs; the parson sits at home and unravels his vestments, one after another; but the doctor is supposed to be omnipotent with his merciful surgeon's hand. Well, as it pleases them; I have not thrust my services on them; if they misuse me for sacred ends, I let that happen to me too; what better do I want, old country doctor that I am, bereft of my servant girl! And so they came, the family and the village elders, and stripped my clothes off me; a school choir with the teacher at the head of it stood before the house and sang these words to an utterly simple tune:

> Strip his clothes off, then he'll heal us,
> If he doesn't, kill him dead!
> Only a doctor, only a doctor.

Then my clothes were off and I looked at the people quietly, my fingers in my beard and my head cocked to one side. I was altogether composed and equal to the situation and remained so, although it was no help to me, since they now took me by the head and feet and carried me to the bed. They laid me down in it next to the wall, on the side of the wound. Then they all left the room; the door was shut; the singing stopped; clouds covered the moon; the bedding was warm around me; the horses' heads in the open windows wavered like shadows. "Do you know," said a voice in my ear, "I have very little confidence in you. Why, you were only blown in here, you didn't come on your own feet. Instead of helping me, you're cramping me on my deathbed. What I'd like best is to scratch your eyes out." "Right," I said, "it is a shame. And yet I am a doctor. What am I to do? Believe me, it is not too easy for me either." "Am I supposed to be content with this apology? Oh, I must be, I

can't help it. I always have to put up with things. A fine wound is all I brought
into the world; that was my sole endowment." "My young friend," said I,
"your mistake is: you have not a wide enough view. I have been in all the
sickrooms, far and wide, and I tell you: your wound is not so bad. Done in
a tight corner with two strokes of the ax. Many a one proffers his side and
can hardly hear the ax in the forest, far less that it is coming nearer to him."
"Is that really so, or are you deluding me in my fever?" "It is really so, take
the word of honor of an official doctor." And he took it and lay still. But now
it was time for me to think of escaping. The horses were still standing faith-
fully in their places. My clothes, my fur coat, my bag were quickly collected;
I didn't want to waste time dressing; if the horses raced home as they had
come, I should only be springing, as it were, out of this bed into my own.
Obediently a horse backed away from the window; I threw my bundle into the
gig; the fur coat missed its mark and was caught on a hook only by the sleeve.
Good enough. I swung myself on to the horse. With the reins loosely trailing,
one horse barely fastened to the other, the gig swaying behind, my fur coat
last of all in the snow. "Gee up!" I said, but there was no galloping; slowly,
like old men, we crawled through the snowy wastes; a long time echoed behind us the new but faulty song of the children:

> O be joyful, all you patients,
> The doctor's laid in bed beside you!

Never shall I reach home at this rate; my flourishing practice is done for; my
successor is robbing me, but in vain, for he cannot take my place; in my house
the disgusting groom is raging; Rose is his victim; I do not want to think about
it any more. Naked, exposed to the frost of this most unhappy of ages, with
an earthly vehicle, unearthly horses, old man that I am, I wander astray. My
fur coat is hanging from the back of the gig, but I cannot reach it, and none
of my limber pack of patients lifts a finger. Betrayed! Betrayed! A false alarm
on the night bell once answered—it cannot be made good, not ever.

Translated by Willa and Edwin Muir

ROBERT LOWELL

The Hospital

We're lost here if we follow what we read,
worse lost if hearsay is our common voice;
we need courses in life and death and what's alive;
trips to the hospital. . . . One has seen stiffs
that look alive, they mostly look alive,
twitched by green fingers till they turn to flowers;
they are and are not—some poor candidate,
the stone-deaf ear no felon's sledge will wake—
others are strapped to their cots, thrust out in hallways,
browner, dirtier, flatter than the dead leaves,
they are whatever crinkles, plugged to tubes,
and plugged to jugs of dim blue doctored water,
held feet above them to lift their eyes to God—
these look dead, unlike the others, they are alive.

ANNE SEXTON

Unknown Girl in the Maternity Ward

Child, the current of your breath is six days long.
You lie, a small knuckle on my white bed;
lie, fisted like a snail, so small and strong
at my breast. Your lips are animals; you are fed
with love. At first hunger is not wrong.
The nurses nod their caps; you are shepherded
down starch halls with the other unnested throng
in wheeling baskets. You tip like a cup; your head
moving to my touch. You sense the way we belong.
But this is an institution bed.
You will not know me very long.

The doctors are enamel. They want to know
the facts. They guess about the man who left me,
some pendulum soul, going the way men go

and leave you full of child. But our case history
stays blank. All I did was let you grow.
Now we are here for all the ward to see.
They thought I was strange, although
I never spoke a word. I burst empty
of you, letting you learn how the air is so.
The doctors chart the riddle they ask of me
and I turn my head away. I do not know.

Yours is the only face I recognize.
Bone at my bone, you drink my answers in.
Six times a day I prize
your need, the animals of your lips, your skin
growing warm and plump. I see your eyes
lifting their tents. They are blue stones, they begin
to outgrow their moss. You blink in surprise
and I wonder what you can see, my funny kin,
as you trouble my silence. I am a shelter of lies.
Should I learn to speak again, or hopeless in
such sanity will I touch some face I recognize?

Down the hall the baskets start back. My arms
fit you like a sleeve, they hold
catkins of your willows, the wild bee farms
of your nerves, each muscle and fold
of your first days. Your old man's face disarms
the nurses. But the doctors return to scold
me. I speak. It is you my silence harms.
I should have known; I should have told
them something to write down. My voice alarms
my throat. "Name of father—none." I hold
you and name you bastard in my arms.

And now that's that. There is nothing more
that I can say or lose.
Others have traded life before
and could not speak. I tighten to refuse
your owling eyes, my fragile visitor.
I touch your cheeks, like flowers. You bruise
against me. We unlearn. I am a shore
rocking you off. You break from me. I choose
your only way, my small inheritor
and hand you off, trembling the selves we lose.
Go child, who is my sin and nothing more.

SYLVIA PLATH

The Surgeon at 2 A.M.

The white light is artificial, and hygienic as heaven.
The microbes cannot survive it.
They are departing in their transparent garments, turned
    aside
From the scalpels and the rubber hands.
The scalded sheet is a snowfield, frozen and peaceful.
The body under it is in my hands.
As usual there is no face. A lump of Chinese white
With seven holes thumbed in. The soul is another light.
I have not seen it; it does not fly up.
Tonight it has receded like a ship's light.

It is a garden I have to do with—tubers and fruits
Oozing their jammy substances,
A mat of roots. My assistants hook them back.
Stenches and colors assail me.
This is the lung-tree.
These orchids are splendid. They spot and coil like snakes.
The heart is a red bell-bloom, in distress.
I am so small
In comparison to these organs!
I worm and hack in a purple wilderness.

The blood is a sunset. I admire it.
I am up to my elbows in it, red and squeaking.
Still it seeps up, it is not exhausted.
So magical! A hot spring
I must seal it off and let fill
The intricate, blue piping under this pale marble.
How I admire the Romans—
Aqueducts, the Baths of Caracalla, the eagle nose!
The body is a Roman thing.
It has shut its mouth on the stone pill of repose.

It is a statue the orderlies are wheeling off.
I have perfected it.
I am left with an arm or a leg,

A set of teeth, or stones
To rattle in a bottle and take home,
And tissues in slices—a pathological salami.
Tonight the parts are entombed in an icebox.
Tomorrow they will swim
In vinegar like saints' relics.
Tomorrow the patient will have a clean, pink plastic limb.

Over one bed in the ward, a small blue light
Announces a new soul. The bed is blue.
Tonight, for this person, blue is a beautiful color.
The angels of morphia have borne him up.
He floats an inch from the ceiling,
Smelling the dawn drafts.
I walk among sleepers in gauze sarcophagi.
The red night lights are flat moons. They are dull with blood.
I am the sun, in my white coat,
Grey faces, shuttered by drugs, follow me like flowers.

D. H. LAWRENCE

The Horse Dealer's Daughter

"Well, Mabel, and what are you going to do with yourself?" asked Joe, with foolish flippancy. He felt quite safe himself. Without listening for an answer, he turned aside, worked a grain of tobacco to the tip of his tongue, and spat it out. He did not care about anything, since he felt safe himself.

The three brothers and the sister sat round the desolate breakfast-table, attempting some sort of desultory consultation. The morning's post had given the final tap to the family fortunes, and all was over. The dreary dining-room itself, with its heavy mahogany furniture, looked as if it were waiting to be done away with.

But the consultation amounted to nothing. There was a strange air of ineffectuality about the three men, as they sprawled at table, smoking and reflecting vaguely on their own condition. The girl was alone, a rather short, sullen-looking young woman of twenty-seven. She did not share the same life as her brothers. She would have been good-looking, save for the impressive fixity of her face, "bull-dog," as her brothers called it.

There was a confused tramping of horses' feet outside. The three men all sprawled round in their chairs to watch. Beyond the dark holly bushes that separated the strip of lawn from the high-road, they could see a cavalcade of shire horses swinging out of their own yard, being taken for exercise. This was the last time. These were the last horses that would go through their hands. The young men watched with critical, callous look. They were all frightened at the collapse of their lives, and the sense of disaster in which they were involved left them no inner freedom.

Yet they were three fine, well-set fellows enough. Joe, the eldest, was a man of thirty-three, broad and handsome in a hot, flushed way. His face was red, he twisted his black moustache over a thick finger, his eyes were shallow and restless. He had a sensual way of uncovering his teeth when he laughed, and his bearing was stupid. Now he watched the horses with a glazed look of helplessness in his eyes, a certain stupor of downfall.

The great draught-horses swung past. They were tied head to tail, four of them, and they heaved along to where a lane branched off from the high-road, planting their great hoofs floutingly in the fine black mud, swinging their great rounded haunches sumptuously, and trotting a few sudden steps as they were led into the lane, round the corner. Every movement showed a massive, slumbrous strength, and a stupidity which held them in subjection. The groom at the head looked back, jerking the leading rope. And the cavalcade moved out of sight up the lane, the tail of the last horse, bobbed up tight and stiff, held out taut from the swinging great haunches as they rocked behind the hedges in a motion-like sleep.

Joe watched with glazed hopeless eyes. The horses were almost like his own body to him. He felt he was done for now. Luckily he was engaged to a woman as old as himself, and therefore her father, who was steward of a neighbouring estate, would provide him with a job. He would marry and go into harness. His life was over, he would be a subject animal now.

He turned uneasily aside, the retreating steps of the horses echoing in his ears. Then, with foolish restlessness, he reached for the scraps of bacon-rind from the plates, and making a faint whistling sound, flung them to the terrier that lay against the fender. He watched the dog swallow them, and waited till the creature looked into his eyes. Then a faint grin came on his face, and in a high, foolish voice he said:

"You won't get much more bacon, shall you, you little b——?"

The dog faintly and dismally wagged its tail, then lowered its haunches, circled round, and lay down again.

There was another helpless silence at the table. Joe sprawled uneasily in his seat, not willing to go till the family conclave was dissolved. Fred Henry, the second brother, was erect, clean-limbed, alert. He had watched the passing of the horses with more *sang-froid*. If he was an animal, like Joe, he was an animal which controls, not one which is controlled. He was master of any horse, and he carried himself with a well-tempered air of mastery. But he was not master of the situations of life. He pushed his coarse brown moustache upwards, off his lip, and glanced irritably at his sister, who sat impassive and inscrutable.

"You'll go and stop with Lucy for a bit, shan't you?" he asked. The girl did not answer.

"I don't see what else you can do," persisted Fred Henry.

"Go as a skivvy," Joe interpolated laconically.

The girl did not move a muscle.

"If I was her, I should go in for training for a nurse," said Malcolm, the youngest of them all. He was the baby of the family, a young man of twenty-two, with a fresh, jaunty *museau*.

But Mabel did not take any notice of him. They had talked at her and round her for so many years, that she hardly heard them at all.

The marble clock on the mantelpiece softly chimed the half-hour, the dog rose uneasily from the hearth-rug and looked at the party at the breakfast-table. But still they sat on in ineffectual conclave.

"Oh, all right," said Joe suddenly, apropos of nothing. "I'll get a move on."

He pushed back his chair, straddled his knees with a downward jerk, to get them free, in horsey fashion, and went to the fire. Still he did not go out of the room; he was curious to know what the others would do or say. He began to charge his pipe, looking down at the dog and saying in a high, affected voice:

"Going wi' me? Going wi' me are ter? Tha'rt goin' further than tha counts on just now, dost hear?"

The dog faintly wagged its tail, the man stuck out his jaw and covered his pipe with his hands, and puffed intently, losing himself in the tobacco, looking down all the while at the dog with an absent brown eye. The dog looked up at him in mournful distrust. Joe stood with his knees stuck out, in real horsey fashion.

"Have you had a letter from Lucy?" Fred Henry asked of his sister.

"Last week," came the neutral reply.

"And what does she say?"

There was no answer.

"Does she *ask* you to go and stop there?" persisted Fred Henry.

"She says I can if I like."

"Well, then, you'd better. Tell her you'll come on Monday."

This was received in silence.

"That's what you'll do then, is it?" said Fred Henry, in some exasperation.

But she made no answer. There was a silence of futility and irritation in the room. Malcolm grinned fatuously.

"You'll have to make up your mind between now and next Wednesday," said Joe loudly, "or else find yourself lodgings on the kerbstone."

The face of the young woman darkened, but she sat on immutable.

"Here's Jack Fergusson!" exclaimed Malcolm, who was looking aimlessly out of the window.

"Where?" exclaimed Joe loudly.

"Just gone past."

"Coming in?"

Malcolm craned his neck to see the gate.

"Yes," he said.

There was a silence. Mabel sat on like one condemned, at the head of the table. Then a whistle was heard from the kitchen. The dog got up and barked sharply. Joe opened the door and shouted:

"Come on."

After a moment a young man entered. He was muffled up in overcoat and a purple woollen scarf, and his tweed cap, which he did not remove, was pulled down on his head. He was of medium height, his face was rather long and pale, his eyes looked tired.

"Hello, Jack! Well, Jack!" exclaimed Malcolm and Joe. Fred Henry merely said: "Jack."

"What's doing?" asked the newcomer, evidently addressing Fred Henry.

"Same. We've got to be out by Wednesday. Got a cold?"

"I have—got it bad, too."

"Why don't you stop in?"

"*Me* stop in? When I can't stand on my legs, perhaps I shall have a chance." The young man spoke huskily. He had a slight Scotch accent.

"It's a knock-out, isn't it," said Joe, boisterously, "if a doctor goes round croaking with a cold. Looks bad for the patients, doesn't it?"

The young doctor looked at him slowly.

"Anything the matter with *you*, then?" he asked sarcastically.

"Not as I know of. Damn your eyes, I hope not. Why?"

"I thought you were very concerned about the patients, wondered if you might be one yourself."

"Damn it, no, I've never been patient to no flaming doctor, and hope I never shall be," returned Joe.

At this point Mabel rose from the table, and they all seemed to become aware of her existence. She began putting the dishes together. The young doctor looked at her, but did not address her. He had not greeted her. She went out of the room with the tray, her face impassive and unchanged.

"When are you off then, all of you?" asked the doctor.

"I'm catching the eleven-forty," replied Malcolm. "Are you goin' down wi' th' trap, Joe?"

"Yes, I've told you I'm going down wi' th' trap, haven't I?"

"We'd better be getting her in then. So long, Jack, if I don't see you before I go," said Malcolm, shaking hands.

He went out, followed by Joe, who seemed to have his tail between his legs.

"Well, this is the devil's own," exclaimed the doctor, when he was left alone with Fred Henry. "Going before Wednesday, are you?"

"That's the orders," replied the other.

"Where, to Northampton?"

"That's it."

"The devil!" exclaimed Fergusson, with quiet chagrin.

And there was silence between the two.

"All settled up, are you?" asked Fergusson.

"About."

There was another pause.

"Well, I shall miss yer, Freddy, boy," said the young doctor.

"And I shall miss thee, Jack," returned the other.

"Miss you like hell," mused the doctor.

Fred Henry turned aside. There was nothing to say. Mabel came in again, to finish clearing the table.

"What are *you* going to do, then, Miss Pervin?" asked Fergusson. "Going to your sister's, are you?"

Mabel looked at him with her steady, dangerous eyes, that always made him uncomfortable, unsettling his superficial ease.

"No," she said.

"Well, what in the name of fortune *are* you going to do? Say what you mean to do," cried Fred Henry, with futile intensity.

But she only averted her head, and continued her work. She folded the white table-cloth, and put on the chenille cloth.

"The sulkiest bitch that ever trod!" muttered her brother.

But she finished her task with perfectly impassive face, the young doctor watching her interestedly all the while. Then she went out.

Fred Henry stared after her, clenching his lips, his blue eyes fixing in sharp antagonism, as he made a grimace of sour exasperation.

"You could bray her into bits, and that's all you'd get out of her," he said, in a small, narrowed tone.

The doctor smiled faintly.

"What's she *going* to do, then?" he asked.

"Strike me if *I* know!" returned the other.

There was a pause. Then the doctor stirred.

"I'll be seeing you to-night, shall I?" he said to his friend.

"Ay—where's it to be? Are we going over to Jessdale?"

"I don't know. I've got such a cold on me. I'll come round to the Moon and Stars, anyway."

"Let Lizzie and May miss their night for once, eh?"

"That's it—if I feel as I do now."

"All's one——"

The two young men went through the passage and down to the back door together. The house was large, but it was servantless now, and desolate. At the back was a small bricked house-yard and beyond that a big square, gravelled fine and red, and having stables on two sides. Sloping, dank, winter-dark fields stretched away on the open sides.

But the stables were empty. Joseph Pervin, the father of the family, had been a man of no education, who had become a fairly large horse dealer. The stables had been full of horses, there was a great turmoil and come-and-go of horses and of dealers and grooms. Then the kitchen was full of servants. But of late things had declined. The old man had married a second time, to retrieve his fortunes. Now he was dead and everything was gone to the dogs, there was nothing but debt and threatening.

For months, Mabel had been servantless in the big house, keeping the home together in penury for her ineffectual brothers. She had kept house for ten years. But previously it was with unstinted means. Then, however brutal and coarse everything was, the sense of money had kept her proud, confident. The men might be foul-mouthed, the women in the kitchen might have bad reputations, her brothers might have illegitimate children. But so long as there was money, the girl felt herself established, and brutally proud, reserved.

No company came to the house, save dealers and coarse men. Mabel had no associates of her own sex, after her sister went away. But she did not mind. She went regularly to church, she attended to her father. And she lived in the memory of her mother, who had died when she was fourteen, and whom she had loved. She had loved her father, too, in a different way, depending upon him, and feeling secure in him, until at the age of fifty-four he married again. And then she had set hard against him. Now he had died and left them all hopelessly in debt.

She had suffered badly during the period of poverty. Nothing, however, could shake the curious, sullen, animal pride that dominated each member of the family. Now, for Mabel, the end had come. Still she would not cast about her. She would follow her own way just the same. She would always hold the keys of her own situation. Mindless and persistent, she endured from day to day. Why should she think? Why should she answer anybody? It was enough that this was the end, and there was no way out. She need not pass any more darkly along the main street of the small town, avoiding every eye. She need not demean herself any more, going into the shops and buying the cheapest food. This was at an end. She thought of nobody, not even of herself. Mindless and persistent, she seemed in a sort of ecstasy to be coming nearer to her fulfilment, her own glorification, approaching her dead mother, who was glorified.

In the afternoon she took a little bag, with shears and sponge and a small scrubbing-brush, and went out. It was a grey, wintry day, with saddened, dark green fields and an atmosphere blackened by the smoke of foundries not far off. She went quickly, darkly along the causeway, heeding nobody, through the town to the churchyard.

There she always felt secure, as if no one could see her, although as a matter of fact she was exposed to the stare of everyone who passed along under the churchyard wall. Nevertheless, once under the shadow of the great looming church, among the graves, she felt immune from the world, reserved within the thick churchyard wall as in another country.

Carefully she clipped the grass from the grave, and arranged the pinky white, small chrysanthemums in the tin cross. When this was done, she took an empty jar from a neighbouring grave, brought water, and carefully, most scrupulously sponged the marble headstone and the coping-stone.

It gave her sincere satisfaction to do this. She felt in immediate contact with the world of her mother. She took minute pains, went through the park in a state bordering on pure happiness, as if in performing this task she came into a subtle, intimate connection with her mother. For the life she followed here in the world was far less real than the world of death she inherited from her mother.

The doctor's house was just by the church. Fergusson, being a mere hired assistant, was slave to the country-side. As he hurried now to attend to the out-patients in the surgery, glancing across the graveyard with his quick eye, he saw the girl at her task at the grave. She seemed so intent and remote, it was like looking into another world. Some mystical element was touched in him. He slowed down as he walked, watching her as if spellbound.

She lifted her eyes, feeling him looking. Their eyes met. And each looked again at once, each feeling, in some way, found out by the other. He lifted his cap and passed on down the road. There remained distinct in his consciousness, like a vision, the memory of her face, lifted from the tombstone in the churchyard, and looking at him with slow, large, portentous eyes. It *was* portentous, her face. It seemed to mesmerise him. There was a heavy power in her eyes which laid hold of his whole being, as if he had drunk some powerful drug. He had been feeling weak and done before. Now the life came back into him, he felt delivered from his own fretted, daily self.

He finished his duties at the surgery as quickly as might be, hastily filling up the bottles of the waiting people with cheap drugs. Then, in perpetual haste, he set off again to visit several cases in another part of his round, before tea-time. At all times he preferred to walk if he could, but particularly when he was not well. He fancied the motion restored him.

The afternoon was falling. It was grey, deadened, and wintry, with a slow, moist, heavy coldness sinking in and deadening all the faculties. But why should he think or notice? He hastily climbed the hill and turned across the dark green fields, following the black cinder-track. In the distance, across a shallow dip in the country, the small town was clustered like smouldering ash, a tower, a spire, a heap of low, raw, extinct houses. And on the nearest fringe of the town, sloping into the dip, was Oldmeadow, the Pervins' house. He could see the stables and the outbuildings distinctly, as they lay towards him on the slope. Well, he would not go there many more times! Another resource would be lost to him, another place gone: the only company he cared for in the alien, ugly little town he was losing. Nothing but work, drudgery, constant hastening from dwelling to dwelling among the colliers and the iron-workers. It wore him out, but at the same time he had a craving for it. It was a stimulant to him to be in the homes of the working people, moving, as it were, through the innermost body of their life. His nerves were excited and gratified. He could come so near, into the very lives of the rough, inarticulate, powerfully emotional men and women. He grumbled, he said he hated the hellish hole. But as a matter of fact it excited him, the contact with the rough, strongly-feeling people was a stimulant applied direct to his nerves.

Below Oldmeadow, in the green, shallow, soddened hollow of fields, lay a square, deep pond. Roving across the landscape, the doctor's quick eye detected a figure in black passing through the gate of the field, down towards the pond. He looked again. It would be Mabel Pervin. His mind suddenly became alive and attentive.

Why was she going down there? He pulled up on the path on the slope above, and stood staring. He could just make sure of the small black figure moving in the hollow of the failing day. He seemed to see her in the midst of such obscurity, that he was like a clairvoyant, seeing rather with the mind's eye than with ordinary sight. Yet he could see her positively enough, whilst he kept his eye attentive. He felt, if he looked away from her, in the thick, ugly falling dusk, he would lose her altogether.

He followed her minutely as she moved, direct and intent, like something transmitted rather than stirring in voluntary activity, straight down the field towards the pond. There she stood on the bank for a moment. She never raised her head. Then she waded slowly into the water.

He stood motionless as the small black figure walked slowly and deliberately towards the centre of the pond, very slowly, gradually moving deeper into the motionless water, and still moving forward as the water got up to her breast. Then he could see her no more in the dusk of the dead afternoon.

"There!" he exclaimed. "Would you believe it?"

And he hastened straight down, running over the wet, soddened fields, pushing through the hedges, down into the depression of callous wintry obscurity. It took him several minutes to come to the pond. He stood on the bank, breathing heavily. He could see nothing. His eyes seemed to penetrate the dead water. Yes, perhaps that was the dark shadow of her black clothing beneath the surface of the water.

He slowly ventured into the pond. The bottom was deep, soft clay, he sank in, and the water clasped dead cold round his legs. As he stirred he could smell the cold, rotten clay that fouled up into the water. It was objectionable in his lungs. Still, repelled and yet not heeding, he moved deeper into the pond. The cold water rose over his thighs, over his loins, upon his abdomen. The lower part of his body was all sunk in the hideous cold element. And the bottom was so deeply soft and uncertain, he was afraid of pitching with his mouth underneath. He could not swim, and was afraid.

He crouched a little, spreading his hands under the water and moving them round, trying to feel for her. The dead cold pond swayed upon his chest. He moved again, a little deeper, and again, with his hands underneath, he felt all around under the water. And he touched her clothing. But it evaded his fingers. He made a desperate effort to grasp it.

And so doing he lost his balance and went under, horribly, suffocating in the foul earthy water, struggling madly for a few moments. At last, after what seemed an eternity, he got his footing, rose again into the air and looked around. He gasped, and knew he was in the world. Then he looked at the water. She had risen near him. He grasped her clothing, and drawing her nearer, turned to take his way to land again.

He went very slowly, carefully, absorbed in the slow progress. He rose higher, climbing out of the pond. The water was now only about his legs; he was thankful, full of relief to be out of the clutches of the pond. He lifted her and staggered on to the bank, out of the horror of wet, grey clay.

He laid her down on the bank. She was quite unconscious and running with water. He made the water come from her mouth, he worked to restore her. He did not have to work very long before he could feel the breathing begin again in her; she was breathing naturally. He worked a little longer. He could feel her live beneath his hands; she was coming back. He wiped her face, wrapped her in his overcoat, looked round into the dim, dark grey world, then lifted her and staggered down the bank and across the fields.

It seemed an unthinkably long way, and his burden so heavy he felt he would never get to the house. But at last he was in the stable-yard, and then in the house-yard. He opened the door and went into the house. In the kitchen he laid her down on the hearth-rug and called. The house was empty. But the fire was burning in the grate.

Then again he kneeled to attend to her. She was breathing regularly, her eyes were wide open and as if conscious, but there seemed something missing in her look. She was conscious in herself, but unconscious of her surroundings.

He ran upstairs, took blankets from a bed, and put them before the fire to warm. Then he removed her saturated, earthy-smelling clothing, rubbed her dry with a towel, and wrapped her naked in the blankets. Then he went into the dining-room, to look for spirits. There was a little whiskey. He drank a gulp himself, and put some into her mouth.

The effect was instantaneous. She looked full into his face, as if she had been seeing him for some time, and yet had only just become conscious of him.

"Dr. Fergusson?" she said.

"What?" he answered.

He was divesting himself of his coat, intending to find some dry clothing upstairs. He could not bear the smell of the dead, clayey water, and he was mortally afraid for his own health.

"What did I do?" she asked.

"Walked into the pond," he replied. He had begun to shudder like one sick, and could hardly attend to her. Her eyes remained full on him, he seemed to be going dark in his mind, looking back at her helplessly. The shuddering became quieter in him, life came back to him, dark and unknowing, but strong again.

"Was I out of my mind?" she asked, while her eyes were fixed on him all the time.

"Maybe, for the moment," he replied. He felt quiet, because his strength had come back. The strange fretful strain had left him.

"Am I out of my mind now?" she asked.

"Are you?" he reflected a moment. "No," he answered truthfully, "I don't see that you are." He turned his face aside. He was afraid now, because he felt dazed, and felt dimly that her power was stronger than his, in this issue. And she continued to look at him fixedly all the time. "Can you tell me where I shall find some dry things to put on?" he asked.

"Did you dive into the pond for me?" she asked.

"No," he answered. "I walked in. But I went in overhead as well."

There was silence for a moment. He hesitated. He very much wanted to go upstairs to get into dry clothing. But there was another desire in him. And she seemed to hold him. His will seemed to have gone to sleep, and left him, standing there slack before her. But he felt warm inside himself. He did not shudder at all, though his clothes were sodden on him.

"Why did you?" she asked.

"Because I didn't want you to do such a foolish thing," he said.

"It wasn't foolish," she said, still gazing at him as she lay on the floor, with a sofa cushion under her head. "It was the right thing to do. *I* knew best, then."

"I'll go and shift these wet things," he said. But still he had not the power to move out of her presence, until she sent him. It was as if she had the life of his body in her hands, and he could not extricate himself. Or perhaps he did not want to.

Suddenly she sat up. Then she became aware of her own immediate condition. She felt the blankets about her, she knew her own limbs. For a moment it seemed as if her reason were going. She looked round, with wild eye, as if seeking something. He stood still with fear. She saw her clothing lying scattered.

"Who undressed me?" she asked, her eyes resting full and inevitable on his face.

"I did," he replied, "to bring you round."

For some moments she sat and gazed at him awfully, her lips parted.

"Do you love me, then?" she asked.

He only stood and stared at her, fascinated. His soul seemed to melt.

She shuffled forward on her knees, and put her arms round him, round his legs, as he stood there, pressing her breasts against his knees and thighs, clutching him with strange, convulsive certainty, pressing his thighs against her, drawing him to her face, her throat, as she looked up at him with flaring, humble eyes of transfiguration, triumphant in first possession.

"You love me," she murmured, in strange transport, yearning and triumphant and confident. "You love me. I know you love me, I know."

And she was passionately kissing his knees, through the wet clothing, passionately and indiscriminately kissing his knees, his legs, as if unaware of everything.

He looked down at the tangled wet hair, the wild, bare, animal shoulders. He was amazed, bewildered, and afraid. He had never thought of loving her. He had never wanted to love her. When he rescued her and restored her, he was a doctor, and she was a patient. He had had no single personal thought of her. Nay, this introduction of the personal element was very distasteful to him, a violation of his professional honour. It was horrible to have her there embracing his knees. It was horrible. He revolted from it, violently. And yet—and yet—he had not the power to break away.

She looked at him again, with the same supplication of powerful love, and that same transcendent, frightening light of triumph. In view of the delicate flame which seemed to come from her face like a light, he was powerless. And yet he had never intended to love her. He had never intended. And something stubborn in him could not give way.

"You love me," she repeated, in a murmur of deep, rhapsodic assurance. "You love me."

Her hands were drawing him, drawing him down to her. He was afraid, even a little horrified. For he had, really, no intention of loving her. Yet her hands were drawing him towards her. He put out his hand quickly to steady himself, and grasped her bare shoulder. A flame seemed to burn the hand that grasped her soft shoulder. He had no intention of loving her: his whole will was against his yielding. It was horrible. And yet wonderful was the touch of her shoulders, beautiful the shining of her face. Was she perhaps mad? He had a horror of yielding to her. Yet something in him ached also.

He had been staring away at the door, away from her. But his hand remained on her shoulder. She had gone suddenly very still. He looked down at her. Her eyes were now wide with fear, with doubt, the light was dying from her face, a shadow of terrible greyness was returning. He could not bear the touch of her eyes' question upon him, and the look of death behind the question.

With an inward groan he gave way, and let his heart yield towards her. A sudden smile came on his face. And her eyes, which never left his face, slowly, slowly filled with tears. He watched the strange water rise in her eyes, like some slow fountain coming up. And his heart seemed to burn and melt away in his breast.

He could not bear to look at her any more. He dropped on his knees and caught her head with his arms and pressed her face against his throat. She was very still. His heart, which seemed to have broken, was burning with a kind of agony in his breast. And he felt her slow, hot tears wetting his throat. But he could not move.

He felt the hot tears wet his neck and the hollows of his neck, and he remained motionless, suspended through one of man's eternities. Only now it had become indispensable to him to have her face pressed close to him; he could never let her go again. He could never let her head go away from the close clutch of his arm. He wanted to remain like that for ever, with his heart hurting him in a pain that was also life to him. Without knowing, he was looking down on her damp, soft brown hair.

Then, as it were suddenly, he smelt the horrid stagnant smell of that water. And at the same moment she drew away from him and looked at him. Her eyes were wistful and unfathomable. He was afraid of them, and he fell to kissing her, not knowing what he was doing. He wanted her eyes not to have that terrible, wistful, unfathomable look.

When she turned her face to him again, a faint delicate flush was glowing, and there was again dawning that terrible shining of joy in her eyes, which really terrified him, and yet which he now wanted to see, because he feared the look of doubt still more.

"You love me?" she said rather faltering.

"Yes." The word cost him a painful effort. Not because it wasn't true. But because it was too newly true, the *saying* seemed to tear open again his newly-torn heart. And he hardly wanted it to be true, even now.

She lifted her face to him, and he bent forward and kissed her on the mouth, gently, with the one kiss that is an eternal pledge. And as he kissed her his heart strained again in his breast. He never intended to love her. But now it was over. He had crossed over the gulf to her, and all that he had left behind had shrivelled and become void.

After the kiss, her eyes again slowly filled with tears. She sat still, away from him, with her face drooped aside, and her hands folded in her lap. The tears fell very slowly. There was complete silence. He too sat there motionless and silent on the hearth-rug. The strange pain of his heart that was broken seemed to consume him. That he should love her? That this was love! That he should be ripped open in this way! Him, a doctor! How they would all jeer if they knew! It was agony to him to think they might know.

In the curious naked pain of the thought he looked again to her. She was sitting there drooped into a muse. He saw a tear fall, and his heart flared hot. He saw for the first time that one of her shoulders was quite uncovered, one arm bare, he could see one of her small breasts; dimly, because it had become almost dark in the room.

"Why are you crying?" he asked, in an altered voice.

She looked up at him, and behind her tears the consciousness of her situation for the first time brought a dark look of shame to her eyes.

"I'm not crying, really," she said, watching him, half frightened.

He reached his hand, and softly closed it on her bare arm.

"I love you! I love you!" he said in a soft, low vibrating voice, unlike himself.

She shrank, and dropped her head. The soft, penetrating grip of his hand on her arm distressed her. She looked up at him.

"I want to go," she said. "I want to go and get you some dry things."

"Why?" he said. "I'm all right."

"But I want to go," she said. "And I want you to change your things."

He released her arm, and she wrapped herself in the blanket, looking at him rather frightened. And still she did not rise.

"Kiss me," she said wistfully.

He kissed her, but briefly, half in anger.

Then, after a second, she rose nervously, all mixed up in the blanket. He watched her in her confusion as she tried to extricate herself and wrap herself up so that she could walk. He watched her relentlessly, as she knew. And as she went, the blanket trailing, and as he saw a glimpse of her feet and her white leg, he tried to remember her as she was when he had wrapped her in the blanket. But then he didn't want to remember, because she had been nothing to him then, and his nature revolted from remembering her as she was when she was nothing to him.

A tumbling, muffled noise from within the dark house startled him. Then he heard her voice: "There are clothes." He rose and went to the foot of the stairs, and gathered up the garments she had thrown down. Then he came back to the fire, to rub himself down and dress. He grinned at his own appearance when he had finished.

The fire was sinking, so he put on coal. The house was now quite dark, save for the light of a street-lamp that shone in faintly from beyond the holly trees. He lit the gas with matches he found on the mantelpiece. Then he emptied the pockets of his own clothes, and threw all his wet things in a heap into the scullery. After which he gathered up her sodden clothes, gently, and put them in a separate heap on the copper-top in the scullery.

It was six o'clock on the clock. His own watch had stopped. He ought to go back to the surgery. He waited, and still she did not come down. So he went to the foot of the stairs and called:

"I shall have to go."

Almost immediately he heard her coming down. She had on her best dress of black voile, and her hair was tidy, but still damp. She looked at him—and in spite of herself, smiled.

"I don't like you in those clothes," she said.

"Do I look a sight?" he answered.

They were shy of one another.

"I'll make you some tea," she said.

"No, I must go."

"Must you?" And she looked at him again with the wide, strained, doubtful

eyes. And again, from the pain of his breast, he knew how he loved her. He
went and bent to kiss her, gentle, passionately, with his heart's painful kiss.

"And my hair smells so horrible," she murmured in distraction. "And I'm
so awful, I'm so awful! Oh no, I'm too awful." And she broke into bitter,
heart-broken sobbing. "You can't want to love me, I'm horrible."

"Don't be silly, don't be silly," he said, trying to comfort her, kissing her,
holding her in his arms. "I want you, I want to marry you, we're going to be
married, quickly, quickly—to-morrow if I can."

But she only sobbed terribly, and cried:

"I feel awful. I feel awful. I feel I'm horrible to you."

"No, I want you, I want you," was all he answered, blindly, with that terrible intonation which frightened her almost more than her horror lest he
should *not* want her.

JOYCE CAROL OATES

Doctor's Wife

Doctor, what is this joy you bring to marriage?
Unruly disorder in beds and the constant odor
        of sterilized nails
and the muffled ringing of telephones presage
another thirty years for us. . . . The gauge
of our love's guilt is the pain of others.

Observe that the language was invented to lie.
Fluid and skilled as a dancer no longer young
        moving mouth and eyes
you arrange words air-tight and your enormous wage
never seems quite enough. . . . Observe
that one scream is like another
and ten thousand screams are one.

The mattresses are lumpy crosses, you might say.
The spasm and glut of so much dying without death
        is enough to outrage
what's untouched in you, and which is the way
out from all of this? Whose mistake?
Your lips speak and never say "Enough, enough—"

though your body has understood for years.
Memorize, sympathize, abbreviate and prescribe
    and along with widows age
to be worthy of two hundred yards of textbooks
and two thousand years of living.
In the fluorescent-humming corridors are flying fears
that cannot be your fault.

Your face is now a grainy mass, Doctor,
and on it are fossils of real faces, got
    by magic, by crime
not your fault. Someone is eternally present
in the wonder of your 1000-watt
burning. . . . What agony, what last demand
that can't be emptied in bucketfuls?
In your brain is a mess of tubes' knots.

Everything can be emptied by shining nurses.
Let them pad forward to do it, staunch girls
    in bodies' indifference begot
to bodies' indifferent service. . . . Let them
tape to my veins bulging tubes of sorrow
straw-colored and paid-for, expensive sorrow
pumping to my heart, the hiss of faint curses
attending. . . . There is no joke
possible at extremes. No fire
burns clean enough. Lying, a liar,
you are king and devil in the folk-
ways, and caged in your body's sleeping.

WILLIAM MELVIN KELLEY

The Dentist's Wife

In Harlem, there once lived a dentist who didn't love his wife. In fact, he was sure she was insane. Even though he'd given her a fantastic wardrobe, a brownstone on the Hill and a cottage on Long Island, she still wasn't satisfied. She wanted one more thing—to cruise around the world. And so he asked her for a divorce.

    She refused to give it to him.

He kept asking; she kept refusing; he began to feel trapped. He imagined himself cutting her face up or pouring lye under each eyelid while she slept. He imagined ridding himself of her in many ways, but realized finally only one way was open: He would have to catch her committing adultery.

Not that he was certain she was cheating on him. But he was certain she might be; long before he asked for his divorce, he'd stopped making love to her. Common sense told him that if he was not between her legs, then some other black man could be.

But he could not catch her at it and so decided to hire someone to get under his wife's clothes and to have pictures taken of the event. Someone was Carlyle Bedlow.

Carlyle was sitting in the dentist's chair—two small leather pillows messing his straightened hair—when the dentist made his proposal. Carlyle's mind said yes immediately, but he wanted to see if the dentist was serious and just how much he was offering. He pretended reluctance and also that such a job was beneath him. "Man, you must be crazy. I don't do no shit like that." He pretended to be someone else so well that, for a moment, he forgot the dentist had just pulled his tooth.

"You don't let me finish." The dentist stood over him, Carlyle's molar clamped between the prongs of his silver pliers. He inspected the tooth, held it so Carlyle could look into its black hole. "You got to take better care of your mouth, Carlyle." He shook his head. "This is a disgrace." He put the pliers and the tooth into a metal dish. "Look, I'm in a spot and it's my only ex-cape. Besides, I ain't mentioned money yet."

"You're hurting me, man, but don't mention it. I don't go in for that kind of stuff. I stick to numbers and warm fur coats." He leaned forward, as if to get up, but the dentist pushed him deeper into his great chair, fingered Carlyle's wound and inserted fresh cotton between cheek and gum.

"The bleeding's stopping." He paused. "Did you ever realize I ain't asking you to do nothing illegal?" He smiled now; the dentist himself had a good dentist. "It's got to be done by somebody and I was just throwing the money your way. All you do is get her clothes off and someone to break in and take pictures."

"Why don't you just ask her for a divorce?" Of course, Carlyle knew, the dentist had already done that.

"You think I hasn't? She won't hear nothing like that. Look, man, I'm in prison with a crazy warden, trying to get me to do all kinds of crazy things." Then he told about his wife's obsession with sailing all around the world.

Carlyle agreed. That did sound crazy. But he still pretended hesitation. "Suppose she really ain't got nobody else? Some women wait. I heard about them. Besides, it ain't my thing."

"She ain't waiting. She's getting some fun somewhere. You don't understand how bad it is." He went to the glass door and opened it. "Jean, come in here, will you, baby?"

Entering the office, hand against jaw, Carlyle had noticed Jean's legs even through his pain. He had tried his smile on her, but her lips had not softened, had remained stretched across her teeth. Now she came in almost suspiciously, but smiled at the dentist after she'd closed the door.

"This is my girl."

"Pleased to meet you." Her eyes were black. She was younger, darker and much better built up than the dentist's wife, whom Carlyle had seen once or twice, with the dentist, in Jack O'Gee's Silver Goose Bar and Restaurant.

"I want to marry Jean." The dentist sat down. "And I thought you might help me, out of friendship."

Carlyle nodded, leaned into the small basin beside him and spat. He did not consider the dentist his friend. He did not even have his home phone number. And if he'd had it, Carlyle would never have listed it among his first five choices as a number to call when he was being arrested. He and the dentist met two or three times a month, by accident only, in the Silver Goose.

The dentist waited for Carlyle to straighten up before he continued. "Now I found me a sane woman and can't live with a crazy one no more. I need those grounds!"

Carlyle glanced at Jean to see if the scheme was new to her. She leaned against the wall near the door, her face empty except for make-up, which was lighter than her skin. "How much you paying?"

"We ain't got no kids." The dentist hesitated and Carlyle knew this, too, was part of the trouble. Carlyle wasn't married, but already he had two children and visited their mothers when he had some money. "That means no support," the dentist hadn't stopped, "and if I get her on adultery, I can cut the alimony down low. So it's worth a thousand if I get my pictures."

It was a better offer than he had expected, but he didn't tell that to the dentist. "Will you throw in my teeth?"

The dentist agreed.

Carlyle climbed out of the dentist's leather chair. "Then, I guess I'll turn legal for a while."

They agreed to meet that night in the Silver Goose. The dentist would bring his wife. Carlyle would sit at their table. After that, they could only hope that the dentist's wife was ready for another new man.

Carlyle was standing at the bar, over his second drink, when they came in. He had seen her only a few times before and his memory had been kind: She looked even less appetizing than he remembered her—in a dull pink dress that hung loosely from narrow shoulders, drowned high, hard breasts and sharp-edged hips. Her face was the color of milk mixed with orange juice, the features squeezed into its center.

Passing by him on the way to the booths at the rear of the Goose, the dentist had not spoken or nodded. But after helping her into a seat and ordering her drink, he returned to the bar and Carlyle. "Bitch didn't want to come, but I told her I sure didn't want to stare at her all night."

Carlyle looked beyond the dentist at his wife. The glass in front of her, a brandy alexander, was already half empty. "What happens to her when she gets drunk?"

"She cries."

Carlyle told the dentist the truth: It couldn't hurt him. "I like your money, but we'll never make it."

"Well, go ahead and try. One thousand dollars is a lot of money."

"You're right." He pushed away from the bar, leaving his drink, which had been stinging the dentist's work, and started toward the booth, the dentist close behind him.

She looked up at them, light-brown eyes in her light-orange face, but she did not speak.

"I ain't seen this nigger in years, Robena." The dentist suddenly pretended great excitement. "We was in the Army together." He introduced them.

Carlyle smiled. "Pleased to meet you." Her hand was cold, filled with tiny bones.

"Have a seat." The dentist motioned him into the booth, next to his wife. As Carlyle was getting settled, she finished her drink, pushed the foamed glass a few inches across the table.

"You want another?" After she nodded the dentist went on selling Carlyle. "We was in Asia. Right, Carlyle?"

"That's right." But so far, Carlyle had been lucky enough to avoid wearing any uniforms.

She looked at him now, seemed not to believe him.

"So how you been, Carlyle?" The dentist did not let him answer. "You do want another drink, don't you?"

She nodded, continuing to study Carlyle.

"What you been doing, man?"

"A little of a lot of things." He reached for his cigarettes, wishing he had smoked for this meeting, trying to decide what to say if she wanted a more precise definition of his livelihood. But then she turned away.

The dentist did not give up. "Carlyle was a male nurse in the dental corps, even pulled some teeth when we had lots of work. He was pretty good at it. I remember the first time I asked him to swing the hammer while I held the chisel. Cat's tooth'd broken off at the root." He started to laugh. "I had to keep telling Carlyle to hit harder. Finally got that sucker out, though. Right, Carlyle?"

"That's right."

The waiter came with her drink. She drained half right away.

"She drinks that like lemonade, huh, Carlyle?"

He did not know what to answer. The dentist had been stupid to ask it. But he forced himself to speak, watching her eyes. "Some people take it better than others."

"And some get falling-down nasty drunk."

She snorted, a short laugh, leaving Carlyle with a silence to fill. "Your wife don't look like that kind." He tried a broad smile.

"Yeah." The dentist finished his drink, put ten dollars on the table and stood up. "I'll be right back." He went toward the rest rooms; but when, 15 minutes later, he had not returned, Carlyle realized he was on his own.

Weather did not interest her, nor Asia, nor even hemlines. She would not speak, gave him no handle. When the ten-dollar bill had dwindled to seven pennies and a dime, he helped her out of the booth, up the stairs to the street and into a taxi.

On the Hill, she handed him a key and he opened her door. He stepped aside, knowing in this situation she would have to ask him inside. "Can you make it all right?"

She nodded and started into the dark house, with his $1000. Then her heels stopped and turned back, but he could not see her pinched face. "You seem too nice to be his friend, Mr. Bedlow." She closed the door in his face.

The next day, he paid the dentist a visit. "Man, that was the wrongest thing you could've did, leaving like that. I got to sell myself under your nose."

Bent over his worktable, the dentist was inspecting his tools. "What happened?"

"Nothing. She just sat there and filled up on that ten you left." He was in the dentist's chair, and his jaw, remembering, began to throb. "We worse off than when we started."

"How you figure that?"

"Because now she connects me with an unhappy time. I got to have a chance to sympathize with her. But she didn't tell me nothing. I didn't have the chance to call you a bastard."

The dentist turned around, a small knife in his hand. "I couldn't sit there with that crazy bitch no more. I went to Jean's."

"You have to hold that back if you want this to work. You educated and all, but that was dumb."

"I couldn't help it." He looked unhappy. "So you didn't make progress?"

"Nothing, man. As a matter of fact, I think she knows we ain't Army buddies, because at the end, she sticks her head out the door and tells me I'm too nice to be your friend—Mr. Bedlow."

"She did?" The dentist brightened. "Goddamn! You made it, Carlyle." He jumped, the knife shining in his fist. "Why didn't you tell me that before?"

Carlyle cleared his throat. "Remember you said you wanted to get out before you got crazy, too?" He shook his head. "You too late."

"Listen." The dentist came toward him, waving the knife. "You're too nice to be my friend. That's a compliment."

Just then, Carlyle very much wished he was on his way to a steady customer with a fur coat fresh from some white woman's unlocked car, perfume still strong in its silk lining. "That ain't no compliment. Not the way she said it. She was just getting you."

"You're wrong. I know my wife, man. I'm a bad guy. But you're too nice to be my friend. She's going for it. Time for stage number two." The weekend was coming, he went on. Friday night, Carlyle, Jean, the dentist and his wife would go down to the cottage at the end of Long Island. Jean would pretend to be Carlyle's date. But once they had arrived, Jean and the dentist would have lots of paperwork. Carlyle would be free to seduce the dentist's wife. He was so sure it would work that he told Carlyle to arrange to have someone there to take pictures on Saturday night. He would put the photographer up at a small motel nearby.

There was no arguing with him. Carlyle agreed to come to the office at six that Friday with a suitcase full of attractive sports clothes, the better to trap the dentist's wife.

The dentist owned a very big automobile. Carlyle and Jean—her big, beautiful thighs crossed—sat in the back. The dentist's wife stared out of the open right front window at cemeteries, airports, rows of pink and gray houses and, finally, sandy hills covered with stubby Christmas trees and hard, dull-green bushes. Two hours from Harlem, they turned onto a dirt road. Then, even over the engine, Carlyle heard the music, as if they had made a giant circle and returned to the summer jukeboxes of the Avenue.

The community was crowded in the dusk light around a small, bright bay. It did not look like Harlem, but if he had come on it by accident, Carlyle would've known that black people lived there. The music was loud and there was the smell of good food, barbecuing ribs, frying chickens. Carlyle had always believed that black people like the dentist and his wife tried very hard to act white. If so, their music and food gave them away.

The dentist's house was glass and lacquered wood, 30 yards from the beach. They sat around an empty yellow-brick fireplace, flicking their ashes into ceramic trays, while the dentist's wife fixed dinner. Behind her back, the dentist winked, smiled, waved at Jean. Carlyle read a magazine, trying to give them privacy—and wondered if the dentist's wife actually did not know about Jean and the dentist. They ate, drank two or three Scotches apiece, tried to talk and, at 11, gave up and went to bed.

Carlyle had not been in bed at 11 in years, and he awoke in the middle of the night. Listening to the waves, he missed Harlem: cars racing lights on the Avenue, drunks indicting the white man, someone still up and playing music. Unable to get sleep back, he climbed out of bed, removed his black pressing rag and went out into the front yard. Something made him look up and he discovered the stars. In Harlem, he could see only the brightest, strongest ones. But now he saw more stars than sequins on a barmaid's dress, and liked them. He sat, then lay down, careful to keep his hands between the wet grass and his hair.

At first he did not hear her thumping toward him. Then her pinched orange-gray face was peering down at him, her hair wrapped around tiny spiked metal rollers. "You didn't like your bed?" She wore only a nightgown, drab in the starlight.

He sat up quickly. "I couldn't sleep, not enough noise." That sounded funny to him and he laughed quietly.

"I know what you mean." She hesitated for a moment, then sat down next to him. It was going to work, after all. The man did know his wife. Maybe she had some men but was very careful about it.

Lowering herself down beside him, she'd gathered up the nightgown to show him knees as square and hard as fist-sized ivory dice. "It's a nice night, though."

"Yeah." He had not finished judging her legs.

"They're not much, are they? Maybe that's why—" She stopped. "No, that's not why." Then she looked at him. "Mr. Bedlow—"

He did not let her finish, had pushed her onto her back while his name was still soft in the air. It was business, like opening a car door, going through a glove compartment, tossing the road maps aside, hoping to find a portable radio or a wallet. She wrapped her thin arms and legs around him, gasping as if in pain.

On hands and knees, he pulled away from her and discovered she had begun to cry. "Oh, this is bad. This is bad. But . . . I was so hot!" She rolled onto her stomach, muffling sobs in the grass. "This is really bad. I can't do *this.*"

He patted her shoulder blades, pulled her nightgown over her buttocks, realizing, as he tried to comfort her, that the dentist had lied to him. If she had been cheating, Carlyle could hope to be President of the United States. Of course, it did not matter, only that he did not want it known that he believed everything people told him.

Finally, he got her to stop crying and sit up. She would not look at him but huddled on the grass, her back to him. "I'm sorry, Mr. Bedlow. I guess you could tell we was having troubles. But I didn't mean to bring you into it."

"Come on, Robena, the sky won't fall down. And call me Carlyle. Mr. Bedlow don't make it now." He moved closer to her, spoke over her shoulder. "What kind of trouble you people got? You own everything, two houses, a big car and all that. So it can't be money." He believed what he said but had asked because now he wanted to know the dentist's weaknesses.

She lowered her chin to her chest. "No, it's not money. Yes, it's money." She raised her head and turned toward him. "How old are you?"

He gave himself a few years.

"I'm thirty-six." She waited, let the number die. "Me and my husband, when we went to school, in Washington, it was different, even from your time. We always thought, at least I did—I mean, now I don't know what he really thought—I mean, we thought it was enough for him to be a dentist. You know what I mean?"

All this had little to do with marriage, the kind he knew. He had expected the usual story, the dentist in the street, running after the many Jeans he'd had before this one. Or perhaps she would think the dentist cheap. He waited.

"But that's not enough anymore. I mean, he's a good dentist, he really is, but they don't care if he's good or not. I always thought they'd care."

They? Carlyle thought. Then he realized she was talking about white people.

"But they don't. It took me a long time to see that; and after, I didn't want to believe it." She paused. "We was raised to believe we had to be best. My momma was always telling me, you got to be best in your class."

Carlyle, too, remembered those words.

"But I was a girl and was only supposed to be the best wife I could be. So when we got married, I worked so he could go to school full time. He's a good dentist, but it didn't do any good. When he should've been on the staff of a good clinic, he ended up in Harlem. And when he should've—" She stopped, shook her head. "This isn't very interesting, is it?"

One quality Carlyle had developed in his work was patience; he told her to go on, still hoping she would give him something important.

"The point is, when I saw they was lying about caring, I looked into everything they said, and you know what? They lied about everything." She spoke as if still bewildered by her discovery.

"Hell, I known that since I was seven."

She shook her head several times. "No, listen, everything. Even about food. You ever read the small print on a box of ice cream? It's not even ice cream."

"You sound like my little brother." He started to laugh. "He's a Black Jesuit. And you know they crazy."

She ignored him. "What I want is for him to stop working for a year and go around the world. I want to see if what I think is true really is. And I want him to see it. And if it is, maybe we can do just something small. It's not enough for us to sit out here on a little pile of money. I mean, we was supposed to do something good for our race, too." She stopped talking then, sat with her chin on her knees, her nightgown bunched around her thighs, leaving Carlyle disappointed.

Then she stood up. "Well, that's my sad tale. Maybe you'll tell me yours one time." She smiled, for the first time.

In the kitchen, she gave him a cup of instant coffee. He read the label and wondered what kind of chemicals the Xs and Ys were, and what they did to his stomach. When he had finished the coffee, he returned to his room, retied his head and climbed into bed.

The dentist knocked at his door at nine the next morning but did not wait for Carlyle to ask him in. "You made it, didn't you? I knew you could crack it open. Been done before. I hope your man is a good picture taker. My prints got to come out clear!"

Carlyle propped himself against the bed's headboard. "She may not do it again." He had decided he would let the dentist think himself still in charge.

"Go on, man. Everybody knows the first nut is the hardest."

"Maybe so. How you know, anyway?"

"I woke up at three and she wasn't in bed. And neither was you. I figured you was together someplace. What'd you think of it?"

"Ain't the best I ever had."

"Me, too." The dentist came to the bed's foot. "But with the money, you can buy something better." The dentist smiled, good, even white teeth, one gold covered—then closed his lips. "You better drive over to that motel and tell your friend to load his camera."

Carlyle nodded. "What's your plan for today?"

"We're invited to a party. In the late afternoon. We get her drunk, you bring her home, naked, and in bed. I'll make sure you got the house to yourselves." He smiled again. "Me and my Jean'll make sure, someplace." He laughed, turning to the door. "Get your hook in deep."

"I might toss this one back."

He opened the door. "Not in my creek, you won't."

But Carlyle was not so sure.

As he dressed—in short-sleeved pink silk shirt, white bell-bottoms—he tried to decide exactly what to do. Obviously, he wanted to come out the other end with the dentist's $1000. But then the dentist would have to get his pictures. What Carlyle most wanted was to get his money but leave the dentist married to his crazy wife. That would sound good when told in the bars. "That dentist thought he had Carlyle, but then Carlyle Bedlow got down to business, do you hear, business!" That meant he had to get the money before the dentist saw the pictures, bad ones. Pictures in which the woman's face was not quite clear. When he paid the money, the dentist would have to believe the pictures were good. Carlyle heard himself talking: "She passed out, man. I just sat there beside her in my shorts: we pulled back the covers and Hondo snapped away. They so good we might even sell some." But the pictures wouldn't show a thing. He rehearsed his speech while he finished dressing.

He avoided breakfast, wanting the dentist to suffer through a morning with both of his women, imagining that as he drove between the trees on his way to see his friend, the photographer, Hondo Johnson.

"Wait a minute. You saying you don't want the pictures to come out?"

"Right."

"Well, why don't you just give him a blank roll?" Hondo was still in his pajamas, a pullover top, shorts. They were lemon yellow and his legs were brown and shiny. He was sitting on the edge of his motel bed.

"Because, if he ever finds me, I can tell him it was a surprise to me, too. I'll offer to do it again." He was looking into Hondo's mirror, checking his hair. "But he won't go for it, because no man could do it two times to the same woman. And I'm sorry, Doc, but I already spent that money. He ain't got no boys to send after me."

"Come on, man. Why can't we just do it simple? Take the pictures and get the money." Once Hondo thought it was going one way, he did not like to change his plans. He couldn't improvise. But if he knew exactly what to do, it was done. "We'll mess up, man. And I could've used the money."

"We won't lose the money. We'll take insurance pictures. Good ones, with her legs open and all. I know a man downtown'll buy them." And it would be good to have the pictures, just in case the dentist did have some boys. "You satisfied now?"

Hondo nodded but did not look happy. His lips were poked out under his mustache. "Tell me the signal."

"When I turn out the lights." Carlyle hadn't really thought about it.

Hondo started to laugh. "And how'm I supposed to shoot pictures in the dark?" He was pleased to have caught Carlyle.

"You're all right, man." He adjusted his shirt, turned from the mirror. "What about the blinds?"

"That's good. Pull down the blinds, and if they already down, pull them up. Just do something with them blinds." He stood up. "You got that?"

"OK." He liked Hondo. "But I'll try to get her falling-down, so we'll have plenty of time and she won't know nothing. Then we leave. I don't like no drunken broads, anyway."

It was working. She might even pass out before he got her off the dirt road, into the house and out of her clothes. The party had started at five and now, at ten, was still going. They had eaten—potato salad, fried chicken and greens, on paper plates—drinking steadily. The doctors, lawyers, dentists, big-time hustlers got very loud about baseball, the white man, Harlem after the War, when they were all starting careers. Their children, teenagers, had finally gained control of the phonograph and were dancing hard on the lawn. Carlyle had filled her empty glasses. Finally, he asked her if she wanted to go home. Winking at the dentist, he led her out of the house.

In the moonlight, the dirt of the road, half sand, shone gray. He was supporting her with a hand on her bony rib cage. "How you doing?" He did not really want her to answer and disturb herself.

"I'm doing fine. What did you say?"

"Nothing." They were on the dentist's grass now, circling a clump of lawn chairs and an umbrella table, a few steps from the porch. He saw the bushes move and waved at Hondo.

Taking her straight to her bedroom, he turned on the dim table lamp and began to undress her. She did not resist but was so still that he was not sure she was awake. He put her clothes onto a chair, returned to the bed and pulled the bed-covers from under her. "Thanks, baby." It sounded strange the way she said it. It was meant not for him but for the dentist.

He undressed to his shorts, went to the window and pulled down the blinds. "What's that?" She raised her head, but it weighed too much.

He tried to imitate the dentist. "Nothing, baby. We need some air, is all."

Hondo was coming. He had banged open the front door, was making his way through the living room, bumping into things. He slid the coffee table out of his way. Carlyle went to the bedroom door. "Hey, man, quiet down. Follow my voice."

"Why didn't you turn on some lights, nigger?" He had almost reached the hallway. Carlyle was at the other end.

"Follow my voice, man."

Now Hondo ran toward him, appeared, in Bermuda shorts and sneakers. Carlyle backed into the room.

Hondo popped into the doorway, stopped. "You expect me to take pictures in this light?" He was disgusted.

"Quiet down, man," Carlyle whispered. "She ain't out yet."

"I got to have more light. I ain't got no infrared attachment." He began to focus his camera on the dentist's naked wife.

"Baby?" She rolled to her side, then back. "Who's that?"

"Ain't nobody. Close your eyes. I'm turning on the top light."

She did not answer. He waited, then switched it on. It was very bright. For a few seconds, he could not see Hondo. "OK now?"

"I think so." He put the camera to his face again. "But I can't be sure until I read the meter."

"Come on, man. We ain't got time for that." She was going to wake up. Somehow he knew it.

"Always got time. What if we ain't got our insurance pictures?" He took a light meter from his pocket, advanced on her, held it over her navel.

Carlyle sat down on the bed. "How you doing, baby?" He patted her shoulder.

Her eyes were closed. "Who was that just now?"

"Just a guy." He leaned over, kissed her cheek.

"I got it now, man." Hondo had moved to the foot of the bed. "One point four. But I got to do it in seconds, so you can't move."

"Who's that voice?" She raised herself to her elbows, looked up into Hondo's lens. "Who's he?"

"OK, now hold it."

But she was already moving, realizing she was with Carlyle, scrambling to the edge of the bed. "He got you to do this."

Carlyle reached out for her, but she broke away and jumped for the closet, "He'll never get one now." She pulled the door behind her.

Carlyle did not follow her. He could easily open the closet door, but that would be useless. She had to be in bed with a man, looking either surprised or happy, but not struggling. "You better come out of there, Robena." He put a threat into his voice but did not mean it. She had to imprison herself while he thought. He knew what he had to do now: convince her to pose for the pictures.

He looked at Hondo, still busy with final adjustments, then stood up. "Listen, baby, you can't stay in there all night. And nobody's coming to rescue you." His mouth was close to the door.

"And nobody's getting a divorce, either." She started to scold him. "I thought you was nice."

"I am. We ain't even into how nice I really am. Come on out."

Hondo sat down on the bed, camera waiting.

"You're not nice." She paused, cleared her nose. "You make love to women for money." She sniffled again.

"That ain't the way it is. I came out here with Jean. Your husband's nurse?"

"I know her. She got a crush on him."

"No, she don't." He waited; she did not speak. "She's with me, but then last night you and me got into something special. But your husband found out. And he said he'd make a lot of trouble for me if I didn't get his pictures. He got me in a terrible spot."

She paused for a moment. "First of all, you didn't even talk to Jean all the way out in the car. And second, where did you get a cameraman so fast?"

The dentist's wife was very smart. "You being real stupid. What you want with a man who don't want you?"

"He does so want me." She did not believe herself.

"No, he don't. He wants Jean. He wants to marry Jean." His voice was cold, the way he talked to white policemen as long as their guns were buried under blue winter coats. "And he's paying me lots of money to get him a divorce."

She waited again, crying behind the closet door. "Well, he's not getting one."

"Listen to me, Robena." He bent closer, softened his tone. "Face it, baby. He don't want you. He don't want anything about you. He don't want to go around the world with you. He thinks you're crazy to want to do that. Give the man his pictures."

And she did.

They were the clearest pictures any judge would ever see. The woman sat on the bed, bare to the waist. She looked sad, her infidelity uncovered. The young black hoodlum, his hair shiny and slightly waved, was certainly not her husband.

Hondo took no others. Carlyle had decided against trying for the extra money. One thousand was enough. The dentist paid him, in cash, the following Monday evening.

Carlyle had long since turned the money into clothes, a good camel's-hair overcoat, shoes, a few suits, when next he heard from the dentist's wife. She had mailed a postcard to him, care of the Silver Goose. It came from Europe:

Hello. We're here on our honeymoon. My husband is a dentist from [the ink had been smudged] in Africa. Best wishes, Robena (the dentist's wife, remember?).

At first Carlyle did not remember. When he did, he thought about it for a while. . . .

A. J. CRONIN

"Doctor, I can't . . . I won't have a child"

"Doctor, I can't . . . I won't have a child."

It was four o'clock in the afternoon, the hour of my "best" consultations, and the woman who spoke so vehemently was tall, distinguished, and handsome, fashionably dressed in a dark grey costume, with an expensive diamond clip in her smart black hat.

I had just examined her, and now, having dried my hands methodically, I put away the towel and turned toward her. "It's a little late to make that decision now. You should have thought of it two months ago. You are exactly nine weeks pregnant. Your baby will be born toward the middle of July."

"I won't have it. . . . You've got to help me, Doctor. You simply must."

How often had I heard these words before. I had heard them from frightened little shopgirls in trouble; from a shamed spinster, aged thirty-five, who told me in a trembling voice, exactly like the heroine of old-time melodrama, that she had been "betrayed"; from a famous film actress defiantly resolved that her career should not be ruined; above all had I heard them from selfish and neurotic wives, afraid of the pangs of childbirth, afraid of losing their figure, their health, their life, afraid—most specious pretext of all—of "losing their husband's love."

This case was somewhat different. I knew my patient, Beatrice Glendenning, socially; knew also her husband, Henry, and her two grown-up sons. They were wealthy people, with a town house in Knightsbridge and a large estate in Hampshire, where the pheasant shooting was excellent and where, indeed, I had spent several pleasant week ends.

"You understand . . . , it isn't just money, Doctor. . . . I must get out of this business, and to do so I'll give anything." She looked me full in the face.

There was no mistaking her meaning. Indeed, that same offer, indescribable in its implications, had been made to me before, though perhaps never so blatantly. It had been made by a young French modiste, estranged from her husband, who had compromised herself with another man and who, slim, elegant, and bewitching, with affected tears in her beautiful eyes, leaned forward and tried to take my hands in hers.

Doctors are only human, they have the same difficulty in repressing their instincts as other men. Yet, if not for moral reasons, from motives of sheer common sense, I had never lost my head. Once a doctor embarks upon a career as abortionist he is irretrievably lost.

There were, however, many such illicit practitioners in the vicinity, both men and women, plying their perilous undercover trade at exorbitant rates, until one day, inevitably, the death of some wretched girl brought them exposure, ruin, and a long term of imprisonment. Perhaps desperation blinded such patients as came to me, yet it always struck me as amazing how few of them were conscious of the infinite danger involved in illegal abortion. Under the best hospital conditions the operation holds a definite risk. Performed hastily in some backstairs room with a septic instrument by some brutal or unskilled practitioner, the result almost inevitably is severe haemorrhage, followed by infection and acute peritonitis.

There were others too, among these women who believed it was within my power to relieve them of their incubus by such a simple expedient as an ergot pill or a mixture of jalap and senna. Others, too, who confessed to having tried the weirdest expedients, from boiling-hot baths to such eccentric gymnastics as descending the stairs backward, in a crouching position. Poor creatures, some were almost comic in their distress, and there were among them many who needed sympathy and comfort. This they got from me, with much good advice, but nothing more.

Beatrice Glendenning, however, was neither comic nor ignorant, but a strong-minded, intelligent woman of the world who moved with considerable éclat in the best society.

My only possible attitude was not to take her seriously. So I reasoned mildly:

"I daresay it's rather inconvenient . . . , with these two grown-up sons of yours. And it'll spoil your London season. But Henry will be pleased."

"Don't be a fool, Doctor. Henry isn't the father."

Although I had half expected this, it silenced me.

During these country week ends I had met the inevitable family intimate, a close friend of Henry's, who went fishing and shooting with him, a sporting type, one of these "good fellows," whom I had disliked on sight and who obviously was on confidential terms with Henry's wife.

"Well," I said at last, "it's a bad business. But there's nothing I can do about it."

"You won't help me?"

"I can't."

There was a pause. The blood had risen to her cheeks and her eyes flashed fire at me. She drew on her gloves, took up her bag. A rejected woman is an enemy for life.

"Very well, Doctor, there's no more to be said."

"Just one thing before you go. . . . Don't put yourself in the hands of a quack. You may regret it."

She gave no sign of having heard, but swept out of the room without another word.

The interview left me not only with a bad taste in my mouth, but in a thoroughly bad mood. I felt that I had lost an excellent patient, an agreeable hostess, and the half dozen brace of admirable pheasants which I had come to regard as my annual autumnal perquisite. I never expected to see Mrs. Glendenning again. How wrong I was—how little I knew of that invincible woman's character!

About ten days later the telephone rang. It was Henry Glendenning himself. Beatrice, he told me, had a frightful cold, an attack of influenza, in fact. Would I be a dear chap and pop round to Knightsbridge as soon as convenient? Pleased by this *rapprochement,* I arrived within the hour at the Glendenning town house and was shown directly to Beatrice's room.

Attended by a nurse, a heavily built, middle-aged woman with a face like a trap, the patient was in bed. She appeared, at first sight, rather more ill than I had expected—fearfully blanched, with bloodless lips and every indication of a raging fever. Puzzled, I drew back the sheet . . . , and then the truth burst upon me. The thing had been done—botched and bungled—she was thoroughly septic and had been haemorrhaging for at least twelve hours.

"I have everything ready for you, Doctor." The nurse was addressing me in a toneless voice, proffering a container of swabs and gauze.

I drew back in a cold fury. I wanted, there and then, to walk out of the room. But how could I? She was *in extremis.* I must do something for this damned woman, and at once. I was fairly trapped.

I began to work on her. My methods, I fear, were not especially merciful, but she offered no protest, suffered the severest pangs without a word. At last the bleeding was under control. I prepared to go.

All this time, as she lay there, Mrs. Glendenning's eyes had never left my face. And now, with an effort, she spoke:

"It's influenza, Doctor. Henry knows it's influenza. I shall expect you this evening."

Downstairs, in the library, Henry had a glass of sherry ready for me, concerned, naturally, about his wife, whom he adored, yet hospitable, as always. He was in stature quite a small man, shy and rather ineffectual in manner, who had inherited a fortune from his father and spent much of it in making others happy. As I gazed at his open, kindly face, all that I had meant to say died upon my tongue. I could not tell him. I could not.

"Nasty thing, this influenza, Doctor."

I took a quick breath.

"Yes, Henry."

"Quite a severe attack she has, too."

"I'm afraid so."

"You'll see her through, Doctor."

A pause.

"Yes, Henry, I'll see her through."

I called again that evening. I called twice a day for the next ten days. It was a thoroughly unpleasant case, demanding constant surgical attention. I suppose I did my part in maintaining the deception. But the real miracles of strategy were performed by Beatrice and the nurse. For Henry Glendenning, who lived all that time in the same house, who slept every night in the bedroom adjoining the sickroom, *never for a moment suspected the true state of affairs.* The thing sounds incredible, but it is true.

At the end of that month I made my final visit. Mrs. Glendenning was up, reclining on the drawing-room sofa, looking ethereal and soulful in a rose-coloured tea gown with pure white lace at cuff and collar. Flowers were everywhere. Henry, delighted, still adoring, was dancing attendance. Tea was brought, served by a trim maid—the grim-visaged nurse had long since departed.

Toying with a slice of teacake, Beatrice gazed at me with wide and wistful eyes.

"Henry is taking me to Madeira next week, Doctor. He feels I need the change."

"You do indeed, darling."

"Thank you, sweetheart."

Oh God, the duplicity, the perfidy of woman . . . the calm, deep, premeditated, and infernal cunning!

"We'll be alone together for the first week," she concluded, sweetly. "A second honeymoon. Then we expect George to join us. We're both very fond of George."

Her eye sought mine, held it, and did not for an instant falter.

"More tea, Doctor, dear? You must come and shoot with us when we get back."

When I rose to go, Henry saw me to the door, shook my hand warmly.

"Thank you for all you've done, Doctor." And he added, "Confoundedly nasty thing, that influenza."

I walked all the way home across Kensington Gardens, gritting my teeth and muttering, "That creature, oh that damned, that most damnable creature!"

But in September I got my half-dozen brace of pheasants. They were nice, tender birds!

Topics for Discussion and Writing

1. The medical examination can be a frightening experience, as Miller's "On the Examination Table" aptly illustrates. Describe a single recent experience *you* have had as an examinee. Did you see the examination ritual as positive or negative? Why?

2. Selzer's physician-lover and the prostitute both realize that the newly discovered lump may indicate cancer. Discuss the Selzer story in light of recent newspaper and magazine accounts of breast-cancer surgery among women. Is a woman still whole or complete after the removal or loss of a part of her body? Explain your position.

3. Why is it so important to realize that in "The Consultation" the early paragraph beginning "Gloria Snurkowski was the name he had been given to look up" necessarily reflects *only* the surgeon's point of view (the "he" of the story) rather than Selzer's point of view?

4. In the first part of "Diabetes," the speaker learns of his disease and what regimen he should follow to control it; but in the second part, he grows agitated, rebellious, and somewhat morbid. Can you explain these lines from the penultimate stanza: "how hard it [the body] works / For its medical books is not / Everything: everything is how / Much glory is in it"? What, then, is the significance of his having "a long drink of beer" at the end? Does this diabetic (or anyone with a chronic disease) have the right to ignore his physician's instructions and court possible death? Defend your response.

5. Write a short but well-organized essay that compares or contrasts the little girl's reactions and feelings at being examined in Williams' "The Use of Force" with those of someone (perhaps even yourself as a child) who has undergone a similar examination.

6. Consumerism is not a completely new criterion to apply to medical care. What slightly ironic detail appears in the third paragraph of Williams' "The Use of Force," written in 1938? In what ways has the doctor truly earned his fee by the story's conclusion?

7. While we may be surprised to see the examiner (Dr. Williams) express some very human feelings throughout "The Use of Force," it may be more important to notice how he later justifies his behavior toward the child. Does the consideration of community health require his getting an immediate diagnosis? Should he have "desisted and come back in an hour or more"? Or is the question irrelevant because the era of the house call has ended?

8. Kafka's "A Country Doctor" may be read as a dream in which the district doctor is used (or misused) by the people "for sacred ends" and then is cast off once he has fulfilled his sacrificial role. If we are indeed

reading the story as a dream or nightmare, what significance could there be in juxtaposing (a) the servant girl named "Rose" whom we last see fleeing from the brutish man in the pigsty and (b) the boy's eventually discovered wound in his right side, "Rose-red" with worms "themselves rose-red and blood-spotted as well"?

9.   Obviously, in focusing in part 1 primarily on the doctor-patient relationship, we are telling but an incomplete story of medicine in literature. In which selections have nurses and other health-care personnel appeared thus far? List and discuss their roles and functions, citing specific examples from the text.

10. Why are the poems "The Hospital," "Unknown Girl in the Maternity Ward," and "The Surgeon at 2 A.M." grouped together? Do you have an inpatient hospital experience that could serve as the basis for a poem or short story? Does your experience have anything in common with the overall tone or atmosphere of these poems?

11. In Lawrence's "The Horse Dealer's Daughter," point of view or focus of narration (that is, the position or positions from which the story is told) is crucial for determining theme or meaning. First we focus on the general scene, then on Mabel, and finally on the doctor. Whose story is this? Defend your interpretation in an essay that makes use of supporting quotations from the text. Be prepared to summarize your case in a brief panel presentation.

12. How dedicated to healing patients can or should a physician be? There seems to be constant conflict between a doctor's personal life and professional career. Do "The Surgeon at 2 A.M.," "The Horse Dealer's Daughter," and "Doctor's Wife" shed any light on the issue? Can any of the other selections in this part help out here?

13. How exactly does the dentist in Kelley's story violate the customary if not ethical boundaries implicit in the doctor-patient relationship? Write an evaluative character sketch of the dentist. Do the same for Carlyle, the patient. How are these two men similar? How are they different? What of their attitudes toward women?

14. What precisely does the dentist's wife, Robena, want? Does she ever get it? Can we be sure?

15. Is the ending of "The Dentist's Wife" at all contrived? Develop and support your conclusions.

16. Contrast the Kelley story with the interview from Studs Terkel's book *Working* of a sensitive West Indian practical nurse in an old people's home, "Carmelita Lester," in part 5 of this anthology.

17. How do you react to Cronin's "common sense" motives and "moral reasons" for refusing the abortion request? Is sexism evident in Cronin's attitude toward Mrs. Glendenning?

18. Did Cronin do the right thing in treating the woman only after she "was *in extremis*" and in also hiding Mrs. Glendenning's real malady from

her concerned husband? Take a stand and defend it. Do changes in abortion laws since Cronin's earlier twentieth-century setting make any difference in addressing the moral issue at hand?

19. Do you detect instances of humor or at least a lighter side in any of the selections in this part? How does that humor function?

Part 2

Medicine
and Humor

Creative works dealing with medicine-in-literature themes do not always tell a sad, serious, or morbid story. In several selections from the first part, we can discover flashes of humor and some definite emphases on the lighter side of a situation. For the most part, however, the humor there functions as comic relief and is not the main focus. Thus the final conversation between the surgeon and the prostitute in Selzer's "The Consultation" breaks the ice in a very tense situation; the banter in their farewell exchange concludes the story on a somewhat positive note, even though she still has the menacing lump that he has just discovered. Williams' "The Use of Force" depicts a struggle between the doctor-examiner and the child-examinee that is often punctuated by seriocomic events and accidents, as when she reduces to splinters his wooden tongue depressor. Even Kelley's "The Dentist's Wife," a story set in Harlem that raises many moral and ethical questions, presents characters who are flip, smart, or witty as they act out their little drama; the scenes where the dentist tries to match up his wife with his patient, Carlyle, are funny yet at the same time sad. In these three stories, therefore, humor functions as a kind of temporary diversion or comic relief. It has a decidedly adjunct role to play, though a necessary one.

But in the selections in this part humor is *the* major focus and has a primary role. Sometimes writers will aim to poke fun at the medical profession in general. Sometimes they will paint satiric portraits of the relationships possible in a medical setting, whether ancient or modern. The six selections in this part, then, can help us understand and appreciate more fully the lighter side of medicine in literature.

The satiric description of a medical man that appears as part of the "Prologue" to *The Canterbury Tales* by fourteenth-century British poet Geoffrey Chaucer provides insight into how a medieval physician practiced among his patients. His general plan for healing the human body was based on "astronomy" (that is, astrology), the elements, and the "humours." The human body was for a long time thought to be composed of four elements—earth, air, fire, water— in the appropriate proportions; diseases, medieval physicians reasoned, resulted from some imbalance within one or more of these elements. Each element was associated with a specific temperature and degree of moisture. For example, earth was cold and dry, air was hot and moist, fire was hot and dry, and water was cold and moist. One's "humour" or disposition was related to this concept of the four elements. The relative relationship of the elements determined the character of the person. For instance, a man who was melancholy was considered to be cold and dry. It was also possible to be phlegmatic (cold and moist), choleric (hot and dry), and sanguine (hot and moist) in this scheme.

According to Chaucer, a physician could work his "charms and magic effigies" when his patient's "favourable star" was in the right place. Moreover, Chaucer's doctor is aided by being "well-versed" in a long (in fact, too long) list of medical authorities from the mythical Aesculapius through the ancient Hippocrates and Galen to the medieval Gilbertine—though, significantly, "He did not read the Bible very much." Chaucer ironically points out the quite common financial relationship between a doctor and his apothecaries as being mutually beneficial; even today this problem of an unholy alliance between M.D. and druggist persists in some places. Chaucer's physician has made a great deal of money from the plagues—there were many in the Middle Ages—and as a final cut, we learn why "He therefore had a special love of gold."

Ben Jonson, the seventeenth-century British poet and dramatist, follows Chaucer's example with a clever, glib, yet terse four-line epigram, "To Doctor Empirick," that gives double thanks for the freedom the speaker has obtained both from his disease and from Doctor Empirick, his quack physician. Jonson also makes reference to Aesculapius, the Greek god of medicine and healing, in the second line of the epigram. Clearly, in Jonson's time, medicine was far from being as precise or dependable as it is now.

The French playwright Molière was so fond of attacking the hypocrisy of the physician's world that he wrote four comedies with medical themes, including *The Doctor in Spite of Himself,* which we here reprint in its entirety. This rollicking seventeenth-century farce contains many of the same humorous themes that have been carried over into much modern literature on our topic. People often want to be ruled over and prescribed to by a physician; in this way, they can feel a certain sense of security. Molière shows how gullible people can be, and he entertainingly exaggerates a bit to drive home his point. Sganarelle, a local woodcutter, is mistaken for a great doctor. He plays the part well and adapts to whatever situation arises—all for his own self-preservation. In act II, scene 4, there is a grand parody of this would-be doctor's knowledge in an incredible speech in which Sganarelle recites Latin phrases that make absolutely no sense. Yet because the doctor's world seems such a learned, mysterious place to the common man, a long string of Latin phrases (even from an imposter) does much to impress the uninitiated.

Further on in the play, Molière attacks the people's credulity, for they do not really test this "pretend" physician until his disguise wears thin late in the comedy. Dispensing useless advice for ready cash, fooling around with nurses,

doing a profitable business with apothecaries, promising "miracle" cures—
these are but a few of Molière's targets in the medical profession. The reasoning in Sganarelle's key speech at the opening of act III on the benefits of
being a doctor ("No, I tell you: they made me a doctor in spite of me . . .") is
still partially valid in the minds of many people. Sganarelle holds that "The
blunders are never ours, and it's always the fault of the person who dies."
Fortunately, the strict licensing regulations of the medical profession make a
Sganarelle-type doctor a rarity in our times.

Nathaniel Hawthorne's "The Haunted Quack" is a nineteenth-century tale
that continues several Molière themes and goes beyond them. Hippocrates
Jenkins—his first name recalls the famous ancient physician, his last name is
paradoxically a very common one—is a troubled young quack. Everything
goes well for him until a woman dies from one of his strong potions. "Hippy"
flees his practice, is haunted by the ghost of the dead woman, and returns to
face the townspeople. Hawthorne sprinkles this comic story with references to
the making of money by practicing quack medicine (no one is licensed here),
to the age-old apothecary-physician connection, to the calling of Aesculapius
and its mysteries, to the gullibility of people and especially patients, and to
experimentation with various drugs in a wholly unscientific manner. At the
end, "Hippy" is restored to "the practice of his profession," for through a
comic reversal, we learn that old Granny Gordon did not die from the potion
after all (she swooned, then got better) and that the town wants him to
stay on!

In "The Stethoscope Song," nineteenth-century writer-physician Oliver
Wendell Holmes focuses his poetic and humorous attention on a young doctor
whose new stethoscope contains two flies. The erroneous diagnoses that follow
are predictably ridiculous and often deadly. Holmes makes good fun of
medical terms used to excess, and his message appears to be that a doctor
should rely on common sense as well as new technology. It would prove
fruitful to compare and contrast Holmes and Molière on how high-flown
medical terminology may confuse but rarely clarify diagnoses, diseases, and
cures.

Lastly, Phyllis McGinley's "Complaint to the American Medical Association" supplies a lively review of "the Medico, / That hero antiseptic." While
at first she wittily praises the doctor for his many exploits, she soon draws
the line at doctors who seek "a Literary Style," that is, doctors who aspire to
be authors and so practice *her* profession without "Their literary license."
In light of the selections seen thus far in this anthology by Drs. Selzer,
Williams, Cronin, and Holmes, and in light of those works yet to appear here
by Drs. Maugham, Chekhov, Doyle, Keats, and Bridges, we might wish to
evaluate McGinley's two-pronged but good-natured attack: (1) "But is it
fair he [the doctor] should lay claim to / The overcrowded writing game,
too?" and (2) "In what brave school did he matriculate / That he should
be so damned articulate?"

GEOFFREY CHAUCER

The Physician

A *Doctor* too emerged as we proceeded;
No one alive could talk as well as he did
On points of medicine and of surgery,
For, being grounded in astronomy,
He watched his patient's favourable star
And, by his Natural Magic, knew what are
The lucky hours and planetary degrees
For making charms and magic effigies.
The cause of every malady you'd got
He knew, and whether dry, cold, moist or hot;
He knew their seat, their humour and condition.
He was a perfect practising physician.
These causes being known for what they were,
He gave the man his medicine then and there.
All his apothecaries in a tribe
Were ready with the drugs he would prescribe,
And each made money from the other's guile;
They had been friendly for a goodish while.
He was well-versed in Esculapius too
And what Hippocrates and Rufus knew
And Dioscorides, now dead and gone,
Galen and Rhazes, Hali, Serapion,
Averroes, Avicenna, Constantine,
Scotch Bernard, John of Gaddesden, Gilbertine.
In his own diet he observed some measure;
There were no superfluities for pleasure,
Only digestives, nutritives and such.
He did not read the Bible very much.
In blood-red garments, slashed with bluish-grey
And lined with taffeta, he rode his way;
Yet he was rather close as to expenses
And kept the gold he won in pestilences.
Gold stimulates the heart, or so we're told.
He therefore had a special love of gold.

Translated by Nevill Coghill

BEN JONSON

To Doctor Empirick

When men a dangerous disease did 'scape
Of old, they gave a cock to Aesculape;
Let me give two, that doubly am got free
From my disease's danger, and from thee.

MOLIÈRE

The Doctor in Spite of Himself

CHARACTERS

SGANARELLE, husband of Martine
MARTINE, wife of Sganarelle
MONSIEUR ROBERT, neighbor of Sganarelle
VALÈRE, servant of Géronte
LUCAS, husband of Jacqueline
GÉRONTE, father of Lucinde
JACQUELINE, wet-nurse at Géronte's and wife of Lucas
LUCINDE, daughter of Géronte
LÉANDRE, in love with Lucinde
THIBAUT, a peasant, father of Perrin
PERRIN, a peasant, son of Thibaut

ACT I

A clearing. The houses of Sganarelle and Monsieur Robert may be seen through the trees.

Scene 1.   SGANARELLE, MARTINE (*who enter quarreling*)

SGANARELLE: No, I tell you I won't do anything of the sort, and I'm the one to say and be the master.

MARTINE: And *I* tell *you* that I want you to live to suit me, and I didn't marry you to put up with your carryings-on.

SGANARELLE: Oh, what a weary business it is to have a wife, and how right Aristotle is when he says a wife is worse than a demon!

MARTINE: Just listen to that smart fellow with his half-wit Aristotle!

SGANARELLE: Yes, a smart fellow. Just find me a woodcutter who knows how to reason about things, like me, who served a famous doctor for six years, and who as a youngster knew his elementary Latin book by heart.

MARTINE: A plague on the crazy fool!

SGANARELLE: A plague on the slut!

MARTINE: Cursed be the day when I went and said yes!

SGANARELLE: Cursed be the hornified notary who had me sign my own ruin!

MARTINE: Really, it's a fine thing for you to complain of that affair! Should you let a single moment go by without thanking Heaven for having me for your wife? And did you deserve to marry a person like me?

SGANARELLE: Oh, yes, you did me too much honor, and I had reason to congratulate myself on our wedding night! Oh, my Lord! Don't get me started on that! I'd have a few things to say . . .

MARTINE: What? What would you say?

SGANARELLE: Let it go at that; let's drop that subject. Enough that we know what we know, and that you were very lucky to find me.

MARTINE: What do you mean, lucky to find you? A man who drags me down to the poorhouse, a debauchee, a traitor, who eats up everything I own?

SGANARELLE: That's a lie: I drink part of it.

MARTINE: Who sells, piece by piece, everything in the house.

SGANARELLE: That's living on our means.

MARTINE: Who's taken even my bed from under me.

SGANARELLE: You'll get up all the earlier in the morning.

MARTINE: In short, who doesn't leave a stick of furniture in the whole house.

SGANARELLE: All the easier to move out.

MARTINE: And who does nothing but gamble and drink from morning to night.

SGANARELLE: That's so I won't get bored.

MARTINE: And what do you expect me to do with my family in the mean-time?

SGANARELLE: Whatever you like.

MARTINE: I have four poor little children on my hands.

SGANARELLE: Set them on the floor.

MARTINE: Who are constantly asking me for bread.

SGANARELLE: Give them the whip. When I've had plenty to eat and drink, I want everyone in my house to have his fill.

MARTINE: And you, you drunkard, do you expect things to go on forever like this?

SGANARELLE: My good wife, let's go easy, if you please.

MARTINE: And me to endure your insolence and debauchery to all eternity?

SGANARELLE: Let's not get excited, my good wife.

MARTINE: And that I can't find a way to make you do your duty?

SGANARELLE: My good wife, you know that my soul isn't very patient and my arm is pretty good.

MARTINE: You make me laugh with your threats.

SGANARELLE: My good little wife, my love, you're itching for trouble, as usual.

MARTINE: I'll show you I'm not afraid of you.

SGANARELLE: My dear better half, you're asking for something.

MARTINE: Do you think your words frighten me?

SGANARELLE: Sweet object of my eternal vows, I'll box your ears.

MARTINE: Drunkard that you are!

SGANARELLE: I'll beat you.

MARTINE: Wine-sack!

SGANARELLE: I'll wallop you.

MARTINE: Wretch!

SGANARELLE: I'll tan your hide.

MARTINE: Traitor, wiseacre, deceiver, coward, scoundrel, gallowsbird, beggar, good-for-nothing, rascal, villain, thief . . .

SGANARELLE (*takes a stick and beats her*):   Ah! So you want it, eh?

MARTINE: Oh, oh, oh, oh!

SGANARELLE: That's the right way to pacify you.

Scene 2.   MONSIEUR ROBERT, SGANARELLE, MARTINE

MONSIEUR ROBERT: Hey there, hey there, hey there! Fie! What's this? What infamy! Confound the rascal for beating his wife that way!

MARTINE (*arms akimbo, forces* MONSIEUR ROBERT *back as she talks, and finally gives him a slap*):   And as for me, I want him to beat me.

MONSIEUR ROBERT: Oh! Then with all my heart, I consent.

MARTINE: What are you meddling for?

MONSIEUR ROBERT: I'm wrong.

MARTINE: Is it any business of yours?

MONSIEUR ROBERT: You're right.

MARTINE: Just look at this meddler, trying to keep husbands from beating their wives.

MONSIEUR ROBERT: I take it all back.

MARTINE: What have you got to do with it?

MONSIEUR ROBERT: Nothing.

MARTINE: Have you any right to poke your nose in?

MONSIEUR ROBERT: No.

MARTINE: Mind your own business.

MONSIEUR ROBERT: I won't say another word.

MARTINE: I like to be beaten.

MONSIEUR ROBERT: All right.

MARTINE: It's no skin off your nose.

MONSIEUR ROBERT: That's true.

MARTINE: And you're a fool to come butting in where it's none of your business. (*Slaps* MONSIEUR ROBERT. *He turns toward* SGANARELLE, *who likewise forces him back as he talks, threatening him with the same stick and finally beating and routing him with it.*)

MONSIEUR ROBERT: Neighbor, I beg your pardon with all my heart. Go on, beat your wife and thrash her to your heart's content; I'll help you if you want.

SGANARELLE: Me, I don't want to.

MONSIEUR ROBERT: Oh well, that's another matter.

SGANARELLE: I want to beat her if I want to; and I don't want to beat her if I don't want to.

MONSIEUR ROBERT: Very well.

SGANARELLE: She's my wife, not yours.

MONSIEUR ROBERT: Undoubtedly.

SGANARELLE: I don't take orders from you.

MONSIEUR ROBERT: Agreed.

SGANARELLE: I don't need any help from you.

MONSIEUR ROBERT: That's fine with me.

SGANARELLE: And you're a meddler to interfere in other people's affairs. Learn that Cicero says that you mustn't put the bark between the tree and your finger. (*Beats* MONSIEUR ROBERT *and drives him offstage, then returns to his wife and clasps her hand.*)
Well now, let's us two make peace. Shake on it.

MARTINE: Oh yes! After beating me that way!

SGANARELLE: That's nothing. Shake.

MARTINE: I will not.

SGANARELLE: Eh?

MARTINE: No.

SGANARELLE: My little wife!

MARTINE: No sir.

SGANARELLE: Come on, I say.

MARTINE: I won't do anything of the kind.

SGANARELLE: Come, come, come.

MARTINE: No, I want to be angry.

SGANARELLE: Fie! It's nothing. Come on, come on.

MARTINE: Let me be.

SGANARELLE: Shake, I say.

MARTINE: You've treated me too badly.

SGANARELLE: All right then, I ask your pardon: give me your hand.

MARTINE: I forgive you; (*aside*) but you'll pay for it.

SGANARELLE: You're crazy to pay any attention to that: those little things are necessary from time to time for a good friendship; and five or six cudgel-blows between people in love only whet their affection. There now, I'm off to the woods, and I promise you more than a hundred bundles of kindling wood today.

Scene 3.   MARTINE (*alone*)

MARTINE: All right, whatever face I put on, I'm not forgetting my resentment; and I'm burning inside to find ways to punish you for the beatings you give me. I know very well that a wife always has in hand means of taking revenge on a husband; but that's too delicate a punishment for my gallowsbird. I want a vengeance that he'll feel a bit more; and that would be no satisfaction for the offense I've received.

Scene 4.   VALÈRE, LUCAS, MARTINE

LUCAS: Doggone it! We sure both tooken on one heck of a job; and me, I don't know what I'm gonna come up with.

VALÈRE: Well, what do you expect as the wet-nurse's husband? We have to obey our master; and then we both have an interest in the health of the mistress, his daughter; and no doubt her marriage, put off by her illness, would be worth some kind of present to us. Horace, who is generous, has the best chances of anyone to win her hand; and although she has shown a fondness for a certain Léandre, you know very well that her father has never consented to accept him as a son-in-law.

MARTINE (*musing, aside*):   Can't I think up some scheme to get revenge?

LUCAS: But what kind of wild idea has the master tooken into his head, now that the doctors have used up all their Latin?

VALÈRE: You sometimes find, by looking hard, what you don't find at first; and often in simple places . . .

MARTINE: Yes, I must get revenge, whatever the price; that beating sticks in my crop, I can't swallow it, and . . . (*She says all this still musing, not noticing the two men, so that when she turns around she bumps into them.*) Oh! Gentlemen, I beg your pardon; I didn't see you, and I was trying to think of something that's bothering me.

VALÈRE: Everyone has his problems in this world, and we too are looking for something we would very much like to find.

MARTINE: Would it be anything I might help you with?

VALÈRE: It just might. We're trying to find some able man, some special doctor, who might give some relief to our master's daughter, ill with a disease that has suddenly taken away the use of her tongue. Several doctors have already exhausted all their learning on her; but you sometimes find people with wonderful secrets, with certain special remedies, who can very often do what the others couldn't; and that's what we're looking for.

MARTINE (*aside*):   Oh! What a wonderful scheme Heaven inspires me with to get revenge on my gallowsbird! (*Aloud*) You couldn't have come to a better place to find what you're looking for; and we have a man here, the most marvelous man in the world for hopeless illnesses.

VALÈRE: And, pray, where can we find him?

MARTINE: You'll find him right now in that little clearing over there, spending his time cutting wood.

LUCAS: A doctor cutting wood?

VALÈRE: Spending his time gathering herbs, do you mean?

MARTINE: No, he's an extraordinary man who enjoys that—strange, fantastic, crotchety—you'd never take him for what he is. He goes around dressed in an eccentric way, sometimes affects ignorance, keeps his knowledge hidden, and every day avoids nothing so much as exercising the marvelous talents Heaven has given him for medicine.

VALÈRE: It's an amazing thing that all great men always have some caprice, some little grain of folly mingled with their learning.

MARTINE: This one's mania is beyond all belief, for it sometimes goes to the point of his wanting to be beaten before he'll acknowledge his capacity; and I'm telling you you'll never get the better of him, he'll never admit he's a doctor, if he's in that mood, unless you each take a stick and beat him into confessing in the end what he'll hide from you at first. That's what *we* do when we need him.

VALÈRE: That's a strange mania!

MARTINE: That's true; but afterward, you'll see he does wonders.

VALÈRE: What's his name?

MARTINE: His name is Sganarelle, but he's easy to recognize. He's a man with a big black beard, wearing a ruff and a green and yellow coat.

LUCAS: A green and yaller coat? So he's a parrot doctor?[1]

VALÈRE: But is it really true that he's as skillful as you say?

MARTINE: What? He's a man who works miracles. Six months ago a woman was abandoned by all the other doctors. They thought she'd been dead for a good six hours, and were getting ready to bury her, when they forced the man we're talking about to come. After he'd looked her over, he put a little drop of something or other in her mouth, and that very moment she got up out of bed and right away started walking around her room as if nothing had happened.

LUCAS: Ah!

VALÈRE: It must have been a drop of elixir of gold.

MARTINE: That might well be. Then again, not three weeks ago a youngster twelve years old fell down from the top of the steeple and broke his head, arms, and legs on the pavement. They had no sooner brought our man in than he rubbed the boy's whole body with a certain ointment he knows how to make; and right away the boy got up on his feet and ran off to play marbles.

LUCAS: Ah!

VALÈRE: That man must have a universal cure.

MARTINE: Who doubts it?

LUCAS: By jingo, that's sure the man we need. Let's go get him quick.

VALÈRE: We thank you for the favor you're doing us.

---

1. In Molière's time, doctors always wore black robes.

MARTINE: But anyway, be sure to remember what I warned you about.

LUCAS: Tarnation! Leave it to us. If a beating is all it takes, she's our cow.

VALÈRE: That certainly was a lucky encounter for us; and for my part, I'm very hopeful about it.

Scene 5.   SGANARELLE, VALÈRE, LUCAS

SGANARELLE (*enters singing, bottle in hand*). La, la, la!

VALÈRE: I hear someone singing and cutting wood.

SGANARELLE: La, la, la . . . ! My word, that's enough work for a while. Let's take a little breather. (*Drinks*) That wood is salty as the devil. (*Sings*)
>Sweet glug-glug,
>How I love thee!
>Sweet glug-glug
>Of my little jug!
>But everybody would think me too smug
>If you were as full as you can be.
>Just never be empty, that's my plea.
>Come, sweet, let me give you a hug.

(*Speaks again*) Come on, good Lord, we mustn't breed melancholy.

VALÈRE: There's the man himself.

LUCAS: I think you're right, and we done stumbled right onto him.

VALÈRE: Let's get a closer look.

SGANARELLE (*seeing them, looks at them, turning first toward one then toward the other, and lowers his voice*). Ah! my little hussy! How I love you, my little jug!
>But everybody . . . would think . . . me . . . too smug, If . . .

What the devil! What do these people want?

VALÈRE: That's the one, no doubt about it.

LUCAS: That's him, his spit an' image, just like they prescribed him to us.

SGANARELLE (*aside*). They're looking at me and consulting. What can they have in mind? (*He puts his bottle on the ground. As* VALÈRE *bows to greet him,* SGANARELLE *thinks he is reaching down to take his bottle away, and so puts it on the other side of him. When* LUCAS *bows in turn, he picks it up again and clutches it to his belly, with much other byplay.*)

VALÈRE: Sir, isn't your name Sganarelle?

SGANARELLE: How's that?

VALÈRE: I'm asking you if you're not the man named Sganarelle?

SGANARELLE (*turning toward* VALÈRE, *then toward* LUCAS):   Yes and no, depending on what you want with him.

VALÈRE: All we want is to pay him all the civilities we can.

SGANARELLE: In that case, my name *is* Sganarelle.

VALÈRE: Sir, we are delighted to see you. We have been addressed to you for something we're looking for; and we come to implore your aid, which we need.

SGANARELLE: If it's something, sirs, connected with my little line of business, I am all ready to serve you.

VALÈRE: Sir, you are too kind. But sir, put on your hat, please; the sun might give you trouble.

LUCAS: Slap it on, sir.

SGANARELLE (*aside*):   These are very ceremonious people.

VALÈRE: Sir, you must not find it strange that we should come to you. Able men are always sought out, and we are well informed about your capability.

SGANARELLE: It is true, gentlemen, that I'm the best man in the world for cutting kindling wood.

VALÈRE: Ah, sir . . . !

SGANARELLE: I spare no pains, and cut it in such a way that it's above criticism.

VALÈRE: Sir, that's not the point.

SGANARELLE: But also I sell it at a hundred and ten sous for a hundred bundles.

VALÈRE: Let's not talk about that, if you please.

SGANARELLE: I promise you I can't let it go for less.

VALÈRE: Sir, we know how things stand.

SGANARELLE: If you know how things stand, you know that that's what I sell them for.

VALÈRE: Sir, you're joking when . . .

SGANARELLE: I'm not joking, I can't take anything off for it.

VALÈRE: Let's talk in other terms, please.

SGANARELLE: You can find it for less elsewhere: there's kindling and kindling; but as for what I cut . . .

VALÈRE: What? Sir, let's drop this subject.

SGANARELLE: I swear you couldn't get it for a penny less.

VALÈRE: Fie now!

SGANARELLE: No, on my conscience, that's what you'll pay. I'm speaking sincerely, and I'm not the man to overcharge.

VALÈRE: Sir, must a person like you waste his time on these crude pretenses and stoop to speaking like this? Must such a learned man, a famous doctor like yourself, try to disguise himself in the eyes of the world and keep his fine talents buried?

SGANARELLE (*aside*): He's crazy.

VALÈRE: Please, sir, don't dissimulate with us.

SGANARELLE: What?

LUCAS: All this here fiddle-faddle don't do no good; we knows what we knows.

SGANARELLE: What about it? What are you trying to tell me? Whom do you take me for?

VALÈRE: For what you are: for a great doctor.

SGANARELLE: Doctor yourself: I'm not one and I've never been one.

VALÈRE (*aside*): That's his madness gripping him. (*Aloud*) Sir, please don't deny things any longer; and pray let's not come to regrettable extremes.

SGANARELLE: To what?

VALÈRE: To certain things that we would be sorry for.

SGANARELLE: Good Lord! Come to whatever you like. I'm no doctor, and I don't know what you're trying to tell me.

VALÈRE (*aside*): I can certainly see we'll have to use the remedy. (*Aloud*) Once more, sir, I beg you to admit what you are.

LUCAS: Dad bust it! No more messin' around; confess franklike that you're a doctor.

SGANARELLE: I'm getting mad.

VALÈRE: Why deny what everyone knows?

LUCAS: Why all this fuss and feathers? And what good does that done you?

SGANARELLE: Gentlemen, I tell you in one word as well as in two thousand: *I'm not a doctor.*

VALÈRE: You're not a doctor?

SGANARELLE: No.

LUCAS: You ain't no doc?

SGANARELLE: No, I tell you.

VALÈRE: Since you insist, we'll have to go ahead.
                              (*They each take a stick and beat him.*)

SGANARELLE: Oh, oh, oh! Gentlemen, I'm whatever you like.

VALÈRE: Why, sir, do you force us to this violence?

LUCAS: Why do you give us the botherment of beating you?

VALÈRE: I assure you that I could not regret it more.

LUCAS: By jeepers, I'm sorry about it, honest.

SGANARELLE: What the devil is this, gentlemen? I ask you, is it a joke, or are you both crazy, to insist I'm a doctor?

VALÈRE: What? You still won't give in, and you deny you're a doctor?

SGANARELLE: Devil take me if I am!

LUCAS: It ain't true that you're a doc?

SGANARELLE: No, plague take me! (*They start beating him again.*) Oh, oh! Well gentlemen, since you insist, I'm a doctor, I'm a doctor; an apothecary too, if you see fit. I'd rather consent to anything than get myself beaten to death.

VALÈRE: Ah! That's fine, sir; I'm delighted to find you in a reasonable mood.

LUCAS: You fair cram my heart with joy when I see you talk thataway.

VALÈRE: I beg your pardon with all my heart.

LUCAS: I begs your excuse for the liberty I done tooken.

SGANARELLE (*aside*):   Well now! Suppose I'm the one that's mistaken? Could I have become a doctor without noticing it?

VALÈRE: Sir, you won't regret showing us what you are; and you'll certainly be satisfied with your treatment.

SGANARELLE: But, gentlemen, aren't you making a mistake yourselves? Is it quite certain that I'm a doctor?

LUCAS: Yup, by jiminy!

SGANARELLE: Honestly?

VALÈRE: Beyond a doubt.

SGANARELLE: Devil take me if I knew it!

VALÈRE: What? You're the ablest doctor in the world.

SGANARELLE: Aha!

LUCAS: A doc which has cureded I don't know how many maladies.

SGANARELLE: My Lord!

VALÈRE: A woman had been taken for dead six hours before; she was ready to be buried, when, with a drop of something or other, you brought her back to life and set her walking around the room right away.

SGANARELLE: I'll be darned!

LUCAS: A little boy twelve years old left himself fall from the top of a steeple, from which he got his head, legs and arms busted; and you, with some kind of ointment or other, you fixed him so he gets right up on his feet and goes off to play marbles.

SGANARELLE: The devil you say!

VALÈRE: In short, sir, you will have every satisfaction with us; and you'll earn whatever you like if you'll let us take you where we mean to.

SGANARELLE: I'll earn whatever I like?

VALÈRE: Yes.

SGANARELLE: Oh! I'm a doctor, there's no denying it. I'd forgotten, but now I remember. What's the problem? Where do we have to go?

VALÈRE: We'll take you. The problem is to go see a girl who's lost her speech.

SGANARELLE: My word! I haven't found it.

VALÈRE: He likes his little joke. Let's go, sir.

SGANARELLE: Without a doctor's gown?

VALÈRE: We'll get one.

SGANARELLE (*presenting his bottle to* VALÈRE):   Hold that, you: that's where
I put my potions. (*Turning toward* LUCAS *and spitting on the ground.*) You
step on that; doctor's orders.

LUCAS: Land's sakes! That's a doctor I like. I reckon he'll do all right, 'cause
he's a real comic.[2]

ACT II

A room in Géronte's house

Scene 1.   GÉRONTE, VALÈRE, LUCAS, JACQUELINE

VALÈRE: Yes, sir, I think you'll be satisfied; and we've brought you the
greatest doctor in the world.

LUCAS: Oh, gee whillikins! You gotta pull up the ladder after that one, and
all the rest ain't good enough to take off his shoon.

VALÈRE: He's a man who has performed wonderful cures.

LUCAS: As has cureded some folk as were dead.

VALÈRE: He's a bit capricious, as I've told you; and sometimes he has moments when his mind wanders and he doesn't seem what he really is.

LUCAS: Yup, he likes to clown; and sometimes you'd say, with no offense,
that he'd been hit on the head with an axe.

VALÈRE: But underneath it, he's all learning, and very often he says quite
lofty things.

LUCAS: When he gets to it, he talks right straight out just like he was reading
out of a book.

VALÈRE: His reputation has already spread hereabouts, and everybody is
coming to see him.

GÉRONTE: I'm dying to meet him. Bring him to me quick.

2. Some have taken this remark as Molière's own disgruntled comment on the mediocre
success of *The Misanthrope*.

VALÈRE: I'll go and get him.

JACQUELINE: Land's sakes, sir, this'un'll do just what the others done. I reckon it'll be just the same old stuff; and the bestest med'cine anyone could slip your daughter, if you're asking me, would be a good handsome husband she had a hankering for.

GÉRONTE: Well now! My good wet-nurse, you certainly meddle in lots of things.

LUCAS: Be quiet, Jacqueline, keep to your housework: you ain't the one to stick your nose in there.

JACQUELINE: I told you before and I'll tell you some more that all these here doctors won't do nothing more for her than plain branch water, that your daughter needs something mighty different from rhubarb and senna, and that a husband is the kind of poultice that'll cure all a girl's troubles.

GÉRONTE: Is she in condition now for anyone to want to take her on, with the infirmity she has? And when I was minded to have her married, didn't she oppose my will?

JACQUELINE: I should think she did: you was wanting to pass her a man she don't love. Why didn't you take that Monsieur Léandre that she had a soft spot for? She would've been real obedient; and I'm gonna bet you he'd take her just like she is, if you'd give her to him.

GÉRONTE: That Léandre is not what she needs; he's not well off like the other.

JACQUELINE: He's got such a rich uncle, and he's his hair.

GÉRONTE: All this property to come is just so much nonsense to me. There's nothing like what you've got; and you run a big risk of fooling yourself when you count on what someone else is keeping for you. Death doesn't always keep her ears open to the wishes and prayers of their honors the heirs; and you can grow a long set of teeth when you're waiting for some-one's death so as to have a livelihood.

JACQUELINE: Anyway I've always heard that in marriage, as elsewhere, hap-piness counts more than riches. The pas and mas, they have that goldarned custom of always asking "How much has he got?" and "How much has she got?" and neighbor Peter married off his daughter Simonette to fat Thomas 'cause he had a quarter vineyard more than young Robin, which she'd set her heart on; and now, poor critter, it's turned her yellow as a quince, and she hasn't got her property in all the time since. That's a fine example for *you*, sir. All we got in this world is our pleasure; and I'd rather give my daughter a good husband which she liked than all the revenues in Beauce.

GÉRONTE: Plague take it, Madame Nurse, how you do spit it out! Be quiet, please; you're getting too involved and you're heating up your milk.

LUCAS (*by mistake, tapping* GÉRONTE *on the chest instead of* JACQUELINE):   Gosh darn it! Shut up, you're just a meddler. The master don't have no use for your speeches, and he knows what he's got to do. You see to nursing the child you're nurse to, and don't give us none of your big ideas. The master is his daughter's father, and he's good enough and wise enough to see what she needs.

GÉRONTE: Easy! Oh! Easy!

LUCAS: Sir, I want to mortify her a bit, and teach her the respect she owes you.

GÉRONTE: Yes, but those gestures aren't necessary.

Scene 2.   VALÈRE, SGANARELLE, GÉRONTE, LUCAS, JACQUELINE

VALÈRE: Sir, prepare yourself. Here comes our doctor.

GÉRONTE: Sir, I'm delighted to have you in my house, and we need you badly.

SGANARELLE (*in a doctor's gown, with a sharply pointed hat*):   Hippocrates says . . . that we should both put our hats on.

GÉRONTE: Hippocrates says that?

SGANARELLE: Yes.

GÉRONTE: In what chapter, if you please?

SGANARELLE: In his chapter on hats.

GÉRONTE: Since Hippocrates says it, we must do it.

SGANARELLE: Sir Doctor, since I have heard the wonderful things . . .

GÉRONTE: Whom are you speaking to, pray?

SGANARELLE: You.

GÉRONTE: I'm not a doctor.

SGANARELLE: You're not a doctor?

GÉRONTE: No, really.

SGANARELLE (*takes a stick and beats him just as he himself was beaten*):   You really mean it?

GÉRONTE: I really mean it. Oh, oh, oh!

SGANARELLE: You're a doctor now. I never got any other license.

GÉRONTE: What the devil kind of a man have you brought me?

VALÈRE: I told you he was a joker of a doctor.

GÉRONTE: Yes, but I'd send him packing with his jokes.

LUCAS: Don't pay no attention to that, sir: that's just for a laugh.

GÉRONTE: I don't like that kind of a laugh.

SGANARELLE: Sir, I ask your pardon for the liberty I took.

GÉRONTE: Your servant, sir.

SGANARELLE: I'm sorry . . .

GÉRONTE: That's nothing.

SGANARELLE: For the cudgeling . . .

GÉRONTE: No harm done.

SGANARELLE: That I had the honor of giving you.

GÉRONTE: Let's say no more about it. Sir, I have a daughter who has caught a strange disease.

SGANARELLE: Sir, I'm delighted that your daughter needs me; and I wish with all my heart that you and your whole family needed me too, just to show you how much I want to serve you.

GÉRONTE: I am obliged to you for those sentiments.

SGANARELLE: I assure you that I'm speaking straight from the heart.

GÉRONTE: You do me too much honor.

SGANARELLE: What's your daughter's name?

GÉRONTE: Lucinde.

SGANARELLE: Lucinde! Oh, what a fine name to prescribe for! Lucinde![3]

GÉRONTE: I'll just go and have a look to see what she's doing.

---

3. Here a theatrical tradition has Sganarelle decline the name: Lucindus, Lucinda, Lucindum.

SGANARELLE: Who's that big buxom woman?

GÉRONTE: She's the wet-nurse of a little baby of mine.

SGANARELLE: Plague take it! That's a pretty piece of goods! Ah, nurse, charming nurse, my medicine is the very humble slave of your nurseship, and I'd certainly like to be the lucky little doll who sucked the milk (*puts his hand on her breast*) of your good graces. All my remedies, all my learning, all my capacity is at your service, and . . .

LUCAS: With your pummission, Mister Doctor, leave my wife be, I beg you.

SGANARELLE: What? Is she your wife?

LUCAS: Yes.

SGANARELLE (*makes as if to embrace* LUCAS, *then, turning toward the nurse, embraces her*):   Oh! really! I didn't know that, and I'm delighted for the sake of you both.

LUCAS (*pulling him away*):   Easy now, please.

SGANARELLE: I assure you I'm delighted that you're united. I congratulate her (*he again makes as if to embrace* LUCAS, *and, passing under his arms, throws himself on* JACQUELINE'S *neck*) on having a husband like you; and you, I congratulate you on having a wife as beautiful, modest, and well-built as she is.

LUCAS (*pulling him away again*):   Hey! Goldarn it! Not so much compliment, I ask you now.

SGANARELLE: Don't you want me to rejoice with you at such a fine assembly?

LUCAS: With me, all you like; but with my wife, let's skip these kind of formalities.

SGANARELLE: I take part in the happiness of you both alike; and (*same business as before*) if I embrace you to attest my joy to you, I embrace her as well to attest my joy to her too.

LUCAS (*pulling him away once more*):   Oh! Dad blast it, Mister Doctor, what a lot of fiddle-faddle!

Scene 3.   SGANARELLE, GÉRONTE, LUCAS, JACQUELINE

GÉRONTE: Sir, they're going to bring my daughter to you. She'll be here right away.

SGANARELLE: I await her sir, and all medicine with me.

GÉRONTE: Where is it?

SGANARELLE (*tapping his forehead*):   In there.

GÉRONTE: Very good.

SGANARELLE (*trying to touch the nurse's breasts*):   But since I am interested in your whole family, I must take a small sample of your nurse's milk, and inspect her bosom.

LUCAS (*pulling him away and spinning him around*):   Nah, nah, I don't want no truck with that.

SGANARELLE: It's the doctor's job to examine nurses' breasts.

LUCAS: Job nor no job, I'm your servant.

SGANARELLE: Do you really have the audacity to set yourself up against the doctor? Begone!

LUCAS: The heck with that!

SGANARELLE (*looking at him askance*):   I'll give you the fever.

JACQUELINE (*taking LUCAS by the arm and spinning him around*):   That's right, get out of there. Ain't I big enough to defend myself if he does something to me as a person hadn't ought?

LUCAS: Well, me, I don't want him a-feeling you.

SGANARELLE: Fie! The peasant! He's jealous of his wife!

GÉRONTE: Here is my daughter.

Scene 4.   LUCINDE, VALÈRE, GÉRONTE, LUCAS, SGANARELLE, JACQUELINE

SGANARELLE: Is this the patient?

GÉRONTE: Yes, she's the only daughter I have, and I'd be heartbroken if she were to die.

SGANARELLE: She'd better not! She mustn't die except on doctor's orders.

GÉRONTE: Come, come, a chair![4]

---

4. Chairs were relatively rare luxuries in Molière's France. By ordering a regular chair, not a folding stool, Géronte shows his respect for the learned doctor.

SGANARELLE: That's not such a bad-looking patient, and I maintain that a really healthy man would make out all right with her.

GÉRONTE: You've made her laugh, sir.

SGANARELLE: That's fine. When the doctor makes the patient laugh, that's the best possible sign. Well! What's the problem? What's wrong with you? Where does it hurt?

LUCINDE (*answers in sign language, putting her hand to her mouth, her head, and under her chin*):   Hah, heeh, hoh, hah.

SGANARELLE: Eh? What's that you say?

LUCINDE (*same gestures as before*):   Hah, heeh, hoh, hah, hah, heeh, hoh.

SGANARELLE: What?

LUCINDE: Hah, heeh, hoh.

SGANARELLE (*imitating her*):   Hah, heeh, hoh, hah, hah: I don't understand you. What the devil kind of language is that?

GÉRONTE: Sir, that's her illness. She's been struck dumb, and up to now no one has been able to learn the reason why; and it's an accident that has put off her marriage.

SGANARELLE: And why so?

GÉRONTE: The man she is to marry wants to wait until she's cured to make things final.

SGANARELLE: And who is the fool that doesn't want his wife to be dumb? Would God mine had that disease! I'd be the last one to want to cure her.

GÉRONTE: Anyway, sir, we beg you to make every effort to relieve her of her trouble.

SGANARELLE: Oh! Don't worry. Tell me now, does this trouble bother her a lot?

GÉRONTE: Yes, sir.

SGANARELLE: Very good. Does she feel great pains?

GÉRONTE: Very great.

SGANARELLE: That's just fine. Does she go—you know where?

GÉRONTE: Yes.

SGANARELLE: Copiously?

GÉRONTE: I don't know anything about that.

SGANARELLE: Does she achieve laudable results?

GÉRONTE: I'm no expert in those matters.

SGANARELLE (*turning to the patient*):   Give me your arm. That pulse shows your daughter is dumb.

GÉRONTE: Why yes, sir, that's her trouble! You found it the very first thing.

SGANARELLE: Aha!

JACQUELINE: Just lookit how he guessed her illness!

SGANARELLE: We great doctors, we know things right away. An ignorant one would have been embarrassed and would have gone and told you "It's this" or "It's that"; but *I* hit the mark on the first shot, and I inform you that your daughter is dumb.

GÉRONTE: Yes; but I wish you could tell me what it comes from.

SGANARELLE: Nothing easier: it comes from the fact that she has lost her speech.

GÉRONTE: Very good; but the reason, please, why she has lost her speech?

SGANARELLE: All our best authors will tell you that it's the stoppage of the action of her tongue.

GÉRONTE: But still, what are your views about this stoppage of the action of her tongue?

SGANARELLE: Aristotle, on that subject, says . . . some very fine things.

GÉRONTE: I believe it.

SGANARELLE: Oh! He was a great man!

GÉRONTE: No doubt.

SGANARELLE (*raising his forearm*):   An utterly great man: a man who was greater than I by all of that! So, to get back to our reasoning, I hold that this stoppage of the action of her tongue is caused by certain humors, which among us scholars we call peccant humors: peccant, that is to say . . . peccant humors; because the vapors formed by the exhalations of the influences arising in the region where the maladies lie, when they come . . . so to speak . . . to . . . Do you understand Latin?

GÉRONTE: Not in the least.

SGANARELLE (*getting up in astonishment*):   You don't understand Latin?

GÉRONTE: No.

SGANARELLE (*assuming various comical poses*): *Cabricias arci thuram, catalamus, singulariter, nominativo haec Musa,* "the Muse," *bonus, bona, bonum, Deus sanctus, estne oratio latinas? Etiam,* "yes." *Quare,* "why?" *Quia substantivo et adjectivum concordat in generi, numerum, et casus.*[5]

GÉRONTE: Oh! Why did I never study?

JACQUELINE: Land! That's an able man!

LUCAS: Yup, that's so purty I can't make out a word of it.

SGANARELLE: Now when these vapors I'm speaking of come to pass from the left side, where the liver is, to the right side, where the heart is, it happens that the lungs, which in Latin we call *armyan,* having communication with the brain, which in Greek we call *nasmus,* by means of the vena cava, which in Hebrew we call *cubile,*[6] on its way encounters the said vapors, which fill the ventricles of the omoplate; and because the said vapors— follow this reasoning closely, I beg you—and because the said vapors have a certain malignity . . . Listen to this carefully, I conjure you.

GÉRONTE: Yes.

SGANARELLE: Have a certain malignity, which is caused . . . Be attentive, please.

GÉRONTE: I am.

SGANARELLE: Which is caused by the acridity of the humors engendered in the concavity of the diaphragm, it happens that these vapors . . . *Ossabandus, nequeys, nequer, potarinum, quipsa milus.* That's exactly what is making your daughter dumb.

JACQUELINE: Oh! That man of ourn! Ain't that well said?

LUCAS: Why ain't *my* tongue that slick?

GÉRONTE: No one could reason any better, no doubt about it. There's just one thing that surprised me: the location of the liver and the heart. It seems to me that you place them otherwise than they are; that the heart is on the left side and the liver on the right side.

SGANARELLE: Yes, it used to be that way; but we have changed all that, and now we practice medicine in a completely new way.

---

5. Traditionally, as Sganarelle winds up this hodge-podge of gibberish and elementary Latin phrases with the word *casus* ("case," or "fall"), he throws himself back in his chair too hard, and falls over in it on his back. He remains in this position during the next two remarks.
6. These are all invented names, except that *cubile* is Latin for *bed.*

GÉRONTE: That's something I didn't know, and I beg your pardon for my ignorance.

SGANARELLE: No harm done, and you're not obliged to be as able as we are.

GÉRONTE: To be sure. But, sir, what do you think needs to be done for this illness?

SGANARELLE: What I think needs to be done?

GÉRONTE: Yes.

SGANARELLE: My advice is to put her back in bed and have her take, as a remedy, a lot of bread steeped in wine.

GÉRONTE: And why that, sir?

SGANARELLE: Because in bread and wine mixed together there is a sympathetic virtue that makes people speak. Haven't you noticed that they don't give anything else to parrots, and that they learn to speak by eating that?

GÉRONTE: That's true. Oh, what a great man! Quick, lots of bread and wine!

SGANARELLE: I'll come back toward evening and see how she is. (*To the nurse*) Hold on, you. Sir, here is a nurse to whom I must administer a few little remedies.

JACQUELINE: Who? Me? I couldn't be in better health.

SGANARELLE: Too bad, nurse, too bad. Such good health is alarming, and it won't be a bad thing to give you a friendly little bloodletting, a little dulcifying enema.

GÉRONTE: But, sir, that's a fashion I don't understand. Why should we go and be bled when we haven't any illness?

SGANARELLE: No matter, it's a salutary fashion; and just as we drink on account of the thirst to come, so we must have ourselves bled on account of the illness to come.

JACQUELINE (*starting to go off*):   My Lord! The heck with that, and I don't want to make my body into a drugstore.

SGANARELLE: You are resistant to remedies, but we'll manage to bring you to reason.   (*Exit* JACQUELINE)
    (*To* GÉRONTE) I bid you good day.

GÉRONTE: Wait a bit, please.

SGANARELLE: What do you want to do?

GÉRONTE: Give you some money, sir.

SGANARELLE (*holding out his hand behind, beneath his gown, while* GÉRONTE *opens his purse*):   I won't take any, sir.

GÉRONTE: Sir . . .

SGANARELLE: Not at all.

GÉRONTE: Just a moment.

SGANARELLE: By no means.

GÉRONTE: Please!

SGANARELLE: You're joking.

GÉRONTE: That's that.

SGANARELLE: I'll do nothing of the sort.

GÉRONTE: Eh?

SGANARELLE: Money is no motive to me.

GÉRONTE: I believe it.

SGANARELLE (*after taking the money*):   Is this good weight?

GÉRONTE: Yes, sir.

SGANARELLE: I'm not a mercenary doctor.

GÉRONTE: I'm well aware of it.

SGANARELLE: I'm not ruled by self-interest.

GÉRONTE: I have no such idea.

Scene 5.   SGANARELLE, LÉANDRE

SGANARELLE (*looking at his money*):   My word! That's not too bad; and if only . . .

LÉANDRE: Sir, I've been waiting for you a long time, and I come to implore your assistance.

SGANARELLE (*taking his wrist*):   That's a very bad pulse.

LÉANDRE: I'm not sick, sir, and that's not why I've come to see you.

SGANARELLE: If you're not sick, why the devil don't you say so?

LÉANDRE: No. To put the whole thing in a word, my name is Léandre, and I'm in love with Lucinde, whom you've just examined; and since, because of her father's bad disposition, I'm denied all access to her, I'm venturing to beg you to serve my love, and give me a chance to carry out a scheme I've thought up to say a word or two to her on which my happiness and my life depend absolutely.

SGANARELLE (*feigning anger*): Whom do you take me for? How can you dare come up and ask me to serve you in your love, and try to degrade the dignity of a doctor to this type of employment?

LÉANDRE: Sir, don't make so much noise.

SGANARELLE: *I* want to make noise. You're an impertinent young man.

LÉANDRE: Ah! Gently, sir.

SGANARELLE: A dunderhead.

LÉANDRE: Please!

SGANARELLE: I'll teach you that I'm not the kind of man for that, and that it's the height of insolence . . .

LÉANDRE (*pulling out a purse and giving it to him*): Sir . . .

SGANARELLE: To want to use me . . . I'm not speaking about you, for you're a gentleman, and I would be delighted to do you a service; but there are some impertinent people in the world who come and take people for what they're not; and I admit that makes me angry.

LÉANDRE: I ask your pardon, sir, for the liberty that . . .

SGANARELLE: Don't be silly. What's the problem?

LÉANDRE: You shall know, then, sir, that this illness that you want to cure is make-believe. The doctors have reasoned in due form about it, and have not failed to say that it came, some say from the brain, some from the intestines, some from the spleen, some from the liver; but it is certain that love is the real cause of it, and that Lucinde hit upon this illness only to deliver herself from a threatened marriage. But, for fear we may be seen together, let's get out of here, and as we walk I'll tell you what I would like from you.

SGANARELLE: Let's go, sir: you've given me an inconceivable fondness for your love; and unless I'm no doctor, either the patient will die or else she'll be yours.

ACT III

Géronte's garden

Scene 1.   SGANARELLE, LÉANDRE

LÉANDRE: It seems to me I don't look bad this way as an apothecary; and since the father has scarcely ever seen me, this change of costume and wig may well succeed, I think, in disguising me to his eyes.

SGANARELLE: No doubt about it.

LÉANDRE: All I could wish would be to know five or six big medical terms to adorn my speech and make me seem like a learned man.

SGANARELLE: Come, come, all that is unnecessary: the costume is enough, and I know more about it than you.

LÉANDRE: What?

SGANARELLE: Devil take me if I know anything about medicine! You're a good sort, and I'm willing to confide in you, just as you are confiding in me.

LÉANDRE: What? You're not really . . . ?

SGANARELLE: No, I tell you: they made me a doctor in spite of me. I had never bothered my head about being that learned; and all my studies went only up to seventh grade. I don't know what put this idea into their heads; but when I saw that they absolutely insisted on my being a doctor, I decided to be one, at the expense of whom it may concern. However, you'd never believe how the mistaken idea has gotten around, and how everybody is hell-bent on thinking me a learned man. They come looking for me from all directions; and if things keep on this way, I believe I'll stick to medicine all my life. I think it's the best trade of all; for whether you do well or badly, you're always paid just the same. Bad work never comes back onto our backs, and we cut the material we work on as we please. A cobbler making shoes could never botch a piece of leather without paying for the broken crockery; but in this work we can botch a man without its costing us anything. The blunders are never ours, and it's always the fault of the person who dies. In short, the best part of this profession is that there's a decency, an unparalleled discretion, among the dead; and you never see one of them complaining of the doctor who killed him.

LÉANDRE: It's true that dead men are very decent folk on that score.

SGANARELLE (*seeing some men coming toward him*): There are some people who look as though they were coming to consult me. Go ahead and wait for me near your sweetheart's house.

Scene 2.   THIBAUT, PERRIN, SGANARELLE

THIBAUT: Sir, we done come to see you, my son Perrin and me.

SGANARELLE: What's the matter?

THIBAUT: His poor mother, her name is Perrette, is sick in bed these six months now.

SGANARELLE (*holding out his hand to receive money*): And what do you expect me to do about it?

THIBAUT: We'd like, sir, for you to slip us some kind of funny business for to cure her.

SGANARELLE: I'll have to see what she's sick of.

THIBAUT: She's sick of a proxy, sir.

SGANARELLE: Of a proxy?

THIBAUT: Yes, that is to say she's all swelled up all over; and they say it's a whole lot of seriosities she's got inside her, and that her liver, her belly, or her spleen, whatever you want to call it, 'stead of making blood don't make nothing but water. Every other day she has a quotigian fever, with pains and lassitules in the muskles of her legs. You can hear in her throat phlegums like to choke her; and sometimes she gets tooken with syncopations and compulsions till I think she done passed away. In our village we got a 'pothecary, all respect to him, who's given her I don't know how many kinds of stuff; and it costs me more'n a dozen good crowns in enemas, no offense, and beverages he had her take, in jacinth confusions and cordial portions. But all that stuff, like the feller said, was just a kind of salve that didn't make her no better nor no worse. He wanted to slip her one certain drug that they call hermetic wine; but me, frankly, I got scared that would send her to join her ancestors; and they do say those big doctors are killing off I don't know how many people with that there invention.[7]

---

7. A big medical controversy of the time concerned the value of emetic wine, which contained antimony.

SGANARELLE (*still holding out his hand and signaling with it for money*):
Let's get to the point, my friend, let's get to the point.

THIBAUT: The fact is, sir, that we done come to ask you to tell us what we
should do.

SGANARELLE: I don't understand you at all.

PERRIN: Sir, my mother is sick; and here be two crowns that we've brung
you so you'll give us some cure.

SGANARELLE: Oh! Now *you*, I understand you. Here's a lad who speaks
clearly and explains himself properly. You say that your mother is ill with
dropsy, that her whole body is swollen, that she has a fever and pains in
her legs, and that she is sometimes seized with syncopes and convulsions,
that is to say, fainting spells?

PERRIN: Oh, yes, sir, that's exactly it.

SGANARELLE: I understood you right away. You have a father who doesn't
know what he's talking about. Now you're asking me for a remedy?

PERRIN: Yes, sir.

SGANARELLE: A remedy to cure her?

PERRIN: That's what we got in mind.

SGANARELLE: Look, here's a piece of cheese that you must have her take.

PERRIN: Cheese, sir?

SGANARELLE: Yes, it's a specially prepared cheese containing gold, coral,
pearls, and lots of other precious things.

PERRIN: Sir, we be much obliged to you; and we'll have her take this right
away.

SGANARELLE: Go ahead. If she dies, don't fail to give her the best burial you
can.

Scene 3.   JACQUELINE, SGANARELLE; LUCAS (*backstage*)

SGANARELLE: Here's that beautiful nurse. Ah, nurse of my heart, I'm delighted that we meet again, and the sight of you is the rhubarb, cassia, and
senna that purge my soul of all its melancholy!

JACQUELINE: Well I swan, Mister Doctor, you say that too purty for me,
and I don't understand none of your Latin.

SGANARELLE: Fall ill, nurse, I beg you; fall ill for my sake; it would give me all the pleasure in the world to cure you.

JACQUELINE: I'm your servant, sir: I'd much rather not have no one cure me.

SGANARELLE: How sorry I am for you, fair nurse, for having a jealous, troublesome husband like the one you have!

JACQUELINE: What would you have me do, sir? It's a penance for my sins. Where the goat is tied, that's where she's got to graze.

SGANARELLE: What? A clod like that! A man who's always watching you, and won't let anyone talk to you!

JACQUELINE: Mercy me, you ain't seen nothin' yet, and that's only a little sample of his bad humor.

SGANARELLE: Is it possible? And can a man have a soul so base as to mistreat a person like you? Ah, lovely nurse, I know people, and not far from here either, who would think themselves happy just to kiss the little tips of your footsies! Why must so lovely a person have fallen into such hands, and must a mere animal, a brute, a lout, a fool . . . ? Pardon me, nurse, if I speak in this way of your husband.

JACQUELINE: Oh, sir, I know good and well he deserves all them names.

SGANARELLE: Yes, nurse, he certainly does deserve them; and he would also deserve to have you plant a certain decoration on his head, to punish him for his suspicions.

JACQUELINE: It's quite true that if I was only thinking about him, he might drive me to some strange carryings-on.

SGANARELLE: My word! It wouldn't be a bad idea for you to take vengeance on him with someone else. He's a man, I tell you, who really deserves that; and if I were fortunate enough, beautiful nurse, to be chosen to . . .
   (*At this point they both notice* LUCAS, *who was in back of them all the time listening to their talk. They go off in opposite directions, the doctor with comical byplay.*)

Scene 4.   GÉRONTE, LUCAS

GÉRONTE: Hey there, Lucas! Haven't you seen our doctor around?

LUCAS: Yup, tarnation take it! I seen him, and my wife too.

GÉRONTE: Then where can he be?

LUCAS: I dunno, but I wish he'd go to the devil in hell.

GÉRONTE: Go take a look and see what my daughter is doing.

Scene 5.   SGANARELLE, LÉANDRE, GÈRONTE

GÉRONTE: Ah, sir! I was just asking where you were.

SGANARELLE: I was busy in your courtyard—expelling the superfluity of my potations. How is the patient?

GÉRONTE: A little worse since taking your prescription.

SGANARELLE: Very good: that's a sign that it's working.

GÉRONTE: Yes; but as it works, I'm afraid it will choke her.

SGANARELLE: Don't worry; I have remedies that make light of everything, and I'll wait for her in her death agony.

GÉRONTE: Who's this man you're bringing with you?

SGANARELLE (*gesturing like an apothecary giving an enema*):   He's . . .

GÉRONTE: What?

SGANARELLE: The one . . .

GÉRONTE: Eh?

SGANARELLE: Who . . .

GÉRONTE: I understand.

SGANARELLE: Your daughter will need him.

Scene 6.   JACQUELINE, LUCINDE, GÉRONTE, LÈANDRE, SGANARELLE

JACQUELINE: Sir, here's your daughter as wants to take a little walk.

SGANARELLE: That will do her good. Mister Apothecary, go along and take her pulse a bit so that I can discuss her illness with you presently.
(At this point he draws GÉRONTE to one side of the stage, and, passing one arm over his shoulders, puts his hand under his chin and turns him

back toward himself whenever GÉRONTE *tries to watch what his daughter and the apothecary are doing together.*) Sir, it's a great and subtle question among the learned whether women are easier to cure than men. I beg you to listen to this, if you please. Some say no, others say yes; and *I* say yes and no: inasmuch as the incongruity of the opaque humors that are found in the natural temperament of women, is the reason why the brutish part always tries to gain power over the sensitive part, we see that the inequality of their opinions depends on the oblique movement of the moon's circle; and since the sun, which darts its rays over the concavity of the earth, finds . . .

LUCINDE: No, I'm utterly incapable of changing my feelings.

GÉRONTE: That's my daughter speaking! Oh, what wonderful virtue in that remedy! Oh, what an admirable doctor! How obliged I am to you for this marvelous cure! And what can I do for you after such a service?

SGANARELLE (*walking around the stage and wiping his brow*): That's an illness that gave me a lot of trouble!

LUCINDE: Yes, father, I've recovered my speech; but I've recovered it to tell you that I shall never have any other husband than Léandre, and that there's no use your trying to give me Horace.

GÉRONTE: But . . .

LUCINDE: Nothing can shake my resolution.

GÉRONTE: What . . . ?

LUCINDE: All your fine objections will be in vain.

GÉRONTE: If . . .

LUCINDE: All your arguments will be no use.

GÉRONTE: I . . .

LUCINDE: It's a thing I'm determined on.

GÉRONTE: But . . .

LUCINDE: There is no paternal authority that can force me to marry in spite of myself.

GÉRONTE: I've . . .

LUCINDE: All your efforts will not avail.

GÉRONTE: He . . .

LUCINDE: My heart could never submit to this tyranny.

GÉRONTE: There . . .

LUCINDE: And I'll cast myself into a convent rather than marry a man I don't love.

GÉRONTE: But . . .

LUCINDE (*in a deafening voice*):   No. By no means. Nothing doing. You're wasting your time. I won't do anything of the sort. That's settled.

GÉRONTE: Oh! What a rush of words! There's no way to resist it. Sir, I beg you to make her dumb again.

SGANARELLE: That's impossible for me. All I can do for your service is to make you deaf, if you want.

GÉRONTE: Many thanks! (*To* LUCINDE) Then do you think . . . ?

LUCINDE: No. All your reasons will make no impression on my soul.

GÉRONTE: You shall marry Horace this very evening.

LUCINDE: I'll sooner marry death.

SGANARELLE: Good Lord! Stop, let me medicate this affair. Her illness still grips her, and I know the remedy we must apply.

GÉRONTE: Is it possible, sir, that you can also cure this illness of the mind?

SGANARELLE: Yes. Leave it to me, I have remedies for everything, and our apothecary will serve us for this cure. (*Calls the apothecary.*) One word. You see that the ardor she has for this Léandre is completely contrary to her father's will, that there is no time to lose, that the humors are very inflamed, and that it is necessary to find a remedy promptly for this ailment, which could get worse with delay. For my part, I see only one, which is a dose of purgative flight, which you will combine properly with two drams of matrimonium in pill form. She may make some difficulty about taking this remedy; but since you are an able man at your trade, it's up to you to persuade her and make her swallow the dose as best you can. Go along and get her to take a little turn around the garden, so as to prepare the humors, while I talk to her father here; but above all don't waste time. The remedy, quickly, the one specific remedy!

Scene 7.   GÉRONTE, SGANARELLE

GÉRONTE: What are those drugs, sir, that you just mentioned? It seems to me I've never heard of them.

SGANARELLE: They are drugs used in great emergencies.

GÉRONTE: Did you ever see such insolence as hers?

SGANARELLE: Daughters are sometimes a little headstrong.

GÉRONTE: You wouldn't believe how crazy she is about this Léandre.

SGANARELLE: The heat of the blood does this to young minds.

GÉRONTE: For my part, ever since I discovered the violence of this love, I've managed to keep my daughter always locked up.

SGANARELLE: You've done wisely.

GÉRONTE: And I've kept them from having any communication together.

SGANARELLE: Very good.

GÉRONTE: Some folly would have resulted if I'd allowed them to see each other.

SGANARELLE: No doubt.

GÉRONTE: And I think she'd have been just the girl to run off with him.

SGANARELLE: That's prudent reasoning.

GÉRONTE: I've been warned that he's making every effort to speak to her.

SGANARELLE: What a clown!

GÉRONTE: But he'll be wasting his time.

SGANARELLE: Ha, ha!

GÉRONTE: And I'll keep him from seeing her, all right.

SGANARELLE: He's not dealing with a dolt, and you know tricks of the game that he doesn't. Smarter than you is no fool.

Scene 8.   LUCAS, GÉRONTE, SGANARELLE

LUCAS: Dad blast it, sir, here's a lot of ruckus: your daughter's done run off with her Léandre. The 'pothecary, that was him; and Mister Doctor here's the one as pufformed that fine operation.

GÉRONTE: What? Assassinate me in that way! Here, get a policeman! Don't let him get out. Ah, traitor! I'll have the law on you.

LUCAS: Hah! By jingo, Mister Doctor, you'll be hung: just don't move outa
there.

Scene 9.   MARTINE, SGANARELLE, LUCAS

MARTINE: Oh, Good Lord! What a time I've had finding this house! Tell me,
what's the news of the doctor I provided for you?

LUCAS: Here he be. Gonna be hung.

MARTINE: What? My husband hanged? Alas! What's he done?

LUCAS: He fixed it for our master's daughter to get run away with.

MARTINE: Alas! My dear husband, is it really true they're going to hang
you?

SGANARELLE: As you see. Oh!

MARTINE: Must you let yourself die in the presence of all these people?

SGANARELLE: What do you expect me to do about it?

MARTINE: At least if you'd finished cutting our wood, I'd have some consolation.

SGANARELLE: Get out of here, you're breaking my heart.

MARTINE: No, I mean to stay to give you courage in the face of death, and
I won't leave you until I see you hanged.

SGANARELLE: Oh!

Scene 10.   GÉRONTE, SGANARELLE, MARTINE, LUCAS

GÉRONTE: The constable will be here soon, and they'll put you in a place
where they'll be answerable for you to me.

SGANARELLE (*hat in hand*):   Alas! Can't this be changed to a modest cudgeling?

GÉRONTE: No, no, justice will take its course . . . But what's this I see?

Scene 11. LÉANDRE, LUCINDE, JACQUELINE, LUCAS, GÉRONTE, SGANARELLE, MARTINE

LÉANDRE: Sir, I come to reveal Léandre to you and restore Lucinde to your power. We both intended to run away and get married; but this plan has given way to a more honorable procedure. I do not aim to steal your daughter from you, and it is only from your hands that I wish to receive her. I will tell you this, sir: I have just received letters informing me that my uncle has died and that I am heir to all his property.

GÉRONTE: Sir, I have the highest consideration for your virtues, and I give you my daughter with the greatest pleasure in the world.

SGANARELLE: That was a close shave for medicine!

MARTINE: Since you're not going to be hanged, you can thank me for being a doctor; for I'm the one who procured you that honor.

SGANARELLE: Yes, you're the one who procured me quite a beating.

LÉANDRE: The result is too fine for you to harbor resentment.

SGANARELLE: All right: I forgive you for the beatings in consideration of the dignity you've raised me to; but prepare henceforth to live in the greatest respect with a man of my consequence, and bear in mind that the wrath of a doctor is more to be feared than anyone can believe.

Translated by Donald M. Frame

NATHANIEL HAWTHORNE

The Haunted Quack

A Tale of a Canal Boat

In the summer of 18—, I made an excursion to Niagara. At Schenectady, finding the roads nearly impassable, I took passage in a canal boat for Utica. The weather was dull and lowering. There were but few passengers on board; and of those few, none were sufficiently inviting in appearance to induce me to make any overtures to a travelling acquaintance. A stupid answer, or a surly monosyllable, were all that I got in return for the few simple questions I hazarded. An occasional drizzling rain, and the wet and slippery condition of the tow-path, along which the lazy beasts that dragged the vessel travelled, rendered it impossible to vary the monotony of the scene by walking. I had neglected to provide myself with books, and as we crept along at the dull rate of four miles per hour, I soon felt the foul fiend *Ennui* coming upon me with all her horrors.

"Time and the hour," however, "run through the roughest day," and night at length approached. By degrees the passengers, seemingly tired of each other's company, began to creep slowly away to their berths; most of them fortifying themselves with a potation, before resigning themselves to the embrace of Morpheus. One called for a glass of hot whiskey punch, because he felt cold; another took some brandy toddy to prevent his taking cold; some took mint juleps; some gin-slings; and some rum and water. One took his dram because he felt sick; another to make him sleep well; and a third because he had nothing else to do. The last who retired from the cabin, was an old gentleman who had been deeply engaged in a well-thumbed volume all day, and whose mental abstraction I had more than once envied. He now laid down his book, and, pulling out a red nightcap, called for a pint of beer, to take the vapors out of his head.

As soon as he had left the cabin, I took up the volume, and found it to be Glanville's marvellous book, entitled the *History of Witches, or the Wonders of the Invisible World Displayed*. I began to peruse it, and soon got so deeply interested in some of his wonderful narrations, that the hours slipped unconsciously away, and midnight found me poring half asleep over the pages. From this dreamy state I was suddenly aroused by a muttering, as of a suppressed voice, broken by groans and sounds of distress. Upon looking round, I saw that they proceeded from the figure of a man enveloped in a cloak who was lying asleep upon one of the benches of the cabin whom I had not previously noticed. I recognized him to be a young man, with whose singular appearance and behavior during the day, I had been struck. He was tall and thin in person, rather shabbily dressed, with long, lank, black hair, and large gray eyes, which gave a visionary character to one of the most pallid and cadaverous countenances I had ever beheld. Since he had come on board, he had appeared restless and unquiet, keeping away from the table at meal times, and seeming averse from entering into conversation with the passengers. Once or twice, on catching my eye, he had slunk away as if, conscience-smitten by the remembrance of some crime, he dreaded to meet the gaze of a fellow mortal. From this behavior I suspected that he was either a fugitive from justice, or else a little disordered in mind; and had resolved to keep my eye on him and observe what course he should take when we reached Utica.

Supposing that the poor fellow was now under the influence of nightmare, I got up with the intention of giving him a shake to rouse him, when the

words "murder," "poison," and others of extraordinary import, dropping un-
connectedly from his lips, induced me to stay my hand. "Go away, go away,"
exclaimed he, as if conscious of my approach, but mistaking me for another.
"Why do you continue to torment me? If I did poison you, I didn't mean
to do it, and they can't make that out more than manslaughter. Besides,
what's the use of haunting me now? Ain't I going to give myself up, and
tell all? Begone! I say, you bloody old hag, begone!" Here the bands of
slumber were broken by the intensity of his feelings, and with a wild expression of countenance and a frame shaking with emotion, he started from the
bench, and stood trembling before me.

Though convinced that he was a criminal, I could not help pitying him
from the forlorn appearance he now exhibited. As soon as he had collected
his wandering ideas, it seemed as if he read in my countenance, the mingled
sentiments of pity and abhorrence, with which I regarded him. Looking anxiously around, and seeing that we were alone, he drew the corner of the
bench towards me, and sitting down, with an apparent effort to command
his feelings, thus addressed me. His tone of voice was calm and distinct; and
his countenance, though deadly pale, was composed.

"I see, Sir, that from what I am conscious of having uttered in my disturbed
sleep, you suspect me of some horrid crime. You are right. My conscience
convicts me, and an awful nightly visitation, worse than the waking pangs of
remorse, compels me to confess it. Yes, I am a murderer. I have been the
unhappy cause of blotting out the life of a fellow being from the page of
human existence. In these pallid features, you may read enstamped, in the
same characters which the first murderer bore upon his brow, Guilt—guilt—
guilt!"

Here the poor young man paused, evidently agitated by strong internal
emotion. Collecting himself, however, in a few moments, he thus continued.

"Yet still, when you have heard my sad story, I think you will bestow
upon me your pity. I feel that there is no peace for me, until I have dis-
burthened my mind. Your countenance promises sympathy. Will you listen to
my unhappy narrative?"

My curiosity being strongly excited by this strange exordium, I told him I
was ready to hear whatever he had to communicate. Upon this, he proceeded
as follows:—

"My name is Hippocrates Jenkins. I was born in Nantucket, but my father
emigrated to these parts when I was young. I grew up in one of the most
flourishing villages on the borders of the canal. My father and mother both
dying of the lake fever, I was bound apprentice to an eminent operative in the
boot and shoe making line, who had lately come from New York. Would that
I had remained content with this simple and useful profession. Would that I
had stuck to my waxed ends and awl, and never undertaken to cobble up
people's bodies. But my legs grew tired of being trussed beneath my haunches;
my elbows wearied with their monotonous motion; my eyes became dim with

gazing forever upon the dull brick wall which faced our shop window; and my whole heart was sick of my sedentary, and, as I foolishly deemed it, particularly mean occupation. My time was nearly expired, and I had long resolved, should any opportunity offer of getting into any other employment, I would speedily embrace it.

"I had always entertained a predilection for the study of medicine. What had given my mind this bias, I know not. Perhaps it was the perusal of an old volume of Doctor Buchan, over whose pages it was the delight of my youthful fancy to pore. Perhaps it was the oddness of my Christian cognomen, which surely was given me by my parents in a prophetic hour. Be this as it may, the summit of my earthly happiness was to be a doctor. Conceive then my delight and surprise, one Saturday evening, after having carried home a pair of new white-topped boots for Doctor Ephraim Ramshorne, who made the care of bodies his care, in the village, to hear him ask me, how I should like to be a doctor. He then very generously offered to take me as a student. From my earliest recollections, the person and character of Doctor Ramshorne had been regarded by me with the most profound and awful admiration. Time out of mind the successful practitioner for many miles around, I had looked upon him as the *beau idéal* of a doctor—a very Apollo in the healing art. When I speak of him, however, as the *successful* practitioner, I mean it not to be inferred that death was less busy in his doings, or funerals scarcer during his dynasty; but only that he had, by some means or other, contrived to force all those who had ventured to contest the palm with him, to quit the field. He was large and robust in person, and his ruby visage showed that if he grew fat upon drugs, it was not by swallowing them himself. It was never exactly ascertained from what college the Doctor had received his diploma; nor was he very forward to exhibit his credentials. When hard pressed, however, he would produce a musty old roll of parchment, with a red seal as broad as the palm of his hand, which looked as if it might have been the identical diploma of the great Boerhaave himself, and some cramped manuscript of a dozen pages, in an unknown tongue, said by the Doctor to be his Greek thesis. These documents were enough to satisfy the doubts of the most sceptical. By the simple country people, far and near, the Doctor was regarded, in point of occult knowledge and skill, as a second Faustus. It is true, the village lawyer, a rival in popularity, used to whisper, that the Doctor's Greek thesis was nothing but a bundle of prescriptions for the bots, wind-galls, spavins, and other veterinary complaints, written in high Dutch by a Hessian horse doctor; that the diploma was all a sham, and that Ephraim was no more a doctor than his jackass. But these assertions were all put down to the score of envy on the part of the lawyer. Be this as it may, on the strength of one or two remarkable cures, which he was said to have performed, and by dint of whee-dling some and bullying others, it was certain that Ramshorne had worked himself into a very good practice. The Doctor united in his own person, the attributes of apothecary and physician; and as he vended, as well as prescribed his own drugs, it was not his interest to stint his patients in their enormous boluses, or nauseous draughts. His former medical student had been worried into a consumption over the mortar and pestle; in consequence of which he had pitched upon me for his successor.

"By the kindness of a few friends I was fitted out with the necessary requisitions for my metamorphosis. The Doctor required no fee, and, in consideration of certain little services to be rendered him, such as taking care of his horse, cleaning his boots, running errands, and doing little jobs about the house, had promised to board and lodge me, besides giving me my professional education. So with a rusty suit of black, and an old plaid cloak, behold equipped the disciple of Aesculapius.

"I cannot describe my elation of mind, when I found myself fairly installed in the Doctor's office. Golden visions floated before my eyes. I fancied my fortune already made, and blessed my happy star, that had fallen under the benign influence of so munificent a patron.

"The Doctor's office, as it was called *par excellence,* was a little nook of a room, communicating with a larger apartment denominated the shop. The paraphernalia of this latter place had gotten somewhat into disorder since the last student had gone away, and I soon learnt that it was to be my task to arrange the heterogeneous mass of bottles, boxes, and gallipots, that were strewed about in promiscuous confusion. In the office, there was a greater appearance of order. A small regiment of musty looking books, were drawn up in line upon a couple of shelves, where, to judge from the superincumbent strata of dust, they appeared to have peacefully reposed for many years. A rickety wooden clock, which the Doctor had taken in part payment from a peddler, and the vital functions of which, to use his own expression, had long since ceased to act, stood in one corner. A mouldy plaster bust of some unknown worthy, a few bottles of pickled, and one or two dried specimens of morbid anatomy, a small chest of drawers, a table, and a couple of chairs, completed the furniture of this *sanctum.* The single window commanded a view of the churchyard, in which, it was said, many of the Doctor's former patients were quietly slumbering. With a feeling of reverence I ventured to dislodge one of the dusty tomes, and began to try to puzzle out the hard words with which it abounded; when suddenly, as if he had been conjured back, like the evil one by Cornelius Agrippa's book, the Doctor made his appearance. With a gruff air, he snatched the volume from my hands, and telling me not to meddle with what I could not understand, bade me go and take care of his horse, and make haste back, as he wanted me to spread a pitch plaster, and carry the same, with a bottle of his patent catholicon, to farmer Van Pelt, who had the rheumatism. On my return, I was ordered by Mrs. Ramshorne to split some wood, and kindle a fire in the parlor, as she expected company; after which Miss Euphemia Ramshorne, a sentimental young lady, who was as crooked in person and crabbed in temper as her own name, despatched me to the village circulating library, in quest of the *Mysteries of Udolpho.* I soon found out that my place was no sinecure. The greater part of my time was occupied in compounding certain quack medicines, of Ramshorne's own invention, from which he derived great celebrity, and no inconsiderable profit. Besides his patent catholicon, and universal panacea, there was his anti-pertusso-balsamico drops, his patent calorific refrigerating anodyne, and his golden restorative of nature. Into the business of compounding these, and other articles with similar high-sounding titles, I was gradually initiated, and soon acquired so much skill in their manipulation, that my services became indispensable to my master; so much so, that he was obliged to hire a little negro to take care of his horse, and clean his boots. What chiefly reconciled me to the drudgery of the shop, was the seeing how well the Doctor got paid for his villainous compounds. A mixture of a little brick dust, rosin, and treacle, dignified with the title of the anthelminthic amalgam, he sold for half a dollar; and a bottle of vinegar and alum, with a little rose water to give it a flavor, yclept the anti-scrofulous abstergent lotion, brought twice that sum. I longed for the day when I should dispense my own medicines, and in my hours of castle-building, looked forward to fortunes far beyond those of the renowned Dr. Solomon. Alas! my fond hopes have been blighted in their bud. I have drunk deeply of the nauseous draught of adversity, and been forced to swallow many bitter pills of disappointment. But I find I am beginning to smell of the shop. I must return to my sad tale. The same accident, which not unfrequently before had put a sudden stop to the Doctor's patients' taking any more of his nostrums, at length prevented him from reaping any longer their golden harvest. One afternoon, after having dined with his friend, Squire Gobbledown, he came home, and complained of not feeling very well. By his directions, I prepared for him some of his elixir sanitatis, composed of brandy and bitters, of which he took an inordinate dose. Shortly after, he was seized with a fit of apoplexy, and before bedtime, in spite of all the drugs in the shop, which I poured down with unsparing hand, he had breathed his last. In three days, Ramshorne was quietly deposited in the churchyard, in the midst of those he had sent there before him.

"Having resided with the Doctor for several years, I had become pretty well known throughout the neighborhood, particularly among the old ladies, whose good graces I had always sedulously cultivated. I accordingly resolved to commence quacking—I mean practising—on my own account. Having obtained my late master's stock of drugs from his widow at an easy rate, and displaying my own name in golden letters as his successor, to work I went, with the internal resolve that where Ramshorne had given one dose, I would give six.

"For a time, Fortune seemed to smile upon me, and everything went on well. All the old women were loud in sounding my praises, far and near. The medicaments of my master, continued to be in demand, and treacle, brick dust, and alum came to a good market. Some drawbacks, however, I occasionally met with. Having purchased the patent right of one of Thompson's steam baths, in my first experiment I came near flaying alive a rheumatic tanner, who had submitted himself to the operation. By an unfortunate mistake in regulating the steam he was nearly parboiled; and it was supposed that the thickness of his hide alone preserved his vitals uninjured. I was myself threatened with the fate of Marsyas, by the enraged sufferer; which he was happily prevented from attempting to inflict, by a return of his malady, which has never since left him. I however after this gave up steaming, and confined myself to regular practice. At length, either the charm of novelty wearing off, or people beginning to discover the inefficacy of the old nostrums, I was obliged to exert my wits to invent new ones. These I generally took the precaution to try upon cats or dogs, before using them upon the human system. They were, however, mostly of an innocent nature, and I satisfied my conscience with the reflection, that if they did no good, they could at least do no harm. Happy would it have been for me, could I always have done thus. Meeting with success in my first efforts, I by degrees ventured upon more active in- gredients. At length in an evil hour, I invented a curious mixture composed of forty-nine different articles. This I dubbed in high-flowing terms 'The Antidote to Death, or the Eternal Elixir of Longevity'; knowing full well that though

'A rose might smell as sweet by any other name,'

yet would not my drugs find as good a sale under a more humble title. This cursed compound proved the antidote to all my hopes of success. Besides forcing me to quit the village in a confounded hurry, it has embittered my life ever since, and reduced me to the ragged and miserable plight in which you see me.

"I dare say you have met with that species of old woman, so frequent in all country towns, who, seeming to have outlived the common enjoyments of life, and outworn the ordinary sources of excitement, seek fresh stimulus in scenes of distress, and appear to take a morbid pleasure in beholding the varieties of human suffering and misery. One of the most noted characters in the village was an old beldame of this description. Granny Gordon, so she was familiarly denominated, was the rib of the village Vulcan, and the din of her eternal tongue was only equalled by the ringing of her husband's anvil. Thin and withered away in person and redolent with snuff, she bore no small resemblance to a newly-exhumed mummy, and to all appearance promised to last as long as one of those ancient dames of Egypt. Not a death, a burial, a fit of sickness, a casualty, nor any of the common calamities of life ever occurred in the vicinity, but Granny Gordon made it her especial business to be present. Wrapped in an old scarlet cloak,—that hideous cloak! the thought of it makes me shudder—she might be seen hovering about the dwelling of the sick. Watching her opportunity, she would make her way into the patient's chamber, and disturb his repose with long dismal stories and ill-boding predictions; and if turned from the house, which was not unfrequently the case, she would depart, muttering threats and abuse.

"As the Indians propitiate the favor of the devil, so had I, in my eagerness to acquire popularity, made a firm friend and ally, though rather a troublesome one, of this old woman. She was one of my best customers, and, provided it was something new, and had a high-sounding name to recommend it, would take my most nauseous compounds with the greatest relish. Indeed the more disgusting was the dose, the greater in her opinion was its virtue.

"I had just corked the last bottle of my antidote, when a message came to tell me that Granny Gordon had one of her old fits, and wanted some new doctor-stuff, as the old physic didn't do her any more good. Not having yet given my new pharmaceutic preparation a trial, I felt a little doubtful about its effects, but trusting to the toughness of the old woman's system, I ventured to send a potion, with directions to take it cautiously. Not many minutes had elapsed, before the messenger returned, in breathless haste, to say that Mrs. Gordon was much worse, and that though she had taken all the stuff, they believed she was dying. With a vague foreboding of evil, I seized my hat, and hastened to the blacksmith's. On entering the chamber my eyes were greeted with a sad spectacle. Granny Gordon, bolstered up in the bed, holding in her hand the bottle I had sent her, drained of its contents, sat gasping for breath, and occasionally agitated by strong convulsions. A cold sweat rested on her forehead, her eyes seemed dim and glazed, her nose, which was usually of a ruby hue, was purple and peaked, and her whole appearance evidently betokened approaching dissolution.

"Around the bed were collected some half dozen withered beldames who scowled upon me, as I entered, with ill-omened visages. Her husband, a drunken brute, who used to beat his better half six times a week, immediately began to load me with abuse, accusing me of having poisoned his dear, dear wife, and threatening to be the death of me, if she died.

"My conscience smote me. I felt stupefied and bewildered, and knew not which way to turn. At this moment, the patient perceiving me, with a hideous contortion of countenance, the expression of which I shall carry to my dying hour, and a voice between a scream and a groan, held up the empty bottle, and exclaimed, 'This is your doing, you villainous quack you' (here she was seized with hiccup);—'you have poisoned me, you have' (here fearful spasms shook her whole frame);—'but I'll be revenged; day and night my ghost shall haunt'—here her voice became inarticulate, and shaking her withered arm at me, she fell back, and to my extreme horror, gave up the ghost. This was too much for my nerves. I rushed from the house, and ran home with the dying curse ringing in my ears, fancying that I saw her hideous physiognomy, grinning from every bush and tree that I passed. Knowing that as soon as the noise of this affair should get abroad, the village would be too hot to hold me, I resolved to decamp as silently as possible. First throwing all my recently manufactured anodyne into the canal, that it should not rise in judgment against me, I made up a little bundle of clothes, and taking my seat in the mail stage, which was passing at the time and fortunately empty, in a couple of days I found myself in the great city of New York. Having a little money with me, I hired a mean apartment in an obscure part of the city, in the hope that I might remain concealed till all search after me should be over, when I might find some opportunity of getting employment, or of resuming my old profession, under happier auspices. By degrees the few dollars I brought with me were expended, and after pawning my watch and some of my clothes, I found myself reduced to the last shilling. But not the fear of impending starvation, nor the dread of jail, are to be compared to the horrors I nightly suffer. Granny Gordon has been as good as her word. Every night, at the solemn hour of twelve" (here he looked fearfully around)—"her ghost appears to me, wrapped in a red cloak, with her gray hairs streaming from beneath an old nightcap of the same color, brandishing the vial, and accusing me of having poisoned her. These visitations have at length become so insupportable, that I have resolved to return and give myself up to justice; for I feel that hanging itself is better than this state of torment."

Here the young man ceased. I plainly saw that he was a little disordered in his intellect. To comfort him, however, I told him that if he had killed fifty old women, they could do nothing to him, if he had done it professionally. And as for the ghost, we would take means to have that put at rest, when we reached Utica.

About the gray of the morning, we arrived at the place of our destination. My *protégé* having unburdened his mind, seemed more at his ease, and taking a mint julep, prepared to accompany me on shore. As we were leaving the boat, several persons in a wagon drove down to the wharf. As soon as my companion observed them, he exclaimed with a start of surprise, "Hang me, if there isn't old Graham the sheriff, and lawyer Dickson, and Bill Gordon come to take me." As he spoke, his foot slipping, he lost his balance, and fell backwards into the canal. We drew him from the water, and as soon as the persons in the wagon perceived him, they one and all sprang out, and ran up with the greatest expressions of joyful surprise. "Why, Hippy, my lad," exclaimed the sheriff, "where have you been? All our town has been in a snarl about you. We all supposed you had been forcibly abducted. Judge Bates offered a reward of twenty dollars for your corpse. We have dragged the canal for more than a mile, and found a mass of bottles, which made us think you had been spirited away. Betsey Wilkins made her affidavit that she heard Bill Gordon swear that he would take your life, and here you see we have brought him down to have his trial. But come, come, jump in the wagon, we'll take you up to the tavern, to get your duds dried, and tell you all about it."

Here a brawny fellow with a smutty face, who I found was Gordon the blacksmith, came up, and shaking Hippocrates by the hand, said, "By goles, Doctor, I am glad to see you. If you hadn't come back I believe it would have gone hard with me. Come, man, you must forgive the hard words I gave you. My old woman soon got well of her fit, after you went away, and says she thinks the stuff did her a mortal sight o' good."

It is impossible to describe the singular expression the countenance of the young man now exhibited. For some time he stood in mute amazement, shaking with cold, and gazing alternately at each of his friends as they addressed him; and it required their reiterated assurance to convince him, that Granny Gordon was still in the land of the living, and that he had not been haunted by a veritable ghost.

Wishing to obtain a further explanation of this strange scene, I accompanied them to the tavern. A plain-looking man in a farmer's dress, who was of the party, confirmed what the blacksmith had said, as to the supposed death of his wife and her subsequent recovery. "She was only in a swoon," said he, "but came to, soon after the Doctor had left her." He added that it was his private opinion that she would now last forever. He spoke of Hippocrates as a " 'nation smart doctor, who had a power of larning, but gave severe doses."

After discussing a good breakfast, my young friend thanked me for the sympathy and interest I had taken in his behalf. He told me he intended returning to the practice of his profession. I admonished him to be more careful in the exhibition of his patent medicines, telling him that all old women had not nine lives. He shook hands with me, and, gayly jumping into the wagon, rode off with his friends.

OLIVER WENDELL HOLMES

The Stethoscope Song

A Professional Ballad

There was a young man in Boston town,
    He bought him a stethoscope nice and new,
All mounted and finished and polished down,
    With an ivory cap and a stopper too.

It happened a spider within did crawl,
    And spun him a web of ample size,
Wherein there chanced one day to fall
    A couple of very imprudent flies.

The first was a bottle-fly, big and blue,
  The second was smaller, and thin and long;
So there was a concert between the two,
  Like an octave flute and a tavern gong.

Now being from Paris but recently,
  This fine young man would show his skill
And so they gave him, his hand to try,
  A hospital patient extremely ill.

Some said that his *liver* was short of *bile,*
  And some that his *heart* was over size,
While some kept arguing, all the while,
  He was crammed with *tubercles* up to his eyes.

This fine young man then up stepped he,
  And all the doctors made a pause;
Said he, The man must die, you see,
  By the fifty-seventh of Louis's laws.

But since the case is a desperate one,
  To explore his chest it may be well;
For if he should die and it were not done,
  You know the *autopsy* would not tell.

Then out his stethoscope he took,
  And on it placed his curious ear;
Mon Dieu! said he, with a knowing look,
  Why, here is a sound that's mighty queer!

The *bourdonnement* is very clear,—
  Amphoric buzzing, as I'm alive!
Five doctors took their turn to hear;
  Amphoric buzzing, said all the five.

There's *empyema* beyond a doubt;
  We'll plunge a *trocar* in his side.
The diagnosis was made out,—
  They tapped the patient; so he died.

Now such as hate new-fashioned toys
  Began to look extremely glum;
They said that *rattles* were made for boys,
  And vowed that his *buzzing* was all a hum.

There was an old lady had long been sick,
    And what was the matter none did know:
Her pulse was slow, though her tongue was quick;
    To her this knowing youth must go.

So there the nice old lady sat,
    With phials and boxes all in a row;
She asked the young doctor what he was at,
    To thump her and tumble her ruffles so.

Now, when the stethoscope came out,
    The flies began to buzz and whiz:
Oh, ho! the matter is clear, no doubt;
    An *aneurism* there plainly is.

The *bruit de râpe* and the *bruit de scie*
    And the *bruit de diable* are all combined;
How happy Bouillaud would be,
    If he a case like this could find!

Now, when the neighboring doctors found
    A case so rare had been descried,
They every day her ribs did pound
    In squads of twenty; so she died.

Then six young damsels, slight and frail,
    Received this kind young doctor's cares;
They all were getting slim and pale,
    And short of breath on mounting stairs.

They all made rhymes with "sighs" and "skies,"
    And loathed their puddings and buttered rolls,
And dieted, much to their friends' surprise,
    On pickles and pencils and chalk and coals.

So fast their little hearts did bound,
    The frightened insects buzzed the more;
So over all their chests he found
    The *râle sifflant* and the *râle sonore*.

He shook his head. There's grave disease,—
    I greatly fear you all must die;
A slight *post-mortem,* if you please,
    Surviving friends would gratify.

The six young damsels wept aloud,
     Which so prevailed on six young men
That each his honest love avowed,
     Whereat they all got well again.

This poor young man was all aghast;
     The price of stethoscopes came down;
And so he was reduced at last
     To practise in a country town.

The doctors being very sore,   ·
     A stethoscope they did devise
That had a rammer to clear the bore,
     With a knob at the end to kill the flies.

Now use your ears, all you that can,
     But don't forget to mind your eyes,
Or you may be cheated, like this young man,
     By a couple of silly, abnormal flies.

PHYLLIS McGINLEY

Complaint to the American Medical Association

Concerning their members' unfair monopoly of best-selling autobiographies and other fiction

Of all God's creatures here below
     Whose feats confound the skeptic
I most admire the Medico,
     That hero antiseptic.
He has my heart, he has my hand,
     He has my utmost loyalties.
(He also has my tonsils and
     A lien on my royalties.)
For from the time he doth begin
His sacred tryst with medicine,
How noble, he! How never-tiring!
Not rain, nor heat, nor maids admiring,

Nor bills unpaid, nor farmers' hounds
Can stay him from his sleepless rounds.
More fleet than winners of the Bendix,
He hastens to the burst appendix,
Or breasts the blizzard cold and shivery
To make some rural free delivery.

Or if to ampler orbits whirled
   (As fate will sometimes toss us),
How he bestrides this narrow world,
   A medical Colossus!
Perhaps, his kit upon his back,
   He dares the jungle thickets,
Intent upon the fevered track
   Of yaws or mumps or rickets.

The chum of kings, the friend of presidents,
He makes the earth his private residence;
One day prescribing pills and pickups
To cure an emperor of hiccups,
The next in stricken cities stranded,
Combating scourges single-handed,
At peril of life, at risk of limb.
Yet do such deeds suffice for him?
No, no. In secret all the while
He's sought a Literary Style.

The pen (so springs the constant hope
   Of all devout physicians)
Is mightier than the stethoscope
   And runs to more editions.
So while he's waged bacillic wars,
   Or sewed a clever suture,
His mind has hummed with metaphors
   Laid up against the future.
Amid the knives and sterile gauzes
He's dreamt of modifying clauses,
And never gone to bed so late
His diary wasn't up to date,
As if he'd sworn an oath to follow
Both Harper Brothers and Apollo.
Oh, more than Einstein, more than Edison
I do admire the man of Medison.
He has my hand, he has my note,

He has those X-rays of my throat,
But is it fair he should lay claim to
The overcrowded writing game, too?

I eye askance those dubious laurels.
Where are his ethics? Where his morals?
In what brave school did he matriculate
That he should be so damned articulate?
And where's the seal to show his betters
He's certified a Man of Letters?

Professional sirs, I gravely doubt,
    In any really nice sense,
Your boys should practice thus without
    Their literary license.

Topics for Discussion and Writing

1. With Chaucer's portrait of a fourteenth-century medical man in mind, compose a short, descriptive, and perhaps satiric poem that focuses on a physician whom you know well enough to write about.

2. In order to learn more about the dynamics of Chaucer's world and about certain key medieval ideas that were passed down to later generations, read your library's copy of E. M. W. Tillyard's concise but interesting book *The Elizabethan World Picture*. In a short report to the class, explain what Tillyard says about "The Stars and Fortune," "The Elements," and "Man." How does the Tillyard discussion help clarify Chaucer's account of his physician's general plan for healing the human body?

3. Much of the humor in Jonson's epigram revolves around its title, "To Doctor Empirick." Look up "empiric," "empirical," and "empiricism" in your library's copy of *The Oxford English Dictionary* in order to discover just what the seventeenth century and Jonson meant by equating "empiric" and "quack." Then explain to the class the results of your brief research trip.

4. With your instructor as director and the class as both cast members and audience, present a book-in-hand performance of act III of *The Doctor in Spite of Himself*. Your director and group will have to decide who will play Sganarelle and the other parts in act III, on what day the class-

room presentation will take place, and which members will serve as the audience for that class period. Since the presentation will allow players to have their books in hand, there will be no need to memorize lines. The emphasis should be on making Molière's farce "come alive" as drama in performance.

5. If you enjoyed Molière's *The Doctor in Spite of Himself*, read another of his comedies on the medical theme, *The Imaginary Invalid*. Compare and contrast these two plays in terms of plot, character, and theme or meaning.

6. What do you think is the point of the comic reversal at the end of "The Haunted Quack"? Could you summarize Hawthorne's theme or message in the story? What is the mental condition of Hippocrates Jenkins when we first see him? Does it change later on? How? Why?

7. Compare and contrast Molière and Hawthorne on the topic of quack physicians and apothecaries.

8. Compare and contrast Molière and Holmes on the topic of the confusing and often humorous role of high-flown medical terminology.

9. Analyze McGinley's poetic and witty "Complaint," paying special attention to diction (both denotation and connotation). Argue for or against the merits of her case in an original thesis-and-support essay.

10. Review the selections by doctors (Selzer, Williams, Cronin, and Holmes). Does the fact that these authors are or were physicians make them better writers on medical themes than lay people? Do their works possess a dimension not found in other pieces? Use the literary texts to support your conclusions.

Part 3

Medicine and Mental Health

The frequent appearance of the topic of mental health in literature reflects the human need not only to express the depression, loneliness, or despair that sometimes fills the soul, but also to try to make sense out of these darker feelings and learn from them. Although the term "mental health" should be a neutral expression that focuses on health, not illness, and on a person's psychic well-being, it is true that in much creative literature concerned with mental health the tendency is toward revealing the anxiety, the fears, and even the neuroses people have suffered. Another issue raised by the selections in this part concerns the similarities and differences between diseases of the body and those of the mind. Can drugs alone cure mental problems? Are not psychological disorders different from, yet equally as important as physical ills such as cancer, diabetes, diphtheria? How are the mind and the body related? Already Hawthorne's "The Haunted Quack" has provided us with a humorous preview of this part's topic. Now we shall probe the matter a bit more deeply.

With Shakespeare's sonnet "My love is as a fever, longing still," we encounter a quasi-medical model from the Renaissance upon which much subsequent therapy for mental illness is indirectly based. Thus, any mental illness (such as depression, suicidal tendencies, or even the kind of madness this poem describes) is presented as being able to be cured with "prescriptions," that is, both the doctor's orders and also his drugs. Shakespeare sets up the analogy of physician/disease versus reason/desire. He employs medical imagery for detailing the madness of love: "Past cure I am, now reason is past care." The speaker realizes the unrelenting madness or crazed passion of his desire, yet he is totally unable to control himself or solve his own problem. Reason, his rational self, has fled somewhat as a physician might give up on a patient who has repeatedly disregarded "his prescriptions." But, paradoxically, there can be no real cure without some kind of special outside intervention.

No one can dispute the tremendous impact Sigmund Freud has had on psychoanalytic theory. This impact was also felt in the literary world, as scores of late nineteenth- and early twentieth-century authors wrote works dealing with mental illness and its cures. Possibly Freud's greatest and most over-emphasized success was in dream therapy and interpretation. The story "Lord Mountdrago" by W. Somerset Maugham (himself a doctor who finished medical school in London, was licensed, but never practiced) is a fine example of a work in which the intertwining of a man's dreams and conscience has disastrous consequences that even fairly modern psychoanalysis cannot prevent.

"Lord Mountdrago" is told primarily through the eyes of Dr. Audlin, a British psychoanalyst who more or less stumbles into this area of medicine during World War I. There are several ironic touches, for Maugham portrays the doctor as giving "the impression of a very sick man" who harbors "the suspicion" that he is "little more than a quack" despite his "extraordinary results" and great healing powers. Audlin's new patient, Lord Mountdrago, is a high government official who cannot concentrate on his sensitive duties as foreign minister because of his progressively disturbing dreams. Despite various treatments, Lord Mountdrago's anxiety, insomnia, and mental anguish continue to worsen, yet he remains Audlin's patient perhaps because the doctor is the only one he can talk to. Maugham's early twentieth-century analyst has much in common with today's psychiatrist or psychologist. Audlin's talking with his patient, helping him to make some sense out of his dreams, using hypnotic suggestion to direct him to specific anxiety-reducing actions, and seeing the patient through his conflict—these techniques might be considered the equivalent of modern "crisis intervention." Unfortunately, Audlin's therapy is not ultimately successful, and the story's haunting climax is unexpected. Indeed, only a very thin line "divides those whom we call sane from those whom we call insane."

The "split self" is a concept that holds great appeal for many modern writers. It appears, for example, in "Lord Mountdrago" when Audlin tells his patient that one of his selves has taken on the semblance of his adversary in government, Owen Griffiths, in order to punish Lord Mountdrago for an earlier injury he once did to Griffiths. And it forms the central thesis of the brief tale "Borges and Myself," by the twentieth-century Argentine author Jorge Luis Borges. Naturally, the aim of the psychiatrist in treating a person with a split personality is to unite all the selves into a cohesive and healthy self. Borges' two selves coexist, apparently with little difficulty; actually, they seem to need each other. But the piece concisely raises the theme of creativity vis-à-vis madness when it concludes: "Which of us is writing this page I don't know."

From Borges it is but an easy transition to the three very personal poems by Anne Sexton, a suburban housewife who took up poetry during a nervous breakdown in the 1950s and whose brilliant literary career was cut short by suicide in 1974. "You, Doctor Martin" is addressed to the speaker's physician: "Your business is people, / you call at the madhouse, an oracular / eye in our nest." Here the doctor assumes a godlike role as he visits his disturbed patients. "Said the Poet to the Analyst" explains, first, how "My business is words" and, second, how "Your business is watching my words." The speaker is still "weak" and unsure of her grounding in reality, but her therapy sessions and poetry writing may be helping. In "Lullaby," we see the poet-speaker on a summer evening "in the best ward at Bedlam"; soon the night nurse passes out the evening medication, and the patient feels that her sleeping pill "floats me out of myself." Sexton makes a movingly dramatic statement in these three poems about the meaning of life, mental health, and creativity. She also offers insight into what it is like to be in a modern mental institution.

Our final work on medicine and mental health is Anton Chekhov's novella "Ward Six." Chekhov, who graduated from the University of Moscow with a medical degree and who practiced medicine briefly during the 1880s before turning to literature, brings this anthology to its midpoint as he tells the story of a doctor's shocking confinement and death in his own hospital's infamous Ward Six, the wing for those whom the state has declared insane. Excellent for asking ironically who is and is not mad and for pointing up what kinds of treatment or abuse may be possible for the mentally ill, this novella rather bleakly maintains that it is a horror to shut up those who act or look differently from what we expect is the norm. In Chekhov's nightmarish world, as contrasted with the picture Sexton paints in her poems, the physician actually avoids as much patient contact as he can. He is a poor general practitioner and an even poorer "psychiatrist," until he comes to deeper self-knowledge (and death) at the end. The medical personnel whom Chekhov and Sexton place before us deserve close comparison and contrast. We might also profitably look back over the Shakespeare, Maugham, Borges, Sexton, and Chekhov selections in this part and ask why these works are so vivid in their emphasis on the mind's various disorders. Is it simply more fascinating to write and read about mental diseases that are at best imperfectly cured? We might also wonder how exact a science psychiatry or psychology is, even when practiced well and with compassion.

WILLIAM SHAKESPEARE

My love is as a fever, longing still

My love is as a fever, longing still
For that which longer nurseth the disease,
Feeding on that which doth preserve the ill,
Th' uncertain sickly appetite to please.
My reason, the physician to my love,
Angry that his prescriptions are not kept,

Hath left me, and I desperate now approve
Desire is death, which physic did except.
Past cure I am, now reason is past care,
And frantic-mad with evermore unrest;
My thoughts and my discourse as madmen's are,
At random from the truth vainly express'd;
> For I have sworn thee fair and thought thee bright,
> Who art as black as hell, as dark as night.

W. SOMERSET MAUGHAM

Lord Mountdrago

Dr. Audlin looked at the clock on his desk. It was twenty minutes to six. He was surprised that his patient was late, for Lord Mountdrago prided himself on his punctuality; he had a sententious way of expressing himself which gave the air of an epigram to a commonplace remark, and he was in the habit of saying that punctuality is a compliment you pay to the intelligent and a rebuke you administer to the stupid. Lord Mountdrago's appointment was for five-thirty.

There was in Dr. Audlin's appearance nothing to attract attention. He was tall and spare, with narrow shoulders and something of a stoop; his hair was grey and thin; his long, sallow face deeply lined. He was not more than fifty, but he looked older. His eyes, pale-blue and rather large, were weary. When you had been with him for a while you noticed that they moved very little; they remained fixed on your face, but so empty of expression were they that it was no discomfort. They seldom lit up. They gave no clue to his thoughts nor changed with the words he spoke. If you were of an observant turn it might have struck you that he blinked much less often than most of us. His hands were on the large side, with long, tapering fingers; they were soft, but firm, cool but not clammy. You could never have said what Dr. Audlin wore unless you had made a point of looking. His clothes were dark. His tie was black. His dress made his sallow lined face paler, and his pale eyes more wan. He gave you the impression of a very sick man.

Dr. Audlin was a psycho-analyst. He had adopted the profession by accident and practised it with misgiving. When the war broke out he had not been long qualified and was getting experience at various hospitals; he offered his services to the authorities, and after a time was sent out to France. It was then that he discovered his singular gift. He could allay certain pains by the touch of his cool, firm hands, and by talking to them often induce sleep in men who were suffering from sleeplessness. He spoke slowly. His voice had no particular colour, and its tone did not alter with the words he uttered, but it was musical, soft and lulling. He told the men that they must rest, that they mustn't worry, that they must sleep; and rest stole into their jaded bones, tranquillity pushed their anxieties away, like a man finding a place for himself on a crowded bench, and slumber fell on their tired eyelids like the light rain of spring upon the fresh-turned earth. Dr. Audlin found that by speaking to men with that low, monotonous voice of his, by looking at them with his pale, quiet eyes, by stroking their weary foreheads with his long firm hands, he could soothe their perturbations, resolve the conflicts that distracted them and banish the phobias that made their lives a torment. Sometimes he effected cures that seemed miraculous. He restored speech to a man who, after being buried under the earth by a bursting shell, had been struck dumb, and he gave back the use of his limbs to another who had been paralysed after a crash in a plane. He could not understand his powers; he was of a sceptical turn, and though they say that in circumstances of this kind the first thing is to believe in yourself, he never quite succeeded in doing that; and it was only the outcome of his activities, patent to the most incredulous observer, that obliged him to admit that he had some faculty, coming from he knew not where, obscure and uncertain, that enabled him to do things for which he could offer no explanation. When the war was over he went to Vienna and studied there, and afterwards to Zurich; and then settled down in London to practise the art he had so strangely acquired. He had been practising now for fifteen years, and had attained, in the specialty he followed, a distinguished reputation. People told one another of the amazing things he had done, and though his fees were high, he had as many patients as he had time to see. Dr. Audlin knew that he had achieved some very extraordinary results; he had saved men from suicide, others from the lunatic asylum, he had assuaged griefs that embittered useful lives, he had turned unhappy marriages into happy ones, he had eradicated abnormal instincts and thus delivered not a few from a hateful bondage, he had given health to the sick in spirit; he had done all this, and yet at the back of his mind remained the suspicion that he was little more than a quack.

It went against his grain to exercise a power that he could not understand, and it offended his honesty to trade on the faith of the people he treated when he had no faith in himself. He was rich enough now to live without working, and the work exhausted him; a dozen times he had been on the point of giving up practice. He knew all that Freud and Jung and the rest of them had written. He was not satisfied; he had an intimate conviction that all their theory was hocus-pocus, and yet there the results were, incomprehensible, but manifest. And what had he not seen of human nature during the fifteen years that patients had been coming to his dingy back room in Wimpole Street? The revelations that had been poured into his ears, sometimes only too willingly, sometimes with shame, with reservations, with anger, had long ceased to surprise him. Nothing could shock him any longer. He knew by now that men were liars, he knew how extravagant was their vanity; he knew far worse than that about them; but he knew that it was not for him to judge or to condemn. But year by year as these terrible confidences were imparted to him his face grew a little greyer, its lines a little more marked and his pale eyes more weary. He seldom laughed, but now and again when for relaxation he read a novel he smiled. Did their authors really think the men and women they wrote of were like that? If they only knew how much more complicated they were, how much more unexpected, what irreconcilable elements co-existed within their souls and what dark and sinister contentions afflicted them!

It was a quarter to six. Of all the strange cases he had been called upon to deal with Dr. Audlin could remember none stranger than that of Lord Mountdrago. For one thing the personality of his patient made it singular. Lord Mountdrago was an able and a distinguished man. Appointed Secretary for Foreign Affairs when still under forty, now after three years in office he had seen his policy prevail. It was generally acknowledged that he was the ablest politician in the Conservative Party and only the fact that his father was a peer, on whose death he would no longer be able to sit in the House of Commons, made it impossible for him to aim at the premiership. But if in these democratic times it is out of the question for a Prime Minister of England to be in the House of Lords, there was nothing to prevent Lord Mountdrago from continuing to be Secretary for Foreign Affairs in successive Conservative administrations and so for long directing the foreign policy of his country.

Lord Mountdrago had many good qualities. He had intelligence and industry. He was widely travelled, and spoke several languages fluently. From early youth he had specialised in foreign affairs, and had conscientiously made himself acquainted with the political and economic circumstances of other countries. He had courage, insight and determination. He was a good speaker, both on the platform and in the House, clear, precise and often witty. He was a brilliant debater and his gift of repartee was celebrated. He had a fine presence: he was a tall, handsome man, rather bald and somewhat too stout, but this gave him solidity and an air of maturity that were of service to him. As a young man he had been something of an athlete and had rowed in the Oxford boat, and he was known to be one of the best shots in England. At twenty-four he had married a girl of eighteen whose father was a duke and her mother a great American heiress, so that she had both position and wealth, and by her he had had two sons. For several years they had lived privately apart, but in public united, so that appearances were saved, and no other attachment on either side had given the gossips occasion to whisper. Lord. Mountdrago indeed was too ambitious, too hard-working, and it must be added too patriotic, to be tempted by any pleasures that might interfere with his career. He had, in short, a great deal to make him a popular and successful figure. He had unfortunately great defects.

He was a fearful snob. You would not have been surprised at this if his

father had been the first holder of the title. That the son of an ennobled lawyer, a manufacturer or a distiller should attach an inordinate importance to
his rank is understandable. The earldom held by Lord Mountdrago's father
was created by Charles II, and the barony held by the first Earl dated from
the Wars of the Roses. For three hundred years the successive holders of the
title had allied themselves with the noblest families of England. But Lord
Mountdrago was as conscious of his birth as a *nouveau riche* is conscious of
his money. He never missed an opportunity of impressing it upon others. He
had beautiful manners when he chose to display them, but this he did only
with people whom he regarded as his equals. He was coldly insolent to those
whom he looked upon as his social inferiors. He was rude to his servants and
insulting to his secretaries. The subordinate officials in the government offices
to which he had been successively attached feared and hated him. His arro-
gance was horrible. He knew that he was a great deal cleverer than most of
the persons he had to do with, and never hesitated to apprise them of the fact.
He had no patience with the infirmities of human nature. He felt himself born
to command and was irritated with people who expected him to listen to their
arguments or wished to hear the reasons for his decisions. He was immeasurably selfish. He looked upon any service that was rendered him as a right due
to his rank and intelligence and therefore deserving of no gratitude. It never
entered his head that he was called upon to do anything for others. He had
many enemies: he despised them. He knew no one who merited his assistance,
his sympathy or his compassion. He had no friends. He was distrusted by his
chiefs, because they doubted his loyalty; he was unpopular with his party,
because he was over-bearing and discourteous; and yet his merit was so great,
his patriotism so evident, his intelligence so solid and his management of
affairs so brilliant that they had to put up with him. And what made it possible
to do this was that on occasion he could be enchanting: when he was with
persons whom he considered his equals, or whom he wished to captivate, in
the company of foreign dignitaries or women of distinction, he could be gay,
witty and debonair; his manners then reminded you that in his veins ran the
same blood as had run in the veins of Lord Chesterfield; he could tell a story
with point, he could be natural, sensible and even profound. You were surprised at the extent of his knowledge and the sensitiveness of his taste. You
thought him the best company in the world; you forgot that he had insulted
you the day before and was quite capable of cutting you dead the next.

Lord Mountdrago almost failed to become Dr. Audlin's patient. A secretary rang up the doctor and told him that his lordship, wishing to consult him,
would be glad if he would come to his house at ten o'clock on the following
morning. Dr. Audlin answered that he was unable to go to Lord Mountdrago's
house, but would be pleased to give him an appointment at his consulting-
room at five o'clock on the next day but one. The secretary took the message
and presently rang back to say that Lord Mountdrago insisted on seeing Dr.
Audlin in his own house and the doctor could fix his own fee. Dr. Audlin re-

plied that he only saw patients in his consulting-room and expressed his regret that unless Lord Mountdrago was prepared to come to him he could not give him his attention. In a quarter of an hour a brief message was delivered to him that his lordship would come not the next day but one, but next day, at five.

When Lord Mountdrago was then shown in he did not come forward, but stood at the door and insolently looked the doctor up and down. Dr. Audlin perceived that he was in a rage; he gazed at him, silently, with still eyes. He saw a big heavy man, with greying hair, receding on the forehead so that it gave nobility to his brow, a puffy face with bold regular features and an expression of haughtiness. He had somewhat the look of one of the Bourbon sovereigns of the eighteenth century.

"It seems that it is as difficult to see you as a Prime Minister, Dr. Audlin. I'm an extremely busy man."

"Won't you sit down?" said the doctor.

His face showed no sign that Lord Mountdrago's speech in any way affected him. Dr. Audlin sat in his chair at the desk. Lord Mountdrago still stood and his frown darkened.

"I think I should tell you that I am His Majesty's Secretary for Foreign Affairs," he said acidly.

"Won't you sit down?" the doctor repeated.

Lord Mountdrago made a gesture, which might have suggested that he was about to turn on his heel and stalk out of the room; but if that was his intention he apparently thought better of it. He seated himself. Dr. Audlin opened a large book and took up his pen. He wrote without looking at his patient.

"How old are you?"

"Forty-two."

"Are you married?"

"Yes."

"How long have you been married?"

"Eighteen years."

"Have you any children?"

"I have two sons."

Dr. Audlin noted down the facts as Lord Mountdrago abruptly answered his questions. Then he leaned back in his chair and looked at him. He did not speak; he just looked gravely, with pale eyes that did not move.

"Why have you come to see me?" he asked at length.

"I've heard about you. Lady Canute is a patient of yours, I understand. She tells me you've done her a certain amount of good."

Dr. Audlin did not reply. His eyes remained fixed on the other's face, but they were so empty of expression that you might have thought he did not even see him.

"I can't do miracles," he said at length. Not a smile, but the shadow of a smile flickered in his eyes. "The Royal College of Physicians would not approve of it if I did."

Lord Mountdrago gave a brief chuckle. It seemed to lessen his hostility. He spoke more amiably.

"You have a very remarkable reputation. People seem to believe in you."

"Why have you come to me?" repeated Dr. Audlin.

Now it was Lord Mountdrago's turn to be silent. It looked as though he found it hard to answer. Dr. Audlin waited. At last Lord Mountdrago seemed to make an effort. He spoke.

"I'm in perfect health. Just as a matter of routine I had myself examined by my own doctor the other day, Sir Augustus Fitzherbert, I daresay you've heard of him, and he tells me I have the physique of a man of thirty. I work hard, but I'm never tired, and I enjoy my work. I smoke very little and I'm an extremely moderate drinker. I take a sufficiency of exercise and I lead a regular life. I am a perfectly sound, normal, healthy man. I quite expect you to think it very silly and childish of me to consult you."

Dr. Audlin saw that he must help him.

"I don't know if I can do anything to help you. I'll try. You're distressed?"

Lord Mountdrago frowned.

"The work that I'm engaged in is important. The decisions I am called upon to make can easily affect the welfare of the country and even the peace of the world. It is essential that my judgment should be balanced and my brain clear. I look upon it as my duty to eliminate any cause of worry that may interfere with my usefulness."

Dr. Audlin had never taken his eyes off him. He saw a great deal. He saw behind his patient's pompous manner and arrogant pride an anxiety that he could not dispel.

"I asked you to be good enough to come here because I know by experience that it's easier for someone to speak openly in the dingy surroundings of a doctor's consulting-room than in his accustomed environment."

"They're certainly dingy," said Lord Mountdrago acidly. He paused. It was evident that this man who had so much self-assurance, so quick and decided a mind that he was never at a loss, at this moment was embarrassed. He smiled in order to show the doctor that he was at ease, but his eyes betrayed his disquiet. When he spoke again it was with unnatural heartiness.

"The whole thing's so trivial that I can hardly bring myself to bother you with it. I'm afraid you'll just tell me not to be a fool and waste your valuable time."

"Even things that seem very trivial may have their importance. They can be a symptom of a deep-seated derangement. And my time is entirely at your disposal."

Dr. Audlin's voice was low and grave. The monotone in which he spoke was strangely soothing. Lord Mountdrago at length made up his mind to be frank.

"The fact is I've been having some very tiresome dreams lately. I know it's silly to pay any attention to them, but—well, the honest truth is that I'm afraid they've got on my nerves."

"Can you describe any of them to me?"

Lord Mountdrago smiled, but the smile that tried to be careless was only rueful.

"They're so idiotic, I can hardly bring myself to narrate them."

"Never mind."

"Well, the first I had was about a month ago. I dreamt that I was at a party at Connemara House. It was an official party. The King and Queen were to be there and of course decorations were worn. I was wearing my ribbon and my star. I went into a sort of cloakroom they have to take off my coat. There was a little man there called Owen Griffiths, who's a Welsh Member of Parliament, and to tell you the truth, I was surprised to see him. He's very common, and I said to myself: 'Really, Lydia Connemara is going too far, whom will she ask next?' I thought he looked at me rather curiously, but I didn't take any notice of him; in fact I cut the little bounder and walked upstairs. I suppose you've never been there?"

"Never."

"No, it's not the sort of house you'd ever be likely to go to. It's a rather vulgar house, but it's got a very fine marble staircase, and the Connemaras were at the top receiving their guests. Lady Connemara gave me a look of surprise when I shook hands with her, and began to giggle; I didn't pay much attention, she's a very silly, ill-bred woman and her manners are no better than those of her ancestors whom King Charles II made a duchess. I must say the reception rooms at Connemara House are stately. I walked through, nodding to a number of people and shaking hands; then I saw the German Ambassador talking with one of the Austrian Archdukes. I particularly wanted to have a word with him, so I went up and held out my hand. The moment the Archduke saw me he burst into a roar of laughter. I was deeply affronted. I looked him up and down sternly, but he only laughed the more. I was about to speak to him rather sharply, when there was a sudden hush and I realised that the King and Queen had come. Turning my back on the Archduke, I stepped forward, and then, quite suddenly, I noticed that I hadn't got any trousers on. I was in short silk drawers, and I wore scarlet sock-suspenders. No wonder Lady Connemara had giggled; no wonder the Archduke had laughed! I can't tell you what that moment was. An agony of shame. I awoke in a cold sweat. Oh, you don't know the relief I felt to find it was only a dream."

"It's the kind of dream that's not so very uncommon," said Dr. Audlin.

"I dare say not. But an odd thing happened next day. I was in the lobby of the House of Commons, when that fellow Griffiths walked slowly past me. He deliberately looked down at my legs and then he looked me full in the face and I was almost certain he winked. A ridiculous thought came to me. He'd been there the night before and seen me make that ghastly exhibition of myself and was enjoying the joke. But of course I knew that was impossible because it was only a dream. I gave him an icy glare and he walked on. But he was grinning his head off."

Lord Mountdrago took his handkerchief out of his pocket and wiped the palms of his hands. He was making no attempt now to conceal his perturbation. Dr. Audlin never took his eyes off him.

"Tell me another dream."

"It was the night after, and it was even more absurd than the first one. I dreamt that I was in the House. There was a debate on foreign affairs which not only the country, but the world, had been looking forward to with the gravest concern. The government had decided on a change in their policy which vitally affected the future of the Empire. The occasion was historic. Of course the House was crowded. All the ambassadors were there. The galleries were packed. It fell to me to make the important speech of the evening. I had prepared it carefully. A man like me has enemies, there are a lot of people who resent my having achieved the position I have at an age when even the cleverest men are content with situations of relative obscurity, and I was determined that my speech should not only be worthy of the occasion, but should silence my detractors. It excited me to think that the whole world was hanging on my lips. I rose to my feet. If you've ever been in the House you'll know how members chat to one another during a debate, rustle papers and turn over reports. The silence was the silence of the grave when I began to speak. Suddenly I caught sight of that odious little bounder on one of the benches opposite, Griffiths the Welsh member; he put out his tongue at me. I don't know if you've ever heard a vulgar music-hall song called 'A Bicycle Made for Two.' It was very popular a great many years ago. To show Griffiths how completely I despised him I began to sing it. I sang the first verse right through. There was a moment's surprise, and when I finished they cried 'Hear, hear,' on the opposite benches. I put up my hand to silence them and sang the second verse. The House listened to me in stony silence and I felt the song wasn't going down very well. I was vexed, for I have a good baritone voice, and I was determined that they should do me justice. When I started the third verse the members began to laugh; in an instant the laughter spread; the ambassadors, the strangers in the Distinguished Strangers Gallery, the ladies in the Ladies' Gallery, the reporters, they shook, they bellowed, they held their sides, they rolled in their seats; everyone was overcome with laughter except the ministers on the Front Bench immediately behind me. In that incredible, in that unprecedented uproar, they sat petrified. I gave them a glance, and suddenly the enormity of what I had done fell upon me. I had made myself the laughing-stock of the whole world. With misery I realised that I should have to resign. I woke and knew it was only a dream."

Lord Mountdrago's grand manner had deserted him as he narrated this, and now having finished he was pale and trembling. But with an effort he pulled himself together. He forced a laugh to his shaking lips.

"The whole thing was so fantastic that I couldn't help being amused. I didn't give it another thought, and when I went into the House on the following afternoon I was feeling in very good form. The debate was dull, but I had to be there, and I read some documents that required my attention. For some reason I chanced to look up and I saw that Griffiths was speaking. He has an unpleasant Welsh accent and an unprepossessing appearance. I couldn't imagine that he had anything to say that it was worth my while to listen to, and I was about to return to my papers when he quoted two lines from 'A Bicycle Made for Two.' I couldn't help glancing at him and I saw that his eyes were fixed on me with a grin of bitter mockery. I faintly shrugged my shoulders. It was comic that a scrubby little Welsh member should look at me like that. It was an odd coincidence that he should quote two lines from that disastrous song that I'd sung all through in my dream. I began to read my papers again, but I don't mind telling you that I found it difficult to concentrate on them. I was a little puzzled. Owen Griffiths had been in my first dream, the one at Connemara House, and I'd received a very definite impression afterwards that he knew the sorry figure I'd cut. Was it a mere coincidence that he had just quoted those two lines? I asked myself if it was possible that he was dreaming the same dreams as I was. But of course the idea was preposterous and I determined not to give it a second thought."

There was a silence. Dr. Audlin looked at Lord Mountdrago and Lord Mountdrago looked at Dr. Audlin.

"Other people's dreams are very boring. My wife used to dream occasionally and insist on telling me her dreams next day with circumstantial detail. I found it maddening."

Dr. Audlin faintly smiled.

"You're not boring me."

"I'll tell you one more dream I had a few days later. I dreamt that I went into a public-house at Limehouse. I've never been to Limehouse in my life and I don't think I've ever been in a public-house since I was at Oxford, and yet I saw the street and the place I went into as exactly as if I were at home there. I went into a room, I don't know whether they call it the saloon bar or the private bar; there was a fireplace and a large leather arm-chair on one side of it, and on the other a small sofa; a bar ran the whole length of the room and over it you could see into the public bar. Near the door was a round marble-topped table and two arm-chairs beside it. It was a Saturday night and the place was packed. It was brightly lit, but the smoke was so thick that it made my eyes smart. I was dressed like a rough, with a cap on my head and a handkerchief round my neck. It seemed to me that most of the people there were drunk. I thought it rather amusing. There was a gramophone going, or the radio, I don't know which, and in front of the fireplace two women were doing a grotesque dance. There was a little crowd round them, laughing, cheering and singing. I went up to have a look and some man said to me: ' 'Ave a drink, Bill?' There were glasses on the table full of a dark liquid which I understand is called brown ale. He gave me a glass and not wishing to be conspicuous I drank it. One of the women who were dancing broke away from the other and took hold of the glass. ' 'Ere, what's the idea?' she said. 'That's my beer you're putting away.' 'Oh, I'm so sorry,' I said, 'this gentleman offered it me and I very naturally thought it was his to offer.' 'All right, mate,' she said, 'I don't mind. You come an' 'ave a dance with me.' Before I could protest she'd caught hold of me and we were dancing together. And then I found myself sitting in the arm-chair with the woman on my lap and we were sharing a glass of beer. I should tell you that sex has never played any great part in my life. I married young because in my position it was desirable that I should marry, but also in order to settle once for all the question of sex. I had the two sons I had made up my mind to have, and then I put the whole matter on one side. I've always been too busy to give much thought to that kind of thing, and living so much in the public eye as I do it would have been madness to do anything that might give rise to scandal. The greatest asset a politician can have is a blameless record as far as women are concerned. I have no patience with the men who smash up their careers for women. I only despise them. The woman I had on my knees was drunk; she wasn't pretty and she wasn't young: in fact, she was just a blowsy old prostitute. She filled me with disgust, and yet when she put her mouth to mine and kissed me, though her breath stank of beer and her teeth were decayed, though I loathed myself, I wanted her—I wanted her with all my soul. Suddenly I heard a voice. 'That's right, old boy, have a good time.' I looked up and there was Owen Griffiths. I tried to spring out of the chair, but that horrible woman wouldn't let me. 'Don't you pay no attention to 'im,' she said, ' 'e's only one of them nosy-parkers.' 'You go to it,' he said. 'I know Moll. She'll give you your money's worth all right.' You know, I wasn't so much annoyed at his seeing me in that absurd situation as angry that he should address me as 'old boy.' I pushed the woman aside and stood up and faced him. 'I don't know you and I don't want to know you,' I said. 'I know you all right,' he said. 'And my advice to you, Molly, is, see that you get your money, he'll bilk you if he can.' There was a bottle of beer standing on the table close by. Without a word I seized it by the neck and hit him over the head with it as hard as I could. I made such a violent gesture that it woke me up."

"A dream of that sort is not incomprehensible," said Dr. Audlin. "It is the revenge nature takes on persons of unimpeachable character."

"The story's idiotic. I haven't told it you for its own sake. I've told it you for what happened next day. I wanted to look up something in a hurry and I went into the library of the House. I got the book and began reading. I hadn't noticed when I sat down that Griffiths was sitting in a chair close by me. Another of the Labour Members came in and went up to him. 'Hullo,

Owen,' he said to him, 'you're looking pretty dicky today.' 'I've got an awful headache,' he answered. 'I feel as if I'd been cracked over the head with a bottle.' "

Now Lord Mountdrago's face was grey with anguish.

"I knew then that the idea I'd had and dismissed as preposterous was true. I knew that Griffiths was dreaming my dreams and that he remembered them as well as I did."

"It may also have been a coincidence."

"When he spoke he didn't speak to his friend, he deliberately spoke to me. He looked at me with sullen resentment."

"Can you offer any suggestion why this same man should come into your dreams?"

"None."

Dr. Audlin's eyes had not left his patient's face and he saw that he lied. He had a pencil in his hand and he drew a straggling line or two on his blotting-paper. It often took a long time to get people to tell the truth, and yet they knew that unless they told it he could do nothing for them.

"The dream you've just described to me took place just over three weeks ago. Have you had any since?"

"Every night."

"And does this man Griffiths come into them all?"

"Yes."

The doctor drew more lines on his blotting-paper. He wanted the silence, the drabness, the dull light of that little room to have its effect on Lord Mountdrago's sensibility. Lord Mountdrago threw himself back in his chair and turned his head away so that he should not see the other's grave eyes.

"Dr. Audlin, you must do something for me. I'm at the end of my tether. I shall go mad if this goes on. I'm afraid to go to sleep. Two or three nights I haven't. I've sat up reading and when I felt drowsy put on my coat and walked till I was exhausted. But I must have sleep. With all the work I have to do I must be at concert pitch; I must be in complete control of all my faculties. I need rest; sleep brings me none. I no sooner fall asleep than my dreams begin, and he's always there, that vulgar little cad, grinning at me, mocking me, despising me. It's a monstrous persecution. I tell you, doctor, I'm not the man of my dreams; it's not fair to judge me by them. Ask anyone you like. I'm an honest, upright, decent man. No one can say anything against my moral character either private or public. My whole ambition is to serve my country and maintain its greatness. I have money, I have rank, I'm not exposed to many of the temptations of lesser men, so that it's no credit to me to be incorruptible; but this I can claim, that no honour, no personal advantage, no thought of self would induce me to swerve by a hair's breadth from my duty. I've sacrificed everything to become the man I am. Greatness is my aim. Greatness is within my reach and I'm losing my nerve. I'm not that mean, despicable, cowardly, lewd creature that horrible little man sees. I've told you three of my dreams; they're nothing; that man has seen me do things that are so beastly, so horrible, so shameful, that even if my life depended on it I wouldn't tell them. And he remembers them. I can hardly meet the derision and disgust I see in his eyes and I even hesitate to speak because I know my words can seem to him nothing but utter humbug. He's seen me do things that no man with any self-respect would do, things for which men are driven out of the society of their fellows and sentenced to long terms of imprisonment; he's heard the foulness of my speech; he's seen me not only ridiculous, but revolting. He despises me and he no longer pretends to conceal it. I tell you that if you can't do something to help me I shall either kill myself or kill him."

"I wouldn't kill him if I were you," said Dr. Audlin, coolly, in that soothing voice of his. "In this country the consequences of killing a fellow-creature are awkward."

"I shouldn't be hanged for it, if that's what you mean. Who would know that I'd killed him? That dream of mine has shown me how. I told you, the day after I'd hit him over the head with a beer-bottle he had such a headache that he couldn't see straight. He said so himself. That shows that he can feel with his waking body what happens to his body asleep. It's not with a bottle I shall hit him next time. One night, when I'm dreaming, I shall find myself with a knife in my hand or a revolver in my pocket, I must because I want to so intensely, and then I shall seize my opportunity. I'll stick him like a pig; I'll shoot him like a dog. In the heart. And then I shall be free of this fiendish persecution."

Some people might have thought that Lord Mountdrago was mad; after all the years during which Dr. Audlin had been treating the diseased souls of men he knew how thin a line divides those whom we call sane from those whom we call insane. He knew how often in men who to all appearance were healthy and normal, who were seemingly devoid of imagination, and who fulfilled the duties of common life with credit to themselves and with benefit to their fellows, when you gained their confidence, when you tore away the mask they wore to the world, you found not only hideous abnormality, but kinks so strange, mental extravagances so fantastic, that in that respect you could only call them lunatic. If you put them in an asylum not all the asylums in the world would be large enough. Anyhow, a man was not certifiable because he had strange dreams and they had shattered his nerve. The case was singular, but it was only an exaggeration of others that had come under Dr. Audlin's observation; he was doubtful, however, whether the methods of treatment that he had so often found efficacious would here avail.

"Have you consulted any other member of my profession?" he asked.

"Only Sir Augustus. I merely told him that I suffered from nightmares. He said I was overworked and recommended me to go for a cruise. That's absurd. I can't leave the Foreign Office just now when the international situation needs constant attention. I'm indispensable, and I know it. On my conduct at the present juncture my whole future depends. He gave me sedatives. They had no effect. He gave me tonics. They were worse than useless. He's an old fool."

"Can you give any reason why it should be this particular man who persists in coming into your dreams?"

"You asked me that question before. I answered it."

That was true. But Dr. Audlin had not been satisfied with the answer.

"Just now you talked of persecution. Why should Owen Griffiths want to persecute you?"

"I don't know."

Lord Mountdrago's eyes shifted a little. Dr. Audlin was sure that he was not speaking the truth.

"Have you ever done him an injury?"

"Never."

Lord Mountdrago made no movement, but Dr. Audlin had a queer feeling that he shrank into his skin. He saw before him a large, proud man who gave the impression that the questions put to him were an insolence, and yet for all that, behind that façade, was something shifting and startled that made you think of a frightened animal in a trap. Dr. Audlin leaned forward and by the power of his eyes forced Lord Mountdrago to meet them.

"Are you quite sure?"

"Quite sure. You don't seem to understand that our ways lead along different paths. I don't wish to harp on it, but I must remind you that I am a Minister of the Crown and Griffiths is an obscure member of the Labour Party. Naturally there's no social connection between us; he's a man of very humble origin, he's not the sort of person I should be likely to meet at any of the houses I go to; and politically our respective stations are so far separated that we could not possibly have anything in common."

"I can do nothing for you unless you tell me the complete truth."

Lord Mountdrago raised his eyebrows. His voice was rasping.

"I'm not accustomed to having my word doubted, Dr. Audlin. If you're going to do that I think to take up any more of your time can only be a waste of mine. If you will kindly let my secretary know what your fee is he will see that a cheque is sent to you."

For all the expression that was to be seen on Dr. Audlin's face you might have thought that he simply had not heard what Lord Mountdrago said. He continued to look steadily into his eyes and his voice was grave and low.

"Have you done anything to this man that *he* might look upon as an injury?"

Lord Mountdrago hesitated. He looked away, and then, as though there were in Dr. Audlin's eyes a compelling force that he could not resist, looked back. He answered sulkily:

"Only if he was a dirty, second-rate little cad."

"But that is exactly what you've described him to be."

Lord Mountdrago sighed. He was beaten. Dr. Audlin knew that the sigh meant he was going at last to say what he had till then held back. Now he had no longer to insist. He dropped his eyes and began again drawing vague geometrical figures on his blotting-paper. The silence lasted two or three minutes.

"I'm anxious to tell you everything that can be of any use to you. If I didn't mention this before, it's only because it was so unimportant that I didn't see how it could possibly have anything to do with the case. Griffiths won a seat at the last election and he began to make a nuisance of himself almost at once. His father's a miner, and he worked in a mine himself when he was a boy; he's been a schoolmaster in the board schools and a journalist. He's that half-baked, conceited intellectual, with inadequate knowledge, ill-considered ideas and impracticable plans, that compulsory education has brought forth from the working-classes. He's a scrawny, grey-faced man, who looks half-starved, and he's always very slovenly in appearance; heaven knows members nowadays don't bother much about their dress, but his clothes are an outrage to the dignity of the House. They're ostentatiously shabby, his collar's never clean and his tie's never tied properly; he looks as if he hadn't had a bath for a month and his hands are filthy. The Labour Party have two or three fellows on the Front Bench who've got a certain ability, but the rest of them don't amount to much. In the kingdom of the blind the one-eyed man is king: because Griffiths is glib and has a lot of superficial information on a number of subjects, the Whips on his side began to put him up to speak whenever there was a chance. It appeared that he fancied himself on foreign affairs, and he was continually asking me silly, tiresome questions. I don't mind telling you that I made a point of snubbing him as soundly as I thought he deserved. From the beginning I hated the way he talked, his whining voice and his vulgar accent; he had nervous mannerisms that intensely irritated me. He talked rather shyly, hesitatingly, as though it were torture to him to speak and yet was forced to by some inner passion, and often he used to say some very disconcerting things. I'll admit that now and again he had a sort of tub-thumping eloquence. It had a certain influence over the ill-regulated minds of the members of his party. They were impressed by his earnestness and they weren't, as I was, nauseated by his sentimentality. A certain sentimentality is the common coin of political debate. Nations are governed by self-interest, but they prefer to believe that their aims are altruistic, and the politician is justified if with fair words and fine phrases he can persuade the electorate that the hard bargain he is driving for his country's advantage tends to the good of humanity. The mistake people like Griffiths make is to take these fair words and fine phrases at their face value. He's a crank, and a noxious crank. He calls himself an idealist. He has at his tongue's end all the tedious blather that the intelligentsia have been boring us with for years. Non-resistance. The brotherhood of man. You know the hopeless rubbish. The worst of it was that it impressed not only his own party, it even shook some of the sillier, more sloppy-minded members of ours. I heard rumours that Griffiths was likely to get office when a Labour Government came in; I even heard it suggested that he might get the Foreign Office. The notion was grotesque but not impossible. One day I had occasion to wind up a debate on foreign affairs which Griffiths had opened. He'd spoken for an hour. I thought it a very good opportunity to cook his goose, and by God, sir, I cooked it. I tore his speech to pieces. I pointed out the faultiness of his reasoning and emphasized the deficiency of his knowledge. In the House of Commons the most devastating weapon is ridicule: I mocked him; I bantered him; I was in good form that day and the House rocked with laughter. Their laughter excited me and I excelled myself. The Opposition sat glum and silent, but even some of them couldn't help laughing once or twice; it's not intolerable, you know, to see a colleague, perhaps a rival, made a fool of. And if ever a man was made a fool of I made a fool of Griffiths. He shrank down in a seat, I saw his face go white, and presently he buried it in his hands. When I sat down I'd killed him. I'd destroyed his prestige for ever; he had no more chance of getting office when a Labour Government came in than the policeman at the door. I heard afterwards that his father, the old miner, and his mother had come up from Wales, with various supporters of his in the constituency, to watch the triumph they expected him to have. They had seen only his utter humiliation. He'd won the constituency by the narrowest margin. An incident like that might very easily lose his seat. But that was no business of mine."

"Should I be putting it too strongly if I said you had ruined his career?" asked Dr. Audlin.

"I don't suppose you would."

"That is a very serious injury you've done him."

"He brought it on himself."

"Have you never felt any qualms about it?"

"I think perhaps if I'd known that his father and mother were there I might have let him down a little more gently."

There was nothing further for Dr. Audlin to say, and he set about treating his patient in such a manner as he thought might avail. He sought by suggestion to make him forget his dreams when he awoke; he sought to make him sleep so deeply that he would not dream. He found Lord Mountdrago's resistance impossible to break down. At the end of an hour he dismissed him. Since then he had seen Lord Mountdrago half a dozen times. He had done him no good. The frightful dreams continued every night to harass the unfortunate man, and it was clear that his general condition was growing rapidly worse. He was worn out. His irritability was uncontrollable. Lord Mountdrago was angry because he received no benefit from his treatment, and yet continued it, not only because it seemed his only hope, but because it was a relief to him to have someone with whom he could talk openly. Dr. Audlin came to the conclusion at last that there was only one way in which Lord

Mountdrago could achieve deliverance, but he knew him well enough to be assured that of his own free will he would never, never take it. If Lord Mountdrago was to be saved from the breakdown that was threatening he must be induced to take a step that must be abhorrent to his pride of birth and his self-complacency. Dr. Audlin was convinced that to delay was impossible. He was treating his patient by suggestion, and after several visits found him more susceptible to it. At length he managed to get him into a condition of somnolence. With his low, soft, monotonous voice he soothed his tortured nerves. He repeated the same words over and over again. Lord Mountdrago lay quite still, his eyes closed; his breathing was regular, and his limbs were relaxed. Then Dr. Audlin in the same quiet tone spoke the words he had prepared.

"You will go to Owen Griffiths and say that you are sorry that you caused him that great injury. You will say that you will do whatever lies in your power to undo the harm that you have done him."

The words acted on Lord Mountdrago like the blow of a whip across his face. He shook himself out of his hypnotic state and sprang to his feet. His eyes blazed with passion and he poured forth upon Dr. Audlin a stream of angry vituperation such as even he had never heard. He swore at him. He cursed him. He used language of such obscenity that Dr. Audlin, who had heard every sort of foul word, sometimes from the lips of chaste and distinguished women, was surprised that he knew it.

"Apologise to that filthy little Welshman? I'd rather kill myself."

"I believe it to be the only way in which you can regain your balance."

Dr. Audlin had not often seen a man presumably sane in such a condition of uncontrollable fury. He grew red in the face and his eyes bulged out of his head. He did really foam at the mouth. Dr. Audlin watched him coolly, waiting for the storm to wear itself out, and presently he saw that Lord Mountdrago, weakened by the strain to which he had been subjected for so many weeks, was exhausted.

"Sit down," he said then, sharply.

Lord Mountdrago crumpled up into a chair.

"Christ, I feel all in. I must rest a minute and then I'll go."

For five minutes perhaps they sat in complete silence. Lord Mountdrago was a gross, blustering bully, but he was also a gentleman. When he broke the silence he had recovered his self-control.

"I'm afraid I've been very rude to you. I'm ashamed of the things I've said to you and I can only say you'd be justified if you refused to have anything more to do with me. I hope you won't do that. I feel that my visits to you do help me. I think you're my only chance."

"You mustn't give another thought to what you said. It was of no consequence."

"But there's one thing you mustn't ask me to do, and that is to make excuses to Griffiths."

"I've thought a great deal about your case. I don't pretend to understand it, but I believe that your only chance of release is to do what I proposed. I have a notion that we're none of us one self, but many, and one of the selves in you has risen up against the injury you did Griffiths and has taken on the form of Griffiths in your mind and is punishing you for what you cruelly did. If I were a priest I should tell you that it is your conscience that has adopted the shape and lineaments of this man to scourge you to repentance and persuade you to reparation."

"My conscience is clear. It's not my fault if I smashed the man's career. I crushed him like a slug in my garden. I regret nothing."

It was on these words that Lord Mountdrago had left him. Reading through his notes, while he waited, Dr. Audlin considered how best he could bring his patient to the state of mind that, now that his usual methods of treatment had failed, he thought alone could help him. He glanced at his clock. It was six. It was strange that Lord Mountdrago did not come. He knew he had intended to because a secretary had rung up that morning to say that he would be with him at the usual hour. He must have been detained by pressing work. This notion gave Dr. Audlin something else to think of: Lord Mountdrago was quite unfit to work and in no condition to deal with important matters of state. Dr. Audlin wondered whether it behooved him to get in touch with someone in authority, the Prime Minister or the Permanent Under-Secretary for Foreign Affairs, and impart to him his conviction that Lord Mountdrago's mind was so unbalanced that it was dangerous to leave affairs of moment in his hands. It was a ticklish thing to do. He might cause needless trouble and get roundly snubbed for his pains. He shrugged his shoulders.

"After all," he reflected, "the politicians have made such a mess of the world during the last five-and-twenty years, I don't suppose it makes much odds if they're mad or sane."

He rang the bell.

"If Lord Mountdrago comes now will you tell him that I have another appointment at six-fifteen and so I'm afraid I can't see him."

"Very good, sir."

"Has the evening paper come yet?"

"I'll go and see."

In a moment the servant brought it in. A huge headline ran across the front page: Tragic Death of Foreign Minister.

"My God!" cried Dr. Audlin.

For once he was wrenched out of his wonted calm. He was shocked, horribly shocked, and yet he was not altogether surprised. The possibility that Lord Mountdrago might commit suicide had occurred to him several times, for that it was suicide he could not doubt. The paper said that Lord Mountdrago had been waiting in a Tube station, standing on the edge of the platform, and as the train came in was seen to fall on the rail. It was supposed that he had had a sudden attack of faintness. The paper went on to

say that Lord Mountdrago had been suffering for some weeks from the effects
of overwork, but had felt it impossible to absent himself while the foreign
situation demanded his unremitting attention. Lord Mountdrago was another
victim of the strain that modern politics placed upon those who played the
more important parts in it. There was a neat little piece about the talents and
industry, the patriotism and vision, of the deceased statesman, followed by
various surmises upon the Prime Minister's choice of his successor. Dr. Audlin
read all this. He had not liked Lord Mountdrago. The chief emotion that his
death caused in him was dissatisfaction with himself because he had been able
to do nothing for him.

Perhaps he had done wrong in not getting into touch with Lord Mountdrago's doctor. He was discouraged, as always when failure frustrated his
conscientious efforts, and repulsion seized him for the theory and practice of
this empiric doctrine by which he earned his living. He was dealing with dark
and mysterious forces that it was perhaps beyond the powers of the human
mind to understand. He was like a man blindfold trying to feel his way to he
knew not whither. Listlessly he turned the pages of the paper. Suddenly he
gave a great start, and an exclamation once more was forced from his lips.
His eyes had fallen on a small paragraph near the bottom of a column. Sudden Death of an M.P., he read. Mr. Owen Griffiths, member for so-and-so,
had been taken ill in Fleet Street that afternoon and when he was brought to
Charing Cross Hospital life was found to be extinct. It was supposed that
death was due to natural causes, but an inquest would be held. Dr. Audlin
could hardly believe his eyes. Was it possible that the night before Lord
Mountdrago had at last in his dream found himself possessed of the weapon,
knife or gun, that he had wanted, and had killed his tormentor, and had that
ghostly murder, in the same way as the blow with the bottle had given him
a racking headache on the following day, taken effect a certain number of
hours later on the waking man? Or was it, more mysterious and more frightful, that when Lord Mountdrago sought relief in death, the enemy he had so
cruelly wronged, unappeased, escaping from his own mortality, had pursued
him to some other sphere there to torment him still? It was strange. The
sensible thing was to look upon it merely as an odd coincidence. Dr. Audlin
rang the bell.

"Tell Mrs. Milton that I'm sorry I can't see her this evening. I'm not well."

It was true; he shivered as though of an ague. With some kind of spiritual
sense he seemed to envisage a bleak, a horrible void. The dark night of the
soul engulfed him, and he felt a strange, primeval terror of he knew not what.

JORGE LUIS BORGES

Borges and Myself

It's to the other man, to Borges, that things happen. I walked along the streets of Buenos Aires, stopping now and then—perhaps out of habit—to look at the arch of an old entranceway or a grillwork gate; of Borges I get news through the mail and glimpse his name among a committee of professors or in a dictionary of biography. I have a taste for hourglasses, maps, eighteenth-century typography, the roots of words, the smell of coffee, and Stevenson's prose; the other man shares these likes, but in a showy way that turns them into stagy mannerisms. It would be an exaggeration to say that we are on bad terms; I live, I let myself live, so that Borges can weave his tales and poems, and those tales and poems are my justification. It is not hard for me to admit that he has managed to write a few worthwhile pages, but these pages cannot save me, perhaps because what is good no longer belongs to anyone— not even the other man—but rather to speech or tradition. In any case, I am fated to become lost once and for all, and only some moment of myself will survive in the other man. Little by little, I have been surrendering everything to him, even though I have evidence of his stubborn habit of falsification and exaggerating. Spinoza held that all things try to keep on being themselves; a stone wants to be a stone and the tiger, a tiger. I shall remain in Borges, not in myself (if it is so that I am someone), but I recognize myself less in his books than in those of others or than in the laborious tuning of a guitar. Years ago, I tried ridding myself of him and I went from myths to the outlying slums of the city to games with time and infinity, but those games are now part of Borges and I will have to turn to other things. And so, my life is a running away, and I lose everything and everything is left to oblivion or to the other man.

Which of us is writing this page I don't know.

Translated by Norman Thomas di Giovanni

ANNE SEXTON

You, Doctor Martin

You, Doctor Martin, walk
from breakfast to madness. Late August,
I speed through the antiseptic tunnel
where the moving dead still talk
of pushing their bones against the thrust
of cure. And I am queen of this summer hotel
or the laughing bee on a stalk

of death. We stand in broken
lines and wait while they unlock
the door and count us at the frozen gates
of dinner. The shibboleth is spoken
and we move to gravy in our smock
of smiles. We chew in rows, our plates
scratch and whine like chalk

in school. There are no knives
for cutting your throat. I make
moccasins all morning. At first my hands
kept empty, unraveled for the lives
they used to work. Now I learn to take
them back, each angry finger that demands
I mend what another will break

tomorrow. Of course, I love you;
you lean above the plastic sky,
god of our block, prince of all the foxes.
The breaking crowns are new
that Jack wore. Your third eye
moves among us and lights the separate boxes
where we sleep or cry.

What large children we are
here. All over I grow most tall
in the best ward. Your business is people,
you call at the madhouse, an oracular
eye in our nest. Out in the hall

the intercom pages you. You twist in the pull
of the foxy children who fall

like floods of life in frost.
And we are magic talking to itself,
noisy and alone. I am queen of all my sins
forgotten. Am I still lost?
Once I was beautiful. Now I am myself,
counting this row and that row of moccasins
waiting on the silent shelf.

ANNE SEXTON

Said the Poet to the Analyst

My business is words. Words are like labels,
or coins, or better, like swarming bees.
I confess I am only broken by the sources of things;
as if words were counted like dead bees in the attic,
unbuckled from their yellow eyes and their dry wings.
I must always forget how one word is able to pick
out another, to manner another, until I have got
something I might have said . . .
but did not.

Your business is watching my words. But I
admit nothing. I work with my best, for instance,
when I can write my praise for a nickel machine,
that one night in Nevada: telling how the magic jackpot
came clacking three bells out, over the lucky screen.
But if you should say this is something it is not,
then I grow weak, remembering how my hands felt funny
and ridiculous and crowded with all
the believing money.

ANNE SEXTON

Lullaby

It is a summer evening.
The yellow moths sag
against the locked screens
and the faded curtains
suck over the window sills
and from another building
a goat calls in his dreams.
This is the TV parlor
in the best ward at Bedlam.
The night nurse is passing
out the evening pills.
She walks on two erasers,
padding by us one by one.

My sleeping pill is white.
It is a splendid pearl;
it floats me out of myself,
my stung skin as alien
as a loose bolt of cloth.
I will ignore the bed.
I am linen on a shelf.
Let the others moan in secret;
let each lost butterfly
go home. Old woolen head,
take me like a yellow moth
while the goat calls hush-
a-bye.

ANTON CHEKHOV

Ward Six

I

In the hospital yard there stands a small annex surrounded by a whole forest of burdock, nettles, and wild hemp. The roof is rusty, the chimney half caved

in, the porch steps rotted and overgrown with grass, and only a few traces
of stucco are left on the walls. The front of the annex faces the hospital and
the back looks onto a field from which it is separated by the gray hospital
fence topped with spikes. These spikes, the fence, and the annex itself all
have that peculiarly desolate, Godforsaken look characteristic of our hospital
and prison buildings.

If you are not afraid of being stung by the nettles, come with me along the
narrow path leading to the annex, and let us see what is going on inside.
Opening the first door, we find ourselves in the entry. Whole mountains of
hospital rubbish are piled against the walls and stove. Mattresses, old tattered
dressing gowns, underdrawers, blue-striped shirts, utterly useless worn-out
boots and shoes—all this litter lying in jumbled, raddled, moldering heaps
and giving off a stifling odor.

Lying on top of this rubbish, his pipe invariably clenched in his teeth, is
the guard Nikita, an old retired soldier still wearing his rusty insignia. He has
a grim haggard face, a red nose, and bushy eyebrows that make him look like
a Russian sheep dog; although small, lean and sinewy, there is nevertheless
something authoritative in his bearing, and his fists are powerful. He is one
of those diligent, simple-minded, dogmatic, and obtuse individuals who love
law and order more than anything else in the world, and as a consequence
are convinced that *they* have to be beaten. He distributes blows indiscriminately on the face, chest, or back, in the certainty that there is no other way
to keep order here.

Next you come into a large spacious room which occupies the whole
building, not counting the entry. The walls are painted a muddy blue, and
the ceiling, as in a peasant's chimneyless hut, is black with soot—obviously
the stoves here smoke in winter, filling the room with charcoal fumes. The
windows are disfigured by an iron grille on the inside. The floor is gray and
splintery. The place stinks of sauerkraut, smoldering wicks, bedbugs, and
ammonia, and for the first moment this stench gives you the impression that
you are entering a menagerie.

The beds in the room are screwed to the floor. Sitting or lying on them are
men in blue hospital gowns and old-fashioned nightcaps. These are the
lunatics.

There are five of them. Only one is of noble birth, the rest are commoners.
The one nearest the door, a tall thin man with a glossy red mustache and eyes
red from weeping, sits with his head in his hands staring fixedly into space.
He grieves day and night, sighing and shaking his head, and smiling bitterly;
he rarely takes part in a conversation and as a rule does not reply to questions;
when given food, he eats and drinks automatically. To judge from his agonizing racking cough, his hectic flush and emaciated body, he is in the early
stages of consumption.

Next to him is a small, sprightly, exceedingly active old man with a pointed
beard and kinky black hair like a Negro's. He spends the day either wandering

up and down the ward, going from window to window, or sitting on the bed, his feet tucked under him Turkish style, restlessly whistling like a bullfinch, singing in a low voice, and chuckling. He manifests the same childish gaiety and lively disposition at night when he gets up to say his prayers, that is, to beat his breast with his fists and pluck at the door with his fingers. This is the Jew Moiseika, a hatter who lost his mind twenty years ago when his workshop burned down.

He alone of the inmates of Ward Six is permitted to go out of the building and even out of the hospital yard and into the street. He has enjoyed this privilege for years, probably as an old resident of the hospital, and as a quiet harmless idiot and town buffoon, whose appearance in the streets surrounded by dogs and little boys has long been a familiar sight. Wearing his ragged hospital robe, a ridiculous nightcap and slippers, sometimes barelegged and even naked under his robe, he roams the streets, stopping at house gates and shops, begging a kopeck. He is given kvass in one place, a bit of bread or a kopeck in another, and generally returns to the annex feeling rich and content. Everything he brings back is taken away from him by Nikita for his own use. This the soldier does roughly and in anger, calling on God to witness that he will never again let the Jew go out into the streets, that for him there is nothing in the world worse than a breach of regulations.

Moiseika loves doing a good turn. He brings his companions water, covers them up when they are asleep, promises to make them new caps and to bring each of them a kopeck when he goes out, and it is he who spoon-feeds his neighbor on the left, a paralytic. He does not act out of compassion or any sort of humane considerations, but simply in imitation of Gromov, his neighbor on the right, automatically submitting to his influence.

Ivan Dmitrich Gromov, a nobleman of about thirty-three, formerly a court bailiff and provincial secretary, suffers from persecution mania. He either lies curled up in bed or paces back and forth as if taking exercise, but seldom sits down. He is always in a state of agitation and excitement, always under the strain of some vague undefined expectation. The slightest rustle in the entry or shout in the yard is enough to make him raise his head and listen: are they coming for him? Is it him they are looking for? At such times his face expresses the most acute anxiety and repugnance.

I like his broad pale face with its high cheekbones, an unhappy face in which a soul tormented by perpetual struggle and fear is reflected as in a mirror. His grimaces are queer and morbid, but the fine lines drawn on his face by deep and genuine suffering denote sensibility and culture, and there is a warm lucid gleam in his eyes. I like the man himself, always courteous, obliging, and extremely considerate in his treatment of everyone except Nikita. When anyone drops a button or a spoon, he leaps from his bed and picks it up. He always greets his companions with a good morning when he gets up and wishes them good night when he goes to bed.

Apart from his grimacing and being continually overwrought, his madness expresses itself in the following ways. Sometimes in the evenings he wraps his robe around him, and, trembling all over, his teeth chattering, begins rapidly pacing up and down like a man in a high fever. From the way he suddenly stops and looks at his companions it is clear that he wants to say something very important, but evidently realizing that nobody will listen to him or understand him, he impatiently shakes his head and continues pacing. Soon, however, the desire to speak overrules all other considerations, and he lets himself go and talks feverishly, passionately. His speech, as in a delirium, is frenzied, spasmodic, disordered, and not always understandable, yet one detects something singularly fine in the words and in his voice. When he talks, both the lunatic and the man are distinguishable in him. It would be difficult to set down on paper his mad tirade. He discourses on human baseness, on violence vanquishing truth, on the glorious life that one day will appear on earth, on the iron grilles on the windows which constantly remind him of the stupidity and cruelty of the oppressors. It makes for a confused and incoherent potpourri of songs which, though old, have yet to be sung to the end.

II

Some twelve or fifteen years ago an official by the name of Gromov, a substantial well-to-do man, lived in his own house on the main street of the town. He had two sons: Sergei and Ivan. When Sergei was a fourth-year student he fell ill with galloping consumption and died, and this death was the prelude to a whole series of misfortunes which suddenly rained down upon the Gromov family. Within a week of Sergei's burial the old man was put on trial for forgery and embezzlement, and soon after died of typhus in the prison hospital. The house and all their personal property was sold at auction, and Ivan Dmitrich and his mother were left entirely without means.

When his father was alive, Ivan Dmitrich, who was living in Petersburg where he was a student at the university, received sixty or seventy rubles a month from home and had absolutely no conception of want, but now he was forced to make drastic changes in his life. He had to work from morning to night giving ill-paid lessons and doing copying, and even so he went hungry, as everything he earned was sent home for the support of his mother. Unable to endure such a life, he lost heart, his health failed, and he left the university and went home. Here in the little town where he had connections, Ivan Dmitrich got work as a teacher in the district school, but he was unable to get along with his colleagues, was not liked by his pupils, and soon gave up teaching. His mother died. He had been out of work for about six months, living on nothing but bread and water, when he obtained the position of court baliff, and he remained in this office till he was dismissed because of ill health.

Even as a young student he had never appeared to be robust. Always pale, thin, and subject to colds, he ate little and slept badly. One glass of wine went to his head and made him hysterical. Although generally drawn to people, thanks to his irritable disposition and mistrustfulness, he never was close to anyone and had no friends. He invariably spoke with contempt of the townspeople, saying that their gross ignorance and sluggish animal life was insufferable and detestable to him. He spoke in a shrill tenor, vehemently, never without either exasperation and indignation or ecstasy and wonder—and always sincerely. No matter what one talked to him about, he always came back to the same thing: the atmosphere of the town is stifling and dull; the people, all devoid of interests, lead dismal meaningless lives diversified only by violence, coarse debauchery, and hypocrisy, scoundrels are well-fed and well-dressed, while honest men live from hand to mouth; there is a need for schools, for a local newspaper with a decent point of view, a theater, public lectures, solidarity of intellectual forces, and for society to be made aware of itself, to be aroused. In judging people he laid the colors on thick, seeing everything as black or white and recognizing no intermediate shades; mankind was divided into honest men and scoundrels, and there was no middle ground. Of women and love he spoke with ardent enthusiasm, but he had never in his life been in love.

Despite the harshness of his judgments and his nervous irritability, he was liked in the town and affectionately referred to as Vanya behind his back. His innate refinement, his complaisance, integrity, and moral purity, together with his shabby coat, sickly appearance, and family misfortunes, combined to inspire a kind, warm, melancholy feeling; moreover he was well-educated and well-read; according to the townspeople there was nothing he did not know and they regarded him as a sort of walking encyclopedia.

He read a great deal. He used to sit in the club, nervously plucking at his beard as he leafed through magazines and books, and from the expression on his face he appeared to be not so much reading as devouring their contents, hardly giving himself time to digest what he read. It makes one think that reading was one of his morbid habits, for he pounced on everything that came to hand with equal avidity, even last year's newspapers and almanacs. At home he always read lying down.

III

One autumn morning Ivan Dmitrich, his overcoat collar turned up, was splashing through the mud of side streets and back yards on his way to the house of some citizen or other to exercise a writ of execution. In one of the side streets he met two convicts in chains accompanied by four armed guards. Ivan Dmitrich had often encountered convicts and they always aroused in him feelings of compassion and discomfort, but this time he was strangely and unaccountably affected. For some reason he suddenly felt that he too could be clapped in irons and led in this same way through the mud to prison. As he passed the post office on his way home he met a police inspector of his acquaintance who greeted him and accompanied him a few paces down the street, and somehow this aroused his suspicion. At home he was haunted all day by these convicts and soldiers with rifles, and an inexplicable mental anxiety prevented him from reading or concentrating. He did not light his lamp in the evening and at night he was unable to sleep, but kept thinking that he too could be arrested, clapped in irons, and thrown into prison. He knew of no crime in his past and was confident that in the future he would never be guilty of murder, arson, or theft, but was it not possible to commit a crime by accident, without meaning to, and was not calumny too, or even a judicial error, conceivable? Not without reason does the age-old experience of the people teach that no one is safe from the poorhouse or prison. And, legal procedures being what they are today, a miscarriage of justice is not only quite possible but would be nothing to wonder at. People who have an official, professional relation to other men's suffering—judges, physicians, the police, for example—grow so callous in the course of time, simply from force of habit, that even if they wanted to they would be unable to treat their clients in any but a formal way; in this respect they are not unlike the peasant who slaughters sheep and calves in his back yard, oblivious to the blood. And once this formal, heartless attitude has been established, only one thing is needed to make a judge deprive an innocent man of all his rights and sentence him to hard labor: time. Just the time necessary for the observation of certain formalities for which a judge receives his salary—and it is all over. Then try to find justice and protection in this filthy little town two hundred versts from a railroad. And, indeed, is it not absurd even to think of justice when society regards every kind of violence as both rational and expedient, while every act of clemency, such as a verdict of acquittal, provokes an outburst of dissatisfaction and feelings of revenge?

In the morning Ivan Dmitrich got up in a state of dread and with cold sweat on his brow, by now absolutely convinced that he could be arrested at any moment. Since the oppressive thoughts of the preceding day had remained with him so long, he thought it meant there was some measure of truth in them. They certainly could not have entered his mind apropos of nothing.

A policeman walked slowly past the window: that could not be without reason. Two men stopped near the house and stood there in silence. Why had they stopped talking?

And for Ivan Dmitrich there now came days and nights of torture. Everyone who passed his windows or entered the yard seemed to him a spy or a detective. The district police inspector was in the habit of driving down the street in a carriage and pair every day at noon on his way to the police department from his estate on the outskirts of town, but now when he passed, Ivan Dmitrich imagined he was driving unusually fast and that his face wore a rather singular expression: obviously he was rushing to announce the appearance of a dangerous criminal in town. Ivan Dmitrich shuddered at every ring and knock at the gate, was in agony if he came upon a new face at his landlady's, smiled and commenced whistling to show how unconcerned he was whenever he encountered a policeman or gendarme. He lay awake whole nights expecting to be arrested, but would sigh and snore loudly to make the landlady think he was sleeping, for, of course, if one could not sleep it meant he was tortured by pangs of conscience—what a piece of evidence that would be! Facts and common sense told him that all these fears were absurd and psychopathic, that there was really nothing so terrible about arrest and imprisonment—so long as one's conscience was clear; but the more sensibly and logically he reasoned, the more acute and agonizing his inner anxiety became. He was like the hermit who tried to make a clearing in the virgin forest: the more zealously he wielded his ax, the denser and mightier grew the forest. Realizing at last that it was futile, Ivan Dmitrich gave up reasoning and abandoned himself to terror and despair.

He commenced to avoid people and to live in solitude. His work, distasteful to him before, now became unbearable. He was afraid someone might get him in trouble, might surreptitiously slip a bribe into his pocket and then expose him; or that he himself would accidentally make some error in the official documents that would be tantamount to fraud, or perhaps lose money that did not belong to him. Oddly, his mind had never before been so flexible and inventive as now when he daily contrived a thousand reasons why he should tremble for his freedom and honor; but, on the other hand, his interest in the outside world, and particularly in books, diminished, and his memory noticeably deteriorated.

In the spring, when the snow had melted, two partly decomposed corpses were found in the ravine near the cemetery—an old woman and a little boy, both bearing marks of a violent death. The whole town talked of nothing but these corpses and the unknown murderers. To prevent people thinking it was he who had killed them, Ivan Dmitrich walked about the streets with a smile on his face, and on meeting one of his acquaintances, would assure him, turning pale then flushing, that there was no more reprehensible crime than murdering the weak and defenseless. But this duplicity soon exhausted him, and after some reflection he decided that the best thing for a man in his position to do was to hide in the landlady's cellar. He spent the whole day and night and the following day in the cellar; then, thoroughly chilled, stole back to his room like a thief when it grew dark. He stood motionless in the middle of his room till daybreak, listening. Early in the morning, before sunrise, some workmen came to the landlady's apartment. Ivan Dmitrich knew perfectly well they had come to reset the stove in the kitchen, but fear prompted him to think they were policemen in disguise. He stealthily crept out of the apartment without stopping to put on his hat and coat and, terror-stricken, ran down the street. Barking dogs tore after him, somewhere behind him a man shouted, the wind whistled in his ears, and it seemed to Ivan Dmitrich that all the violence in the world had gathered together in pursuit of him.

He was stopped and brought home, and the landlady was sent for a doctor. Dr. Andrei Yefimych, of whom more later, prescribed cold compresses and laurel water, then sadly shook his head and left, telling the landlady he would not come again, as one ought not to interfere with people going out of their minds.

Since he had not the means to be taken care of at home, Ivan Dmitrich was sent to the hospital, where he was put into the ward for venereal patients. He did not sleep at night, was capricious, and disturbed the other patients; soon, on Andrei Yefimych's orders, he was transferred to Ward Six.

Within a year Ivan Dmitrich was entirely forgotten in the town, and his books, which the landlady had piled in a sledge in the lean-to, were pilfered by small boys.

IV

Ivan Dmitrich's neighbor on the left, as I have already said, is the Jew Moiseika, and on his right is a peasant so rolling in fat as to be almost spherical, with an inane and totally vacant expression. This inert, gluttonous, slovenly animal, who long ago lost the capacity to think and feel, perpetually exudes a rank, fetid odor.

Nikita, who has to clean up after him, beats him horribly, using all his strength and not even sparing his own fists; and what is awful is not that he is beaten—one can get used to that—but that this stupefied animal does not react to the blows by a sound, a gesture, an expression in the eyes, but merely rocks back and forth like a heavy barrel.

The fifth and last inmate of Ward Six, a former mail sorter in the post office, is a thin little blond man with a kind but rather sly face. Judging by the clear and merry look in his serene intelligent eyes, he harbors some delightful and important secret. Under his pillow and mattress he keeps something he never shows anyone, not from fear of its being taken away or stolen, but from modesty. Sometimes he goes to the window, turns his back to his comrades, and puts this object on his chest, bending his head to look at it; if you go up to him at such a moment he becomes flustered and quickly snatches it off. But his secret is not hard to guess.

"You may congratulate me," he often says to Ivan Dmitrich. "I have been recommended for the Stanislas second grade with a star. The second grade with a star is given only to foreigners, but for some reason they intend to make an exception in my case," he says with a smile, shrugging his shoulders in bewilderment. "That, I must confess, I did not expect!"

"I know nothing about these things," Ivan Dmitrich declares morosely.

"But you know what I'll get sooner or later?" the former mail sorter

continues with a sly wink. "I shall undoubtedly get the Swedish 'Polar Star.'
A decoration like that is worth exerting yourself for. A white cross and black
ribbon. Very handsome."

Probably in no other place is life so monotonous as in the hospital annex.
In the morning the patients, except the paralytic and the fat peasant, wash
at a big tub in the entry, drying themselves on the skirts of their dressing
gowns; after that they drink tea, which is brought by Nikita from the main
building. They are allowed one mugful each. At noon they are given sauerkraut soup and gruel, and in the evening their supper consists of the gruel
left over from dinner. In the intervals they lie on their beds, sleep, gaze out
the windows, and pace up and down. And so it is every day. Even the former
mail sorter talks always of the same decorations.

Rarely is a fresh face seen in Ward Six. The doctor stopped admitting any
new lunatics long ago, and people who are fond of visting insane asylums are
few in this world. Once every two months the barber Semyon Lazarich comes
to the annex. How he cuts the patients' hair, how Nikita assists him, the consternation into which the inmates are thrown at every appearance of the
drunken, grinning barber, are things we shall not speak of.

Apart from the barber no one looks into the ward. The patients are
condemned to seeing no one but Nikita day after day.

Of late, however, a rather strange rumor has been spreading through the
hospital. It is reported that the doctor has been visiting Ward Six.

V

A strange rumor!

Dr. Andrei Yefimych Ragin is a remarkable man in his way. He is said to
have been very religious in his early youth and to have prepared himself for
an ecclesiastical career with the intention of entering the theological academy
on finishing high school in 1863; but it seems that his father, a doctor of
medicine and a surgeon, was virulent in his ridicule and categorically announced that he would no longer consider him his son if he became a priest.
How true this is I do not know, but on more than one occasion Andrei
Yefimych himself confessed that he had never felt a vocation for medicine or
for the exact sciences in general.

However that may be, after graduating from medical school he did not
take Orders. He evinced no special devoutness and was no more like an
ecclesiastic at the beginning of his medical career than he is now.

He is heavy, coarse, and boorish in appearance; his face, beard, and flat
limp hair, and his rugged, ungainly figure, suggest a gruff, overfed, intemper-
ate tavernkeeper. His stern face is covered with blue veins, the eyes small, the
nose red. Being tall and broad-shouldered, with huge hands and feet, he looks
as if one blow of his fist would knock the daylights out of a man. But his
step is soft, his bearing circumspect and ingratiating, and when he meets

anyone in a narrow corridor he is always the first to stop and make way, saying: "Sorry!"—not, as one might expect, in a deep bass, but in a high soft tenor. He has a small tumor on his neck which prevents him from wearing stiff collars, and as a consequence wears only soft linen or cotton shirts. Altogether he does not dress like a doctor. He goes around in the same suit for ten years, and when he does get a new one, which he usually buys in a Jewish shop, it looks just as shabby and rumpled on him as the old one; he receives patients, eats dinner, and visits friends in the same coat, not out of niggardliness, but out of a complete disregard for his personal appearance.

When Andrei Yefimych came to our town to take up his duties, the "charitable institution" was in an appalling state. One could hardly breathe for the stench in the wards, corridors, and hospital yard. The hospital attendants, the nurses, and their children all slept in the wards with the patients. Everyone complained that life was made miserable by cockroaches, bedbugs, and mice. In the surgical section they had not yet got rid of erysipelas. There were only two scalpels in the entire hospital, not a single thermometer, and the bathtubs were used for storing potatoes. The superintendent, matron, and medical assistant all robbed the patients, and the old doctor, Andrei Yefimych's predecessor, was said to have engaged in the illicit sale of hospital alcohol and to have organized a veritable harem for himself among the nurses and patients. The townspeople were well aware of these irregularities and even exaggerated them, but took them calmly; some justified them on the grounds that only peasants and workingmen went to the hospital, and they had nothing to complain of since they were considerably worse off at home —you wouldn't expect to feed them on woodcock! Others made the excuse that the town was unable to support a decent hospital without help from the zemstvo; thank God for any hospital, even a bad one! But the recently formed zemstvo failed to open a hospital either in the town or in the district on the grounds that the town already had one.

After inspecting the hospital, Andrei Yefimych came to the conclusion that it was an infamous institution, highly detrimental to the health of the community. In his opinion the wisest thing to do would be to discharge the patients and close the hospital. But for this, he reasoned, something more than his will would be required, and in any case it would serve no purpose; if physical and moral impurity were driven out of one place they would only move to another; one must wait for it to wither away of itself. Moreover, if the people had opened the hospital and tolerated it, it meant that they needed it; superstition and all the rest of life's filth and abominations are necessary, for in time they are converted into something useful, as dung into black soil. There is nothing on earth so fine that its origin is without foulness.

Once he had taken up his duties, Andrei Yefimych did not appear to be greatly concerned about the irregularities. He only asked the hospital attendants and nurses not to sleep in the wards and installed two cupboards of instruments; but the superintendent and the matron did not change, and the erysipelas in the surgical ward remained.

Andrei Yefimych has an intense love of honesty and reason, but he lacks the will power and self-confidence to organize a reasonable and honest life around him. He is utterly incapable of commanding, forbidding, insisting. It almost seems as if he had taken a vow never to raise his voice or to use the imperative mood. It is hard for him to say: "Give me," or "Bring me"; when he feels hungry he clears his throat and hesitantly says to the cook: "I might have some tea...." or: "I might have dinner now...." As for telling the superintendent to stop stealing, or dismissing him, or abolishing the sinecure—such things are absolutely beyond him. When people deceive him, flatter him, bring him a deliberately falsified account to sign, Andrei Yefimych turns red as a lobster and feels guilty, but signs it; when the patients complain to him of hunger or the rough treatment of the nurses, he is embarrassed and guiltily mumbles:

"Very well, very well, I'll look into it later.... Most likely there is some misunderstanding...."

At first Andrei Yefimych worked assiduously. He received patients daily from morning till dinnertime, performed operations, and even took obstetrical cases. The ladies all said that he was most considerate and an excellent diagnostician, especially of women's and children's diseases. As time went on, however, he became noticeably wearied by the monotony and obvious futility of the work. Thirty patients today, tomorrow thirty-five, the next day forty—and so on, day after day, year after year, but the mortality rate never goes down and the sick never stop coming. To give any real help to forty sick people in the course of a morning is a physical impossibility, and perforce results in fraud. If in a given year you see 12,000 patients, it means, by simple reckoning, that 12,000 people have been deceived. To put the seriously ill in wards and treat them according to the precepts of science is also impossible, for while the precepts exist, there is no science; if, on the other hand, you waive philosophy and pedantically follow the rules as other doctors do, first of all it requires cleanliness and ventilation instead of filth, wholesome nourishment instead of reeking sauerkraut soup, and decent assistants instead of thieves.

And, indeed, why keep people from dying since death is normal, the decreed end for everyone? What if the life of some huckster or official is prolonged by five or ten years? And if one thinks the aim of medicine is the alleviation of suffering by means of drugs, the question inevitably arises: why alleviate it? In the first place, suffering is said to lead to self-perfection, and in the second place, if man learns to ease his suffering with pills and drops he will completely abandon religion and philosophy, wherein till now he has found not only a defense against every adversity, but happiness itself. Pushkin suffered agonies before his death, Heine was a paralytic for years;

why, then, should an Andrei Yefimych or a Matryona Savishna be spared
illness when their insipid lives would be as empty as an amoeba's were it not
for suffering?

Oppressed by such reasoning, Andrei Yefimych grew disheartened and
gave up going to the hospital every day.

VI

This is how he spends his life. Generally, he gets up at eight o'clock,
dresses, and eats breakfast. Then he either sits in his study and reads or goes
to the hospital. In the dark narrow hospital corridor sit the out-patients waiting to be admitted. Attendants and nurses rush by, their heels clattering on
the brick floor; emaciated patients walk by in dressing gowns; corpses and
vessels of waste matter are carried out; children cry; and there is a cold draft.
Andrei Yefimych knows that for feverish, consumptive, or impressionable
patients such conditions are a torture, but what is to be done?

In the consulting room he finds the medical assistant, Sergei Sergeich, a fat
little man with a plump, well-washed, clean-shaven face and mild docile
manners, wearing a new loose-fitting suit and looking more like a senator than
a medical assistant. He has a tremendous practice in the town, wears a white
tie, and considers himself more knowledgeable than the doctor, who has no
practice at all. In one corner of the consulting room there is a large icon in
a case and a heavy icon lamp; near it stands a church candelabra under
a dust cover; the walls are hung with portraits of bishops, a view of the
Svyatogorsk Monastery, and garlands of dried cornflowers. Sergei Sergeich is
religious and loves pomp. The icon was installed at his expense; on Sundays,
by his order, one of the patients reads aloud from the Book of Psalms, after
which Sergei Sergeich himself makes the rounds of the wards carrying a censer
with burning incense.

The patients are numerous and time is short, so the doctor confines himself
to a brief examination and administering medications such as volatile ointment and castor oil. Andrei Yefimych sits lost in thought, his cheek resting
on his fist, and puts his questions mechanically. Sergei Sergeich is also present;
he rubs his hands and occasionally interposes a remark.

"We suffer sickness and want," he says, "because we do not pray to the
merciful Lord as we should. Yes!"

Andrei Yefimych does not perform any operations during this time; he
long ago got out of the habit, and the sight of blood upsets him now. When
he has to open a baby's mouth to look at his throat and the child cries and
defends himself with his little fists, the noise makes his head spin and tears
come to his eyes. He hastily writes a prescription and motions the mother to
take the child away.

He is soon wearied by the timidity and incoherence of the patients, the
presence of the pompous Sergei Sergeich, the portraits on the walls, and his

own questions, which he has not varied in more than twenty years. After seeing five or six patients he goes, leaving the rest to the assistant.

Andrei Yefimych sits down in his study and begins reading as soon as he gets home, enjoying the thought that, thank God, he no longer has a private practice and nobody will disturb him. He reads a great deal and always with pleasure. Half of his salary is spent on books, and three of the six rooms in his apartment are crammed with old magazines and books. He prefers works on history and philosophy; the only medical publication he subscribes to is *The Physician,* which he invariably starts reading from the back. He reads uninterruptedly for hours at a stretch without tiring, not rapidly and passionately as Ivan Dmitrich had once read, but slowly, with penetration, often dwelling on a passage that pleases or puzzles him. There is always a decanter of vodka near his book, and a salted cucumber or pickled apple lying on the cloth without a plate. Every half hour he pours himself a glass of vodka and drinks it down without taking his eyes from the book, then he feels for the cucumber and takes a bite.

At three o'clock he circumspectly approaches the kitchen door, coughs, and says:

"Daryushka, I might have dinner now. . . ."

After a rather poor and badly served dinner, Andrei Yefimych walks from room to room, his arms folded on his chest, thinking. The clock strikes four, then five, and he is still pacing and thinking. From time to time the kitchen door creaks and Daryushka's sleepy red face appears.

"Andrei Yefimych, isn't it time for your beer?" she anxiously inquires.

"No, it's not time yet . . ." he answers. "I'll wait a bit . . . I'll wait. . . ."

Toward evening the postmaster, Mikhail Averyanych, comes in—the only man in the whole town whose company Andrei Yefimych does not find irksome. Mikhail Averyanych was once a very rich landowner and cavalry officer, but was ruined and forced to enter the postal service late in life. He has a hale and hearty look, luxuriant gray side whiskers, a loud but pleasant voice, and the manners of a well-bred man. He is kind and sensitive but irascible. When anyone comes into the post office and protests, disagrees, or merely starts an argument, Mikhail Averyanych turns livid, trembles from head to foot, and in a thunderous voice shouts: "Silence!" so that the post office has a long established reputation for being a formidable institution to visit. Mikhail Averyanych likes and respects Andrei Yefimych for his erudition and nobility of spirit, but he is haughty toward the rest of the town's inhabitants, treating them as though they were his inferiors.

"Well, here I am!" he says, entering the room. "How are you, my friend? Probably getting sick of me by now, eh?"

"On the contrary, I'm delighted," the doctor replies. "Always glad to see you."

The friends sit down on the sofa in the study and smoke in silence for a while.

"Daryushka, what about a little beer?" Andrei Yefimych says.

The first bottle is drunk in the same silence: the doctor musing, Mikhail Averyanych with the merry, animated look of a man who has something very interesting to tell. It is always the doctor who begins the conversation.

"What a pity," he says slowly and softly, shaking his head and not looking his friend in the eye (he never looks anyone in the eye), "what a great pity, my dear Mikhail Averyanych, that our town is devoid of people who enjoy an interesting and intelligent conversation, or who are even capable of one. It's an enormous privation for us. Even the educated classes do not rise above triviality; the level of their development, I assure you, is not a bit higher than that of the lower classes."

"Absolutely true. I agree."

"You are aware, of course," the doctor continues in quiet measured tones, "that everything in this world is insignificant and uninteresting except the higher spiritual manifestations of the human mind. It is the mind which draws a distinct boundary line between the animal and man, giving an intimation of the divinity of the latter, and to some degree even compensating him for a non-existent immortality. From this we may conclude that the intellect is the only possible source of enjoyment. We, however, neither see nor hear any trace of intellect around us—which means we are deprived of enjoyment. True, we have books, but that is not at all the same as living talk and social intercourse. If you will allow me to make a not very apt comparison: books are the printed score, while conversation is the song."

"Absolutely true."

A silence falls. Daryushka comes out of the kitchen and with an expression of blank dejection stands in the doorway listening, her chin propped on her fist.

"Ah!" sighs Mikhail Averyanych, "what can you expect of the present-day mind!"

And he proceeds to tell of how splendid, gay, and interesting life used to be, of how clever the intelligentsia of Russia was then, and what a high value was set on honor and friendship. People used to lend money without promissory notes, and it was considered a disgrace not to extend a helping hand to a friend in need. What campaigns, skirmishes, adventures, what friendships, and what women! And the Caucasus—what a marvelous country! . . . There was the wife of one of the battalion commanders, a strange woman, who used to put on an officer's uniform and drive off into the mountains in the evening alone, without an escort. It was said she had a romance with some prince in one of the native villages.

"Holy Mother!" Daryushka sighs.

"And how we drank! How we ate! What desperate liberals we were!"

Andrei Yefimych listens without hearing; he is lost in thought, sipping his beer.

"I often dream about intelligent people and conversations with them," he suddenly says, interrupting Mikhail Averyanych. "My father gave me an excellent education, but under the influence of the ideas of the sixties, he forced me to become a doctor. I sometimes think that if I had not obeyed him I would now be in the very center of some intellectual movement. I would probably be on the staff of a university. Of course, intellect too is transitory, not immortal, but you know why I have an inclination for it. Life is a miserable trap. As soon as a thinking man reaches maturity and becomes capable of conscious thought, he cannot help feeling that he is in a trap from which there is no escape. When you come to think of it, he has been brought to life from a state of nonexistence against his will, by pure chance. What for? If he tries to find out the meaning and purpose of his existence he either gets no answer or is told all sorts of absurdities; he knocks—no one opens to him; death too comes against his will. And just as men in prison, united by their common misfortune, feel better when they are together, so in life people with a turn for analysis and generalizations do not notice that they are in a trap when they come together and pass the time in the exchange of free and elevating ideas. In this respect the mind is a source of incomparable pleasure."

"Absolutely true."

Without looking his companion in the eye, Andrei Yefimych goes on talking in his soft faltering voice about intellectual people and their conversations, and Mikhail Averyanych listens attentively, agreeing: "Absolutely true."

"But don't you believe in the immortality of the soul?" the postmaster suddenly asks.

"No, my dear Mikhail Averyanych, I do not believe in it, nor do I find grounds for believing in it."

"To tell the truth, I have doubts about it myself. Although, on the other hand, I have a feeling I will never die. Ugh, I think to myself, you old fogy, it's time you were dead! But there is a wee small voice in my soul that whispers: don't believe it, you won't die!"

Soon after nine Mikhail Averyanych leaves. As he stands in the hall putting on his fur coat, he says with a sigh:

"Still, what a hole fate has thrown us into! And the worst of it is, we shall have to die here too. Ugh!"

VII

After seeing his friend out, Andrei Yefimych sits down at the table and resumes his reading. Not a sound breaks the stillness of the night, and time itself seems to have stopped, to be holding its breath with the doctor over his book, as if nothing exists but this book and the lamp with its green globe. Gradually the doctor's coarse rugged face lights up with a smile of impassioned delight at the workings of the human mind. Oh, why is not man immortal? he thinks. Why these brain centers and their convolutions, why vision, speech, feelings, genius, if all this is destined to go into the ground, ultimately to grow cold together with the earth's crust, and then for millions of years to whirl with it around the sun without aim or reason? Surely it is not necessary, merely for the sake of this cooling and whirling, to draw man, with his superior, almost godlike intelligence, out of oblivion, and then, as if in jest, to turn him into clay.

Metabolism! But what cowardice to console oneself with that substitute for immortality! The unconscious processes that take place in nature are beneath even human stupidity, for in stupidity there is at least consciousness and will, while in these processes there is absolutely nothing. Only a coward whose fear of death is greater than his self-respect can solace himself with the thought that his body will go on living in a blade of grass, a stone, a toad. ... To see immortality in the transmutation of matter is as strange as to predict a brilliant future for a violin case after a precious violin has been broken and rendered useless.

When the clock strikes, Andrei Yefimych leans back in his chair and closes his eyes to think a little. And, without realizing it, under the influence of the fine ideas gleaned from his books, he casts a glance at his past and at the present. The past revolts him; better not to think of it. And the present is no different. He knows that while his thoughts are whirling around the sun with the earth's cooling crust, in a large building right next to a doctor's apartment people are languishing in disease and filth; someone is perhaps lying awake trying to combat the vermin, someone else has been infected with erysipelas or is moaning because of a bandage that is wound too tight; patients may be playing cards and drinking vodka with the nurses. Twelve thousand people a year are swindled; the entire hospital system is based on theft, wrangling scandal-mongering, favoritism, and gross quackery, exactly as it was twenty years ago, and remains a vicious institution, in the highest degree detrimental to the health of the community. He knows that behind the bars of Ward No. 6 Nikita beats the patients, and that Moiseika goes through the town begging alms every day.

On the other hand, he knows quite well that during the last twenty-five years a miraculous change has taken place in medicine. When he was studying at the university, it had seemed to him that before long medicine would undergo the fate of alchemy and metaphysics, but now, reading about medicine at night moves him, excites his wonder and enthusiasm. What unforeseen brilliance, what a revolution! Thanks to antiseptics, operations are performed which the great Pirogov had considered impossible even *in spe*. Ordinary zemstvo doctors are not afraid to do a resection of the knee joint; only one in a hundred dies from an abdominal operation; gallstones are considered too trivial to write about; syphilis can be completely cured. And what of hypnotism, the theory of heredity, the discoveries of Pasteur and Koch, the statistics of hygienics, and our Russian zemstvo doctors? Psychiatry, with its modern classification of diseases, its methods of diagnosis and treatment, is a veritable Elborus compared with the past. The insane are no longer doused with cold water or put into strait jackets, but are treated humanely, and, according to what one reads in the newspapers, balls and entertainments are arranged for them. Andrei Yefimych knows that with current views and tastes being what they are, an abomination like Ward Six is possible only in a town two hundred versts from a railroad, where the mayor and the members of the town council are all semiliterate tradesmen who regard a doctor as an oracle to be trusted implicitly, even if he pours molten lead down people's throats; anywhere else the public and the newspapers would have demolished this little Bastille long ago.

"And yet," Andrei Yefimych asks himself, opening his eyes, "what has come of it? Antiseptics, Koch, Pasteur—but the essentials haven't changed in the least. Sickness and mortality remain the same. They organize entertainments and balls for the insane, but they still keep them confined. So it is all futile, senseless, and there is no essential difference between the best Viennese clinic and my hospital."

But mental anguish and a feeling akin to envy disturb his equanimity. This, no doubt, is owing to fatigue. As his heavy head sinks onto the book, he puts his hands over it to make it softer, thinking:

"I am serving a pernicious cause and receiving a salary from the people I deceive. I am dishonest. But, of course, I am nothing of myself, a mere particle in a necessary social evil: all district officials are bad and are paid for doing nothing. . . . Consequently, it is not I who am to blame for my dishonesty, but the times. . . . If I had been born two hundred years later I should have been different."

When the clock strikes three he puts out the lamp and goes to his bedroom. But he does not feel like sleeping.

VIII

A year or two ago the zemstvo magnanimously decided to contribute three thousand rubles a year toward increasing the town's hospital medical staff till such time as a zemstvo hospital should be opened, and the district doctor, Yevgeny Fyodorych Khobotov, was hired as Andrei Yefimych's assistant. Still a young man—not yet thirty—tall, dark, with broad cheekbones and small eyes, he looks as if his ancestors were of an alien race. He arrived in town without a kopeck, bringing with him only a small trunk and a homely young woman with a baby in her arms whom he called his cook. Yevgeny Fyodorych always wears a forage cap and high boots, and in winter goes around in a sheepskin jacket. He soon made friends with the medical assistant, Sergei Sergeich, and with the treasurer, but for some reason he calls the rest of the staff aristocrats and avoids them. There is only one book in his whole apartment—*Latest Prescriptions of the Viennese Clinic for 1881*. He never visits a patient without taking this book with him. At night he plays billiards at the club, but does not care for cards. In conversation he is very keen on using such expressions as "You're dillydallying," or "Don't try to pull the wool over my eyes."

Twice a week he goes to the hospital, makes the rounds of the wards, and receives out-patients. The complete absence of antiseptics and the practice of blood-cupping arouse his indignation, but he avoids introducing any new methods for fear of offending Andrei Yefimych. He considers his colleague Andrei Yefimych an old fraud, suspects him of being a man of great means, and secretly envies him. He would gladly take his place.

IX

One spring evening toward the end of March, when the snow had melted and starlings were singing in the hospital garden, the doctor came out to see his friend the postmaster to the gate. At that moment the Jew Moiseika came into the yard, returning with his booty. He was without a cap and wore only low overshoes on his bare feet; in his hand was a little sack with the alms he had collected.

"Give a little kopeck!" he said to the doctor, smiling and shivering with cold.

Andrei Yefimych, who could never refuse, gave him a ten-kopeck piece.

"How awful that is!" he thought, looking at the man's bare legs and thin raw ankles. "And it's so wet."

Moved by a combination of pity and revulsion, he followed the Jew into the annex, looking now at his bald head, now at his ankles. On seeing the doctor enter, Nikita jumped up from a heap of litter and stood at attention.

"Good evening, Nikita," Andrei Yefimych said in his soft voice. "Perhaps you could give that man a pair of boots . . . otherwise he'll catch cold."

"Yes, sir, Your Honor! I'll report it to the superintendent."

"Please do. Ask him in my name. Say I requested it."

The door leading into the ward was open. Ivan Dmitrich lay on his bed propped up on one elbow listening in alarm to the unfamiliar voice; all at once he recognized the doctor. Trembling with rage he leaped up, his face flushed and wrathful, his eyes starting out of his head, and rushed into the middle of the room.

"The doctor has come!" he cried, and burst out laughing. "At last! I congratulate you, gentlemen. The doctor has deigned to visit us! Dirty dog!" he shrieked in a frenzy such as had never before been seen in the ward. "Kill that damned cur! No, killing's too good for him—drown him in the privy!"

Hearing this, Andrei Yefimych looked into the ward and gently asked: "What for?"

"What for?" shouted Ivan Dmitrich, convulsively pulling his robe around him and approaching the doctor with a threatening look. "What for? Thief!" he uttered the word with disgust, then puckered up his lips as if he were about to spit. "Quack! Hangman!"

"Don't get excited," said Andrei Yefimych with a guilty smile. "I assure you, I have never stolen anything, and as for the rest, you are probably greatly exaggerating. I see you are angry with me. Try to compose yourself, I beg you, and tell me calmly: what is it that makes you so angry?"

"Why do you keep me here?"

"Because you are ill."

"Yes, I am ill. But there are dozens, hundreds, of madmen walking around at liberty, simply because you, in your ignorance, are incapable of distinguishing them from the sane. Why, then, must I, and these other unfortunates, be shut up here as scapegoats for all of them? Morally, you, the medical assistant, the superintendent, and the rest of your hospital rabble are immeasurably inferior to every one of us—why then should we be here and not you? Where's the logic?"

"Morals and logic do not enter into it. Everything depends on chance. Those who are put in here, stay here; those who are not, enjoy their liberty, that's all. And there is no morality or logic in the fact that I am a doctor and you are a mental patient—it's pure chance, nothing more."

"I don't understand that twaddle . . ." Ivan Dmitrich said dully, and sat down on his bed.

Moiseika, whom Nikita had not ventured to search in the doctor's presence, had spread out his crusts, bits of paper, and bones on his bed and, still shivering with cold, began talking to himself in Hebrew in a rapid singsong voice. He probably imagined he had opened a shop.

"Let me out!" said Ivan Dmitrich in a quavering voice.

"I can't."

"But why can't you? Why?"

"Because it is not within my power. Think: what would be the use of my letting you out? You leave—and the townspeople or the police will stop you and bring you back."

"Yes, yes, that's true . . ." Ivan Dmitrich said, rubbing his forehead. "It's awful! What am I to do? Tell me, what?"

His voice and his youthful face, intelligent despite his grimacing, appealed to Andrei Yefimych. He longed to show him some kindness, to soothe him. He sat down on the bed beside him, thought for a moment, and said:

"You ask me what to do? In your position, the best thing you could do would be to run away from here. But, unfortunately, it would be useless. You would be stopped. When society decides to protect itself from criminals, the psychically ill, and other difficult people, it is invincible. There is only one thing left for you: comfort yourself with the thought that your presence here is indispensable."

"It's no good to anyone."

"So long as prisons and insane asylums exist, someone must be put into them. If not you—me; if not me, someone else. Wait for that time, in some distant future, when prisons and insane asylums have ceased to exist, then there will be no bars on the windows, no hospital gowns. Such a time is bound to come sooner or later."

Ivan Dmitrich smiled sardonically.

"You don't mean it," he said, narrowing his eyes. "Gentlemen like you and your right hand, Nikita, have no concern with the future, but you may be sure, my dear sir, that better times will come! I may express myself in a banal way—laugh if you like—but the dawn of a new life is at hand, justice will triumph, and—our day will come! I don't expect to see it, I'll be dead by then, but other men's grandchildren will witness it. I congratulate them with all my heart, and rejoice, rejoice for them! Forward! May God help you, my friends!"

Ivan Dmitrich, his eyes shining, got up, stretched his arms toward the window and went on speaking in an emotional voice.

"From behind these bars I send you my blessing! Long live justice! I rejoice!"

"I see no reason for rejoicing," said Andrei Yefimych, who found Ivan Dmitrich's gesture theatrical, but at the same time very appealing. "There will be no more prisons and lunatic asylums, and justice, as you choose to express it, will triumph, but, you see, the essence of things will not change, the laws of nature will remain the same. People will fall ill, grow old, and die, just as they do now. So, no matter what magnificent dawn illuminates your life, you will, in the end, be nailed up in a coffin and thrown into a pit."

"And immortality?"

"Oh, come now!"

"You don't believe in it; well, I do. Dostoyevsky, or maybe it was Voltaire, said that if there were no God, man would have invented Him. And I firmly believe that if there is no immortality, sooner or later the great human mind will invent it."

"Well said," observed Andrei Yefimych, smiling with pleasure. "It's good that you believe. With such faith one may be well off even sealed up within four walls. But you are an educated man, I see."

"Yes, I attended the university, but I didn't graduate."

"You are a man who knows how to think. In any circumstances you can find solace within yourself. Free and profound thought that strives for an understanding of life, together with a thorough contempt for the vanity of this world—these are two blessings beyond anything man has known. And you can possess them in spite of all the barred windows in the world. Diogenes lived in a barrel, but he was happier than all earthly monarchs."

"Your Diogenes was a blockhead," Ivan Dmitrich remarked sullenly. "Why do you talk to me of Diogenes, and understanding?" All at once he grew anrgy and sprang up. "I love life—love it passionately! I have a persecution mania, a constant, tormenting fear, but there are moments when I am overwhelmed by a thirst for life, and then I am afraid of losing my mind. I want desperately to live, desperately!"

Pacing back and forth in agitation, he lowered his voice and said:

"In my dreams I am visited by phantoms. I hear voices, music, . . . I seem to be walking through a forest, along a seashore, and I long passionately for the bustle and cares of . . . Tell me, what is new there?" asked Ivan Dmitrich. "What is going on in the outside world?"

"Do you want to hear about our town, or things in general?"

"First tell me about the town, and then about the world in general."

"Well . . . it's insufferably boring in town. . . . There's no one to talk to, no one to listen to. There are no new people. Though, as a matter of fact, a young doctor by the name of Khobotov came to us not long ago."

"I was already here when he came. A boor, isn't he?"

"Yes, a man of no culture. It's strange, you know. . . . Judging from what one hears, there is no intellectual stagnation in the big cities, things are going on, which means there must be real people there, but for some reason, they invariably send us people the like of which you've never seen. It's an unfortunate town!"

"Yes, an unfortunate town!" sighed Ivan Dmitrich, and laughed. "But how are things in general? What do they write about in the newspapers and magazines?"

By now it was dark in the ward, and the doctor rose to his feet and stood telling him about what was being written both abroad and in Russia, and of what was now discernible as the modern trend of thought. Ivan Dmitrich listened attentively, asked questions, then suddenly, as if remembering something horrible, clutched his head and lay down on the bed with his back to the doctor.

"What's the matter?" asked Andrei Yefimych.

"You won't get another word out of me," said Ivan Dmitrich rudely. "Leave me alone!"

"But why?"

"Leave me alone, I tell you! Why the hell do you persist?"

Andrei Yefimych shrugged his shoulders, sighed, and went out. As he passed through the entry, he said:

"You might clean up this place, Nikita. . . . There's a terrible strong odor here!"

"Yes, sir, Your Honor!"

"What a nice young man!" thought Andrei Yefimych, as he returned to his own apartment. "In all the time I've been living here, he's the first man I've been able to talk to. He's capable of reasoning, and is interested in just the right things."

While he was reading, and later in bed, he kept thinking about Ivan Dmitrich, and when he woke up the next morning he remembered that he had made the acquaintance of an intelligent and interesting man and decided to pay him another visit at the first opportunity.

X

Ivan Dmitrich was lying in the same position as the day before, his head clutched in his hands and his legs drawn up. His face was not visible.

"Good day, my friend," said Andrei Yefimych. "You're not asleep, are you?"

"In the first place, I am not your friend," Ivan Dmitrich articulated into the pillow, "and in the second place, you are wasting your time: you won't get a single word out of me."

"Strange . . ." murmured Andrei Yefimych, somewhat abashed. "We were having such a harmonious talk yesterday, till all at once you took offense and broke off. . . . I must have made some sort of blunder; perhaps I expressed some idea that is not in accord with your convictions. . . ."

"Do you really expect me to believe that?" said Ivan Dmitrich, raising himself slightly and gazing at the doctor with a mocking and at the same time anxious expression; his eyes were red. "You can do your spying and cross-examining some place else—it won't do you any good here. I knew yesterday what you had come for."

"A strange fantasy!" said the doctor with a wry smile. "So, you think I'm a spy?"

"Yes, I do. . . . A spy or a doctor who has been sent to test me—it's all the same."

"Well, you really are a—forgive me—but you are a queer fellow!"

The doctor sat down on a stool near the bed and shook his head reproachfully.

"But let us suppose that you are right," he said. "Let us suppose that I trick you into saying something in order to betray you to the police. You would be arrested and brought to trial. But would you be any worse off in court, or in prison, than you are here? And if you were deported, even if you were to be sentenced to penal servitude, do you think it would be worse than being locked up in this ward? I don't think it would be any worse. . . . What is there for you to be afraid of then?"

Evidently the words had an effect on Ivan Dmitrich. He quietly sat down.

It was between four and five o'clock in the afternoon, the time of day when Andrei Yefimych was generally pacing up and down in his apartment, and when Daryushka would ask if it were not time for his beer. The day was clear and mild.

"I was taking my after-dinner walk and thought I would drop in and see you," said the doctor. "It's a real spring day."

"What month is it now? March?" asked Ivan Dmitrich.

"Yes, the end of March."

"Very muddy outside?"

"No, not very. The garden paths are already visible."

"It would be nice to drive out of town in an open carriage on a day like this," said Ivan Dmitrich, rubbing his red eyes as if he were just waking up, "and then to return home to a warm comfortable study . . . and have a decent doctor cure one's headache. . . . It's been such a long time since I've lived like a human being. And it's so foul here! Unbearably foul!"

He was enervated and languid after the excitement of the day before, and disinclined to talk. His fingers trembled, and it was evident from his face that he had a severe headache.

"There is no difference between a warm comfortable study and this ward," said Andrei Yefimych. "Peace and contentment do not lie outside a man, but within him."

"What do you mean?"

"The ordinary man looks for good or evil in external things: an open carriage, a study, while the thinking man looks for them within himself."

"Go preach that philosophy in Greece, where it's warm and smells of oranges; it's not suited to the climate here. Who was it I was talking to about Diogenes? Was it you?"

"Yes, it was I . . . yesterday."

"Diogenes didn't need a study or a warm room, it was hot there anyhow. He could sleep in a barrel and eat olives and oranges. But you bring him to Russia to live and he'd be begging for a room, and not just in December, but in May. He'd be doubled up with cold."

"No. One can be impervious to cold, as to any other pain. Marcus Aurelius said: 'Pain is the vivid representation of pain: if, with an effort of will, you change this image, reject it, and stop complaining, the pain will disappear.' This is true. The wise man, or even the merely rational, thinking man, is distinguished precisely by his disdain for suffering; he is always content, and nothing ever surprises him."

"Then I must be an idiot, for I suffer, am discontented, and continually surprised at human baseness."

"But that's all to no purpose. If you will reflect on this more often, you will realize how insignificant the external things which agitate us really are. One must strive for comprehension of life—therein lies the true blessing."

"Comprehension . . ." Ivan Dmitrich frowned. "Internal, external . . . I'm sorry, I don't understand this. All I know is that God created me out of warm blood and nerves—yes! And organic tissue, if it is viable, must react to every irritation. And I do react! To pain I respond with tears and outcries, to baseness with indignation, to vileness with disgust. In my opinion this is exactly what is known as life. The lower the organism, the less sensitive it is, and the more feeble its response to irritation; the higher it is, the more receptive, and the more energetic its reactions to reality. How could you not know this? A doctor, and not know such elementary things! For a man to despise suffering, to be always content, to be surprised at nothing, he would have to reach this state—" and Ivan Dmitrich pointed to the fat, bloated peasant, "or else have become so hardened by suffering as to have lost all sensitivity to it, in other words, to have ceased living. You must excuse me, I am neither a sage nor a philosopher," he continued irascibly, "and I understand nothing of such things. I am in no position to argue."

"On the contrary, you argue exceedingly well."

"The Stoics, whose teaching you travesty, were remarkable men, but their philosophy congealed two thousand years ago and has not advanced a particle, nor will it advance, because it is not practical, not vital. Its success was limited to a minority, which spent its time studying and savoring every sort of teaching, but the majority never understood it. A doctrine that preaches indifference to riches and the comforts of life, and contempt for suffering and death, is absolutely incomprehensible to the vast majority, since this majority has never known either riches or comforts; and to despise suffering would mean to despise one's own life, for man's entire existence is made up of sensations of hunger, cold, humiliation, loss, and a Hamlet-like fear of death. In these sensations lies the whole of life: one may be oppressed by it, one may hate it, but not disdain it. And so, I repeat, the teaching of the Stoics cannot possibly have a future; what has gone on from the beginning of time to our own day, as you see, are struggle, sensibility to pain, and a capacity to respond to irritation."

Ivan Dmitrich suddenly lost the thread of his thoughts, stopped, and rubbed his forehead with vexation.

"I wanted to say something very important, but I'm confused," he said. "What was I saying? Yes! This is what I wanted to say: one of the Stoics sold himself into slavery in order to redeem his neighbor. So, you see, a Stoic reacted to an irritant, for in order to perform such a magnanimous act as destroying oneself for the sake of one's neighbor, one must possess a soul capable of indignation and compassion. Here in this prison I've forgotten everything I ever knew, or I would remember something more. . . . And take Christ! Christ responded to reality by weeping, smiling, being sorrowful, wrathful, and even melancholy; He did not go to meet suffering with a smile, nor did He despise death, but prayed in the garden of Gethsemane that this cup would pass from Him."

Ivan Dmitrich laughed and sat down.

"Let us assume that man's peace and contentment are not external, but within him," he said. "And let us assume that we ought to despise suffering and be surprised at nothing. But what right have you to preach this? Are you a sage? A philosopher?"

"No, I'm not a philosopher, but everyone ought to preach it because it makes sense."

"Yes, but I want to know why you consider yourself competent in the matter of comprehension, disdain for suffering, and so on. Have you ever suffered? Have you any idea what suffering is? Allow me to ask: were you ever whipped as a child?"

"No, my parents had an aversion for corporal punishment."

"My father used to thrash me cruelly. He was a stern hemorrhoidal functionary with a long nose and yellow neck. But let's talk about you. In all your life no one has ever laid a finger on you, intimidated you, or beaten you; you're as strong as an ox. You grew up under your father's wing, were educated at his expense, and then immediately got hold of a sinecure. For more than twenty years you have been living in a warm, well-lighted apartment free of charge; you keep a servant, you have the right to work however you like and as much as you like, or even not to work at all. By nature you are a flaccid, lazy man, and as a consequence have tried to arrange your life so that nothing can disturb you or make you move. You have handed your work over to the medical assistant and the rest of the riffraff, while you yourself sit in peace and warmth, piling up money, reading your books, beguiling yourself with reflections on all sorts of sublime nonsense, and" (Ivan Dmitrich glanced at the doctor's red nose) "drinking. In short, you've never seen life, know absolutely nothing about it, and have only a theoretical acquaintance with reality. And you despise suffering and are surprised at nothing for a very simple reason: your vanity of vanities, external and internal, your contempt for life, suffering, and death, your comprehension and true blessing—all this is a most comfortable philosophy for the Russian sluggard. You see a peasant beating his wife, for instance. Why interfere? Let him beat her, they'll both die sooner or later anyhow; and besides, the one who does the beating wrongs himself, not his victim. Getting drunk is stupid, unseemly; if you drink—you die; and if you don't drink—you die. A woman comes to you with a toothache. . . . Well, what of it? Pain is nothing but the image of pain, and besides, we can't live in this world without sickness, we all die, so run along, my good woman, and don't hinder me from enjoying my thoughts and my vodka. A young man comes to you for advice, he wants to know what to do, how to live: anyone else would stop and think before replying, but you have a ready answer: strive for comprehension, for the true blessing. There is, of course, no answer. . . . We are kept here behind bars, tortured, left to rot, but this is all very fine and rational, because there is absolutely no difference between this ward and a warm comfortable study. A convenient philosophy: you have nothing to do, your conscience is clear, and you feel you're a sage. . . . No, sir, this is not philosophy, not thought, not breadth of vision, but laziness, pretense, mental torpor. . . . Yes!" Ivan Dmitrich grew angry again. "You despise suffering, but if you pinched your little finger in that door, you'd probably start howling at the top of your voice."

"Perhaps I wouldn't howl," said Andrei Yefimych with a gentle smile.

"Oh, no! Look here, if you were suddenly struck down with paralysis, or, let us say, some insolent fool were to take advantage of his rank and position to insult you publicly, and you knew he could do it with impunity—then you would realize what it means to put people off with your 'comprehension' and 'true blessing'!"

"That's very original," said Andrei Yefimych, rubbing his hands and laughing with pleasure. "I admire your turn for generalizations, and the character sketch you have drawn of me is simply brilliant. I must confess that talking with you gives me the greatest pleasure. Well . . . I've heard you out, now be so good as to listen to me. . . ."

XI

They went on talking for about an hour, and apparently the conversation made a deep impression on Andrei Yefimych. He commenced going to the annex every day. He went in the mornings, after dinner, and often dusk would find him in conversation with Ivan Dmitrich. At first Ivan Dmitrich was wary of him, suspecting him of some malicious intent, and openly expressed his hostility; then, as he grew accustomed to him, his fractious manner changed to one of condescending irony.

Soon the rumor spread through the hospital that the doctor had taken to visiting Ward Six. No one—not the medical assistant, the nurses, nor Nikita —could understand why he went, why he sat there for hours at a time, what he could be talking about, why he wrote no prescriptions. His conduct seemed strange. Mikhail Averyanych often failed to find him at home, which had never happened before, and Daryushka did not know what to make of it, for the doctor no longer drank his beer at the proper time and sometimes was even late for dinner.

One day—it was by now the end of June—Dr. Khobotov came to see Andrei Yefimych, and, not finding him at home, went to look for him in the yard; there he was told that the old doctor had gone to visit the mental patients. Going into the annex he stopped in the entry, where he overheard the following conversation.

"We shall never agree, and you will never succeed in converting me to your beliefs," Ivan Dmitrich was saying querulously. "You know nothing of reality, have never suffered, but have only battened on the sufferings of others like a leech; while I have suffered continually from the day I was born till now. Therefore, I tell you frankly, I consider myself superior to you and in all respects more competent. It is not for you to teach me."

"I have absolutely no intention of converting you to my beliefs," said Andrei Yefimych gently, regretting that he was misunderstood. "And that is not the point, my friend. The point is not that you have suffered and I have not. Suffering and joy are transitory; never mind them, they do not matter. The point is that we can think; you and I see in each other men who are capable of thinking and reasoning, and this creates a bond between us, however different our views. If you knew, my friend, how sick I am of the general insanity, mediocrity, and stupidity, and what a pleasure it is to talk to you! You are an intelligent man and I enjoy your company."

Khobotov opened the door an inch and looked into the ward; Andrei Yefimych and Ivan Dmitrich, wearing his nightcap, were sitting side by side on the bed. The insane man was grimacing, shuddering, and convulsively pulling his robe around him, while the doctor sat motionless with bowed head, his flushed face looking helpless and sad. Khobotov shrugged his shoulders, grinned, and exchanged glances with Nikita. Nikita too shrugged his shoulders.

The next day Khobotov went to the annex accompanied by the medical assistant. They both stood in the entry listening.

"Our old man seems to have completely lost his moorings!" said Khobotov as they left the annex.

"Lord have mercy on us sinners!" sighed the pious Sergei Sergeich, carefully avoiding the puddles to keep from soiling his highly polished boots. "To tell you the truth, my dear Yevgeny Fyodorych, I have long been expecting this."

XII

Andrei Yefimych soon became aware of an atmosphere of mystery around him. The attendants, nurses, and patients looked at him inquisitively when they met him and began whispering when he passed. Masha, the superintendent's little girl, whom he used to enjoy meeting in the hospital garden, now for some reason ran away when he smilingly approached, wanting to stroke her hair. The postmaster, Mikhail Averyanych, no longer said: "Absolutely true" when listening to him, but muttered: "Yes, yes, yes . . ." in unaccountable confusion, looking at him thoughtfully and sadly; moreover he was always advising his friend to give up vodka and beer, though, being a tactful man, he never spoke of it directly but always in a roundabout way, telling him, for instance, about a certain battalion commander, an excellent man, or about the regimental priest, also a splendid fellow, both of whom, having fallen ill as a result of drinking, made complete recoveries when they gave it up. Two or three times his colleague Khobotov visited him, and he too advised Andrei Yefimych to give up spirituous liquors, recommending, for no apparent reason, that he take bromine drops.

In August Andrei Yefimych received a letter from the mayor requesting his presence on a very important matter. Arriving at the town hall at the appointed time, he found the military commander, the superintendent of the district school, a member of the town council, Khobotov, and a plump blond gentleman with a difficult Polish name, who lived at the stud farm thirty versts from town and was just passing through.

"We have here a deposition that concerns you, sir," said the councilman to Andrei Yefimych, after everyone had exchanged greetings and sat down at the table. "Yevgeny Fyodorych here says that there's not room enough for the dispensary in the main building, and that it ought to be moved into one of the annexes. This, of course, is no problem, it can be moved, but the main consideration is that the annex is in need of repairs."

"Yes, repairs are inevitable," said Andrei Yefimych, after a moment's thought. "If, for instance, the corner annex were to be fitted up as a dispensary, I suppose a minimum of five hundred rubles would be required. A fruitless expenditure."

Everyone remained silent for a while.

"I have already had the honor of reporting to you ten years ago," Andrei Yefimych went on in his soft voice, "that in its present form this hospital represents a luxury beyond the town's means. It was built in the forties, and things were different then. The town spends too much on unnecessary buildings and superfluous personnel. I think that with a different system it would be possible to maintain two model hospitals for the same money."

"Let's have another system, then!" said the councilman briskly.

"I have already had the honor of submitting my opinion: transfer the medical department to the jurisdiction of the zemstvo."

"Yes, transfer the money to the zemstvo and they'll steal it," said the fair-haired doctor, laughing.

"That's what usually happens," agreed the councilman, also laughing.

Andrei Yefimych turned a dull and apathetic eye on the doctor and said: "We must be fair."

Everyone commenced talking about how boring it was for a decent man to live in such a town. No theater, no music, and at the last club dance there were about twenty women and only two partners for them. The young men did not dance but spent the entire evening swarming around the buffet or playing cards. Andrei Yefimych, without looking at anyone, remarked in his slow quiet way, what a pity, what a great pity it was that the townspeople should squander their life's energy, their hearts and minds, on cards and gossip, and that they should have neither the capacity nor the inclination to spend time in interesting conversation or in reading, should refuse to take advantage of the pleasures of the mind. The mind alone was interesting and remarkable; everything else was base and trivial. Khobotov listened attentively to his colleague and suddenly asked:

"Andrei Yefimych, what is the date today?"

Having received an answer, he and the other doctor, in the tone of examiners who sense their own incompetence, proceeded to ask Andrei Yefimych what day of the week it was, how many days there were in a year, and whether it was true that there was a remarkable prophet living in Ward Six.

In answer to the last question Andrei Yefimych flushed and said:

"Yes, he is ill, but he is an interesting young man."

There were no more questions after that.

When he was putting on his coat in the hall, the military commander came up to him, put his hand on his shoulder, and said with a sigh:

"It's time for us old fellows to take a rest!"

As he came out of the town hall, Andrei Yefimych realized that this was a committee appointed to investigate his mental condition. Remembering the questions that had been put to him, he blushed, and for the first time bitterly deplored the science of medicine.

"My God," he thought, recalling how the doctors had examined him, "only recently they attended lectures on psychiatry and took their examinations— why then this crass ignorance? They haven't the slighest understanding of psychiatry!"

And for the first time in his life he felt insulted and angry.

That same day, toward evening, Mikhail Averyanych came to see him. Without even taking time to greet him, the postmaster went up to him, took both his hands, and with deep feeling said:

"My dear, dear friend, prove to me that you believe in my genuine affection for you and consider me your friend. . . . My dear friend!" and, not letting Andrei Yefimych speak, he went on in great agitation: "I love you for your erudition, for your nobility of soul. Listen to me, my dear. Professional ethics oblige the doctors to hide the truth from you, but I am a soldier, I will be blunt: you are not well! Forgive me, my dear, but this is the truth, and everyone around you noticed it long ago. Dr. Yevgeny Fyodorych has just told me that for the sake of your health it is essential that you have rest and recreation. Absolutely true! Splendid! I am taking a leave of absence in a few days, going away for a change of air. Prove to me that you are my friend and come with me! Come, we'll recapture our youth!"

"I feel perfectly well," said Andrei Yefimych after a moment's thought. "I can't go away. Let me prove my friendship in some other way."

To go somewhere for no reason, without his books, without Daryushka and his beer, suddenly to disturb a routine of life that had been set for twenty years, at first struck him as a wild, fantastic idea. But then he recalled the conversation in the town hall, the feeling of depression he had experienced as he returned home, and the thought of a brief absence from a town where stupid people regarded him as a madman suddenly appealed to him.

"And where exactly do you intend to go?" he asked.

"To Moscow, to Petersburg, to Warsaw. . . . I spent the five happiest years of my life in Warsaw. What an amazing city! Let us go, my dear friend!"

XIII

A week later it was suggested to Andrei Yefimych that he take a rest—in other words, that he send in his resignation—a suggestion he treated with indifference; and a week after that he and Mikhail Averyanych were sitting in a stagecoach on their way to the nearest railway station. It was cool clear weather, the sky was blue, the air transparent. They covered the two hundred versts to the station in two days, twice putting up for the night. At the posting stations, when they were served tea in glasses that had not been properly washed, or when the horses were not harnessed quickly enough, Mikhail

Averyanych became livid and trembled from head to foot. "Silence!" he would shout. "Don't argue!" And in the stagecoach he talked incessantly about his travels in the Caucasus and Poland. What adventures he had had, what encounters! He spoke in a loud voice and with such wide-eyed wonder that it might have been thought he was lying. Moreover he kept breathing into Andrei Yefimych's face and roaring with laughter right next to his ear, which made the doctor extremely uncomfortable and prevented him from concentrating and reflecting.

On the train they traveled third class for the sake of economy, choosing a car for nonsmokers. Half the passengers were quite respectable-looking people. Mikhail Averyanych soon made friends with everyone, moving from one seat to another, saying in a loud voice that no one should travel on these shocking lines. A complete swindle! How different, now, from being on a horse; you cover a hundred versts in a day and feel fresh and healthy afterward. And our crop failure is due, of course, to the draining of the Pinsk marshes. Things are in a bad state everywhere. He got excited, kept talking loudly, and would not let anyone else say a word. His ceaseless chatter interspersed with loud guffaws and vivid gestures wearied Andrei Yefimych.

In Moscow Mikhail Averyanych put on a military jacket without epaulettes, and trousers with red piping. When he went out he wore a military cap and overcoat, and soldiers in the street saluted him. He now appeared to Andrei Yefimych like a man who has dissipated all the good qualities of the country gentleman and kept only the bad. He liked to be waited on, even when there was no need. A box of matches would be lying in plain sight on the table and he would shout for a waiter to bring him matches; he thought nothing of appearing in his underwear in front of the maid; all servants, even old men, he addressed condescendingly, and called them blockheads and fools when he was in a bad temper. This, Andrei Yefimych knew, was typical of men of his class, but it disgusted him.

The first thing Mikhail Averyanych did was to take his friend to the Iverskaya Chapel. He prayed fervently, bowed to the ground with tears in his eyes, afterward saying with a deep sigh:

"Even if you don't believe, it makes you feel better to pray. Kiss the icon, my dear fellow."

Andrei Yefimych was embarrassed but kissed the icon, while Mikhail Averyanych with shaking head and pursed lips whispered a prayer, the tears welling up into his eyes again.

From there they went to the Kremlin, where they saw the Tsar-cannon and Tsar-bell, and even touched them. They admired the view of the river, visited the Cathedral of the Savior, and the Rumyantsev Museum.

They dined at Tyestov's. Mikhail Averyanych studied the menu a long time, stroking his whiskers and speaking to the waiter in the tone of a gourmet who was very much at home in restaurants.

"Let's see what you're going to feed us today, my good man!"

XIV

The doctor walked about, looked at things, ate and drank, the whole time feeling nothing but annoyance with Mikhail Averyanych. He longed for a respite, to get away from him, hide from him, but his friend considered it his duty not to let him out of his sight and to provide him with as many distractions as possible. When there was nothing to look at, he entertained him with conversation. Andrei Yefimych bore it for two days, and on the third day announced that he did not feel well and intended to spend the day in the hotel room. His friend said that in that case he would stay in too. He agreed that they needed a rest, otherwise their legs would give out. Andrei Yefimych lay down on the sofa, his face to the wall, and listened with clenched teeth as his friend vehemently assured him that sooner or later France was bound to crush Germany, that Moscow was full of swindlers, that you cannot judge a horse by its points alone. . . . The doctor was conscious of palpitations and a buzzing in his ears, but he could not bring himself to ask his friend to stop talking or to go away. Fortunately Mikhail Averyanych got tired of sitting in a hotel room and went out for a stroll after dinner.

Left alone, Andrei Yefimych gave himself up to a feeling of relief. How good to lie motionless on a sofa, conscious of being alone in the room! True happiness is impossible without solitude. The fallen angel probably betrayed God out of a longing for that solitude which is denied to angels. Andrei Yefimych wanted to think about the things he had seen and heard in the last few days, but he could not get Mikhail Averyanych out of his mind.

"And to think that he asked for leave and came away with me out of friendship and altruism," thought the doctor with vexation. "There's nothing worse than this benevolent guardianship. He's kind, well-meaning, jolly, but there you are—a bore. An insufferable bore! In the same way there are people who never say a word that isn't sensible and good, yet make you feel how stupid they are."

On the days that followed, Andrei Yefimych professed to be ill and did not leave the room. He lay with his face to the wall and suffered agonies while his friend tried to divert him with talk, and found rest only in his absence. He was angry with himself for having come, as well as with his friend, who daily became more garrulous and unconstrained. Andrei Yefimych was completely unsuccessful in his efforts to raise his thoughts to a serious, elevated plane.

"I'm being called to account by that reality Ivan Dmitrich was talking about," he thought, exasperated by his own pettiness. "However, it's all nonsense. . . . I'll get home, and everything will be as before. . . ."

In Petersburg it was the same: he spent whole days lying on the sofa in the hotel room, getting up only to drink beer.

Mikhail Averyanych was in great haste to reach Warsaw.

"My dear man, why should I go to Warsaw?" Andrei Yefimych said in an imploring voice. "Go without me, and let me go home. I beg you!"

"On no account!" protested Mikhail Averyanych. "It's an amazing city. I spent the five happiest years of my life there."

Andrei Yefimych lacked the will to insist on having his own way, and reluctantly went to Warsaw. Here he kept to his room, lay on the sofa, was furious with himself, his friend, and the hotel servants, who stubbornly refused to understand Russian, while Mikhail Averyanych, as usual, was bursting with good health and high spirits and running about town from morning to night looking up old friends. On several occasions he spent the night out. After one such night he returned early in the morning in a violently agitated state, red-faced and disheveled. He paced the room for a long time, muttering to himself, then stopped and said:

"Honor above all!"

After pacing a little longer, he clutched his head and in a tragic voice proclaimed:

"Yes, honor above all! I curse the moment it entered my head to come to this Babylon! My dear friend," he said, turning to the doctor, "you may well despise me: I have gambled and lost! Give me five hundred rubles!"

Andrei Yefimych counted out five hundred rubles and handed them to his friend without a word. The latter, still red with shame and rage, uttered an incoherent and somewhat unnecessary vow, put on his cap, and went out. When he returned two hours later, he threw himself into an armchair, heaved a loud sigh, and said:

"My honor is saved! Let us go, my friend. I don't want to remain another instant in this cursed city. Swindlers! Austrian spies!"

By the time they reached home it was November and the streets lay under deep snow. Dr. Khobotov had taken Andrei Yefimych's place; he was still living in his old apartment, waiting for Andrei Yefimych to come and vacate the hospital apartment. The homely woman he called his cook was already living in one of the annexes.

A new hospital scandal was going around town. It was said that the homely woman had quarreled with the superintendent, and that he had crawled on his knees before her, begging her forgiveness.

On the very day of his arrival Andrei Yefimych was obliged to look for a new apartment.

"My friend," the postmaster said to him timidly, "forgive an indiscreet question: what means have you at your disposal?"

Andrei Yefimych silently counted his money and replied:

"Eighty-six rubles."

"That's not what I meant," Mikhail Averyanych brought out in embarrassment, having misunderstood the doctor's answer. "I mean, how much money have you got altogether?"

"But that's what I'm telling you: eighty-six rubles. . . . I have nothing more."

Although Mikhail Averyanych regarded the doctor as an honest and upright man, he had always suspected him of having accumulated at least twenty thousand rubles. Now, on learning that Andrei Yefimych was a pauper, that he had absolutely nothing to live on, he burst into tears and threw his arms around his friend.

XV

Andrei Yefimych went to live in a little house with three windows belonging to a woman named Byelova. There were only three rooms in the house, not counting the kitchen. The doctor had the two rooms looking onto the street, and Daryushka, the landlady, and her three children lived in the third room and kitchen. Occasionally the landlady's lover, a drunken peasant who raised an uproar that terrified Daryushka and the children, came to spend the night. When he arrived, settling himself in the kitchen and demanding vodka, everyone felt terribly cramped, and the doctor, who was sorry for the crying children, would take them into his rooms and make up beds for them on the floor; this gave him great satisfaction.

He got up at eight o'clock, as always, and after his morning tea sat down to read his old books and magazines. He had no money to buy new ones. Whether it was because the books were old or because of the change in his surroundings, reading no longer fascinated him, in fact, it tired him. To avoid being idle, he drew up a detailed catalogue of his books and glued labels onto the backs of them, finding this painstaking mechanical work more interesting than reading. In some unaccountable way the monotony of the work seemed to lull his thoughts, and, thinking of nothing, the time passed quickly. Even sitting in the kitchen peeling potatoes or picking over buckwheat with Daryushka seemed interesting now. On Saturdays and Sundays he went to church. Leaning against the wall and closing his eyes, he listened to the choir and thought of his father and mother, of the university, and of various religions; he felt soothed and melancholy, and as he left the church regretted that the service had ended so soon.

Twice he went to the hospital to see Ivan Dmitrich and have a talk with him, but on both occasions found him extraordinarily excited and malicious. He demanded to be left in peace, saying that he had long ago grown sick of empty prattle, and asked only one recompense from these damned scoundrels for all the suffering he had undergone—solitary confinement. Was he to be denied this too? Both times as Andrei Yefimych took his leave and wished him good night, Ivan Dmitrich snarled:

"Go to hell!"

Andrei Yefimych could not make up his mind whether to go a third time or not. He wanted very much to go.

In the old days Andrei Yefimych had been in the habit of pacing the floor after dinner and thinking; now he lay on the sofa with his face to the wall till time for evening tea, indulging in petty thoughts which he could not control.

He was mortified that after more than twenty years of service he had been granted neither a pension nor a bonus. True, he had not done his work honestly, but all civil servants without exception, whether they had served honestly or not, received pensions. Contemporary justice consists precisely in the fact that rank, orders, and pensions are awarded not for any moral quality or ability, but for service, regardless of what it had been. Why should he alone be an exception? He had absolutely no money. He was ashamed to pass a shop and meet the shopkeeper's eye. Thirty-two rubles were owing for beer. And he owed money to Byelova too. Daryushka had been secretly selling his clothes and books, and kept telling the landlady that the doctor was expecting to receive a large sum of money very soon.

He was angry with himself for having spent the thousand rubles he had saved on a trip. How useful that thousand rubles would have been now! And it annoyed him that people would not leave him in peace. Khobotov felt obliged to visit his ailing colleague now and then. Everything about the man was repellent to Andrei Yefimych: his sleek face and horribly condescending tone, his high boots, and the way he used the word "colleague"; but what was most revolting was the fact that he considered it his duty to look after Andrei Yefimych and actually believed he was giving him medical treatment. He never came without bringing a bottle of bromine drops and some rhubarb pills.

Mikhail Averyanych also considered it his duty to visit his friend and divert him. He would enter Andrei Yefimych's room with an exaggerated air of familiarity and forced hilarity, immediately assuring him that he was looking splendid today, and that things were obviously on the mend, thank God—from which one could only conclude that he considered his friend's case hopeless. He had not yet repaid the money he had borrowed in Warsaw and was weighed down by a sense of shame, the strain of which caused him to laugh even louder and to try to tell even funnier stories. His anecdotes and stories now seemed endless and were a torture to both Andrei Yefimych and himself.

During his visits Andrei Yefimych usually lay down on the sofa, turned his back, and listened with clenched teeth; he felt layers of scum forming on the surface of his soul, and after each visit the scum seemed to rise higher, as if it were going to choke him.

In an effort to stifle his contemptible feelings he would try to dwell on the thought that sooner or later he, Khobotov, and Mikhail Averyanych would all die, leaving not the slightest imprint on the world. He tried to imagine some spirit flying through space a million years hence, passing over the globe, looking down and seeing nothing but clay and bare rocks. Everything—culture and moral law—would have vanished, leaving not so much as a burdock growing. Of what consequence then was the insignificant Khobotov, the oppressive friendship of Mikhail Averyanych, or his shame before a shopkeeper? It was all trivial, mere nonsense.

But such reasoning no longer helped. Scarcely had he evoked the image of the globe a million years hence than Khobotov in his high boots would appear from behind the bare rocks, or he would hear the forced laughter of Mikhail Averyanych and his embarrassed whisper: "As for that Warsaw debt, my dear friend, I'll pay you back one of these days . . . without fail."

XVI

One afternoon Mikhail Averyanych came to see Andrei Yefimych after dinner when he was lying on the sofa. Khobotov happened to appear at the same time, with the bromine drops. Andrei Yefimych drew himself up heavily and sat on the sofa supporting himself with both hands.

"Now today, my friend, you have a much better color than you had yesterday. Why, you're fine, just fine! Good for you!"

"It's high time you were improving, my dear colleague," said Khobotov with a yawn. "You're probably getting fed up yourself with all this dilly-dallying."

"We'll get well!" said Mikhail Averyanych jovially. "We'll live to be a hundred, just see if we don't!"

"I don't know about a hundred, but he's certainly good for another twenty," said Khobotov reassuringly. "You're not so bad, my dear colleague, not so bad. . . . Don't look so despondent. . . . You needn't try pulling the wool over our eyes."

"We'll show you what we're made of!" said Mikhail Averyanych, roaring with laughter and slapping his friend on the knee. "We'll show them yet! Next summer, God willing, we'll dash off to the Caucasus and ride all over those mountains on horseback! Trot-trot-trot! And when we come back from the Caucasus, before you know it, we might even be celebrating a wedding!" Mikhail Averyanych winked slyly. "We'll marry you off, my friend, just see if we don't. . . ."

Andrei Yefimych suddenly felt the scum rise to his throat; his heart was pounding violently.

"How vulgar!" he said, rising abruptly and going to the window. "Don't you realize in what bad taste this is?"

He meant to go on mildly and politely, but he involuntarily clenched his fists and raised them over his head.

"Leave me alone!" he shouted, in an unnatural voice, turning red and shaking from head to foot. "Get out! Both of you—get out!"

Mikhail Averyanych and Khobotov stood up and stared at him, first in bewilderment and then in alarm.

"Get out, both of you!" Andrei Yefimych went on shouting. "Stupid people! Fools! I don't want your friendship—nor your medicine, you blockhead! The vulgarity—sickening!"

Khobotov and Mikhail Averyanych exchanged glances, and backed away to the door and out into the passage. Andrei Yefimych snatched up the bottle of bromine drops and threw it after them; the bottle broke with a crash on the threshold.

"You can go to hell!" he shouted in a tearful voice, running out into the passage. "To hell with you!"

When his visitors had gone, Andrei Yefimych, trembling as though in a fever, lay down on the sofa and kept saying over and over again:

"Stupid people! Fools!"

When he had grown calm, the first thing that occurred to him was that poor Mikhail Averyanych must feel terribly humiliated and heavyhearted, and that all this was appalling. Such a thing had never happened to him before. Where was his intelligence, his tact? Where was his comprehension of things, his philosophical detachment?

He was unable to sleep the whole night from shame of vexation with himself, and in the morning, around ten o'clock set out for the post office to apologize to the postmaster.

"We'll forget all about it," said Mikhail Averyanych with a sigh; he was deeply moved and pressed his hand warmly. "Let bygones be bygones. . . . Lyubavkin!" he cried in a voice that made the entire postal staff and everyone else in the post office start. "Bring a chair! And you wait!" he shouted at a peasant woman who was holding out a registered letter to him through the grille. "Can't you see I'm busy? . . . We'll forget what's past," he went on affectionately to Andrei Yefimych. "Do sit down, my dear friend."

He sat for a moment in silence, stroking his knees, and then said:

"It never entered my head to take offense. Illness is no joke, I know. The doctor and I were quite alarmed by your attack yesterday, and we had a long talk about you. My dear friend, why do you refuse to take your illness seriously? You can't go on like this. Forgive me, but as a friend I must tell you frankly," Mikhail Averyanych whispered, "you live in the most unfavorable surroundings: it's cramped, dirty, there's no one to look after you, no money for medical treatment. . . . My dear friend, the doctor and I both implore you with all our hearts to take our advice: go to the hospital! The food there is wholesome, and you'll have nursing and treatment. Although Yevgeny Fyodorych, just between you and me, is *mauvais ton,* he is nevertheless knowledgeable, and you can fully rely on him. He gave me his word he would look after you."

Andrei Yefimych was touched by the postmaster's genuine concern, and by the tears which suddenly glistened on his cheeks.

"My most esteemed friend, don't believe it!" he whispered, laying his hand on his heart. "Don't believe them! It's a trick! All that is wrong with me is that in the course of twenty years I have found only one intelligent man in our whole town, and he is mad. I'm not ill, I've simply been caught in a vicious circle from which there is no way out. And it makes no difference to me now what happens."

"Go to the hospital, my dear friend."

"To the hospital or into a pit—it's all one to me."

"Promise me you will obey Yevgeny Fyodorych in everything."

"Very well, I promise. But I repeat: I've been caught in a vicious circle. Now everything, even the most sincere interest of my friends, leads to only one thing—my ruin. I am going to my ruin, and I have the courage to recognize it."

"You will get better, dear friend."

"What's the use of saying that?" said Andrei Yefimych testily. "There are very few men who, toward the end of their lives, do not experience what I'm going through now. When you are told you have something like diseased kidneys or an enlarged heart and you begin to have medical treatment, or when they tell you you're insane, or a criminal, in other words, when people suddenly start paying attention to you, then you know you are caught in a vicious circle from which you will never escape. If you try to get out you will only get in deeper. You had better give up, for there is no human effort that can save you. So it seems to me."

In the meantime people were crowding around the grille. To avoid keeping them waiting any longer, Andrei Yefimych stood up and began taking his leave. Mikhail Averyanych made him repeat his promise and accompanied him to the door.

That same day toward evening Khobotov, in his sheepskin jacket and high boots, unexpectedly made his appearance and, as if nothing had happened, said to Andrei Yefimych:

"I've come on business, my dear colleague. I want to ask you to join me in a consultation, will you?"

Thinking that Khobotov wanted to divert him with an outing, or perhaps give him a chance to earn a little money, Andrei Yefimych put on his coat and hat and went with him. He was glad of the opportunity to expiate his guilt of the day before and be reconciled with him. In his heart he thanked Khobotov, who made no allusion to the incident, evidently trying to spare his feelings. One would hardly have expected such tact from this uncultivated man.

"And where is your patient?" asked Andrei Yefimych.

"In the hospital. I've been wanting to show you this for a long time now. . . . A most interesting case."

They went into the hospital yard, and, skirting the main building, turned toward the annex where the insane were housed. And all this, for some reason, in silence. As they entered, Nikita, as usual, jumped to attention.

"One of the patients here has developed a complication in the lungs," Khobotov said in an undertone when he and Andrei Yefimych were in the ward. "You wait here, I'll be right back. I'm just going to get a stethoscope."

And he went out.

XVII

It was growing dark. Ivan Dmitrich lay on his bed with his face buried in the pillow; the paralytic sat motionless, quietly weeping and moving his lips.

The fat peasant and the former mail sorter were asleep. It was quiet in the ward.

Andrei Yefimych sat down on Ivan Dmitrich's bed and waited. But when half an hour had passed, instead of Khobotov, Nikita came into the ward carrying a dressing gown, underclothes, and slippers.

"Please change your clothes, Your Honor," he said quietly. "This is your cot here," he added, pointing to an unoccupied bed that obviously had just been brought in. "Don't worry, you'll get well, God willing."

Andrei Yefimych understood everything. Without a word he walked over to the bed Nikita had indicated and sat down; when he saw that Nikita stood there waiting, he completely undressed, feeling horribly embarrassed, and put on the hospital clothing. The drawers were much too short, the shirt long, and the dressing gown smelled of smoked fish.

"You'll get well, God willing," Nikita repeated.

He gathered up the doctor's clothes and went out, shutting the door after him.

"It's all the same . . ." thought Andrei Yefimych, modestly drawing the dressing gown around him and feeling that he looked like a convict in his new costume. "It's all the same . . . whether it's a frockcoat, a uniform, or this robe, it's all the same. . . ."

But what about his watch? And the notebook he kept in his side pocket? His cigarettes? Where had Nikita taken his clothes? Now, perhaps, he would never again, till the day of his death, put on trousers, a waistcoat, and boots. All this seemed strange, even incomprehensible, at first. But Andrei Yefimych was convinced even now that there was no difference between Byelova's house and Ward No. 6, that everything in this world was nonsense, vanity of vanities; and yet his hands trembled, his feet were cold, and the thought that Ivan Dmitrich would soon get up and see him in a hospital robe filled him with dread. He stood up, took a few steps, and sat down again.

Half an hour passed, an hour, and he was sick to death of sitting there; was it really possible to live a day, a week, even years, the way these people lived? Here he had been sitting, getting up and taking a few steps, and sitting down again; he could go and look out the window, walk about once more—and then what? Just sit there like a graven image and think? No, that was hardly possible.

Andrei Yefimych lay down, but immediately got up and wiped the cold sweat from his brow with his sleeve, feeling as he did so that his whole face smelled of smoked fish. He commenced pacing again.

"It's some sort of misunderstanding . . ." he said with a gesture of bewilderment. "I must speak to them, there's some misunderstanding. . . ."

Just then Ivan Dmitrich woke up. He sat up, his cheeks propped on his fists. He spat. Glancing apathetically at the doctor, for a moment he appeared not to understand, then the expression on his sleepy face became mocking and spiteful.

"Aha! So they've locked you up too, my dear!" he said in a hoarse drowsy voice, screwing up one eye. "Delighted! First you sucked other people's blood, now they'll suck yours. Splendid!"

"It's some sort of misunderstanding . . ." mumbled Andrei Yefimych, frightened by Ivan Dmitrich's words; he shrugged his shoulders and repeated: "a misunderstanding of some sort. . . ."

Ivan Dmitrich spat again and lay down.

"This accursed life!" he snarled. "And what makes it so mortifying, so galling, is that life will end, not in any recompense for suffering, not with an apotheosis, as it does in an opera, but in death; a couple of attendants will come, take the corpse by the arms and legs, and drag it down to the cellar. Ugh! Well, it doesn't matter. . . . Our day will come in the next world. I'll come back here as a ghost and haunt these swine. I'll make their hair turn gray."

Moiseika returned from one of his walks, and, seeing the doctor, held out his hand and said:

"Give a little kopeck!"

XVIII

Andrei Yefimych walked to the window and looked out at the field. It was growing dark, and on the horizon at the right rose a cold livid moon. Not far from the hospital fence, some two hundred yards, stood a tall white building surrounded by a stone wall. It was the prison.

"So this is reality!" thought Andrei Yefimych, and he became terrified.

The moon was terrifying, and the prison, and the spikes in the hospital fence, and the distant flames of the bone-black plant. He heard a sigh behind him; turning, he saw a man with stars and decorations sparkling on his chest, who was smiling and slyly winking. And this too was terrifying.

Andrei Yefimych assured himself that there was nothing singular about the moon or the prison, that people who were mentally sound wore decorations, and that in time everything would rot and turn to clay, but he was suddenly overwhelmed with despair, and, clutching the iron grille of the window with both hands, tried with all his might to shake it. But the bars were strong and did not yield.

Then, in an effort to shake off his terror, he went over to Ivan Dmitrich's bed and sat down.

"I've lost courage, dear friend," he murmured, trembling and wiping away the cold sweat. "I've lost courage."

"Try philosophizing," said Ivan Dmitrich derisively.

"My God, my God. . . . Yes, yes. . . . You were once pleased to say that while there is no philosophy in Russia, everyone philosophizes, even the little nobodies. But what harm does their philosophizing do anyone?" Andrei Yefimych's voice sounded as if he were on the verge of tears, as if he wanted to arouse Ivan Dmitrich's pity. "So why this malevolent laugh, dear friend?

And why shouldn't these little people philosophize when they have no other satisfaction? . . . For an intelligent, cultured, proud, freedom-loving man, made in the image of God, to have no alternative to becoming a doctor in a stupid, dirty little town, and spending his whole life applying leeches and mustard plasters! The quackery, narrowness, vulgarity! Oh, my God!"

"You're babbling nonsense. If being a doctor repels you, you could have gone into one of the ministries."

"No, no, there's nothing one can do. We are weak, my friend. . . . I used to be indifferent, I reasoned confidently, soundly, but at the first rude touch of life I lost courage . . . collapsed. . . . We are weak. . . . We are miserable creatures. . . . And you too, my friend. You are intelligent, well-born, you imbibed noble impulses with your mother's milk, but you had hardly embarked on life when you became exhausted and fell ill. . . . Weak, weak! . . ."

With the onset of evening, something other than fear and a sense of ignominy had begun to gnaw at Andrei Yefimych. At last he realized that he was longing for his beer and cigarettes.

"I'm going out, my friend," he said. "I'll tell them to give us some light. . . . I can't stand this. . . . I'm not equal to it. . . ."

Andrei Yefimych went to the door and opened it, but Nikita instantly jumped up and barred his way.

"Where are you going? None of that, none of that!" he said. "It's time you were in bed!"

"But I'm only going out for a minute, just to walk a little in the yard," said Andrei Yefimych, panic-stricken.

"Impossible, not allowed! You know that yourself."

Nikita slammed the door and leaned his back against it.

"But what difference will it make if I go out?" Andrei Yefimych asked, shrugging his shoulders. "I don't understand! Nikita, I must go out!" he said in a trembling voice. "I absolutely must!"

"Don't cause any disorder, now, that's bad," Nikita warned him.

"What in God's name is going on!" screamed Ivan Dmitrich, suddenly jumping up. "What right has he to prevent anyone from going out? How dare they keep us here? The law states quite clearly that no one can be deprived of freedom without a trial. It's coercion! Tyranny!"

"Of course, it's tyranny!" said Andrei Yefimych, encouraged by Ivan Dmitrich's clamor. "I wanted to go out, I must! He has no right to stop me! Let me out, I tell you!"

"Do you hear, you dumb brute?" shouted Ivan Dmitrich, pounding on the door with his fists. "Open the door, or I'll break it down! Butcher!"

"Open it!" shouted Andrei Yefimych, shaking all over. "I insist!"

"Keep it up!" answered Nikita from the other side of the door. "Go on, keep it up!"

"Go and call Yevgeny Fyodorych, at least. Tell him I ask him to please come here . . . for a minute!"

"He'll come tomorrow without being called."

"They'll never let us out!" Ivan Dmitrich was saying meanwhile. "They'll let us rot here! Oh, Lord, can it be that there is no hell in the next world, and that these scoundrels will be forgiven? Where is justice? Open the door, you beast, I'm suffocating!" he cried in a hoarse voice, and threw himself against the door. "I'll beat my brains out! Murderer!"

Nikita quickly opened the door, and using both hands and his knee, roughly knocked Andrei Yefimych to one side, then drew back his fist and punched him in the face. Andrei Yefimych felt as though a huge salty wave had broken over his head and was dragging him back to his bed; there was, in fact, a salty taste in his mouth, probably blood from his teeth. Waving his arms as if trying to emerge, he caught hold of somebody's bed, and at that moment felt two more blows from Nikita's fists in his back.

Ivan Dmitrich screamed loudly. He too was evidently being beaten.

Then all was quiet. The moon shed its pale light through the bars, and on the floor lay a shadow that looked like a net. It was terrible. Andrei Yefimych lay still, holding his breath, waiting in terror to be struck again. He felt as if someone had taken a sickle, thrust it into his body, and twisted it several times in his chest and bowels. He bit the pillow and clenched his teeth with pain; and all of a sudden out of the chaos there clearly flashed through his mind the dreadful, unbearable thought that these people, who now looked like black shadows in the moonlight, must have experienced this same pain day in and day out for years. How could it have happened that in the course of more than twenty years he had not known, had refused to know this? Having no conception of pain, he could not possibly have known it, so he was not guilty, but his conscience, no less obdurate and implacable than Nikita, made him turn cold from head to foot. He jumped up, wanting to shout at the top of his lungs, to rush out and kill Nikita, Khobotov, the superintendent, the medical assistant, and then himself, but no sound came from his mouth and his legs would not obey him; gasping for breath, he tore at his dressing gown and the shirt over his chest, ripped them, and fell back on the bed unconscious.

XIX

The next morning his head ached and there was a buzzing in his ears; he felt ill in every part of his body. The memory of his weakness the day before caused him no shame. He had been cowardly, frightened even of the moon, and had frankly expressed thoughts and feelings he had never suspected in himself; for instance, the notion that lack of satisfaction led the ordinary man to philosophize. But nothing mattered to him now.

He neither ate nor drank, but lay motionless and silent.

"It doesn't matter..." he thought, when he was questioned. "I won't answer.... It doesn't matter."

After dinner Mikhail Averyanych came bringing a quarter of a pound of tea and a pound of fruit candies. Daryushka also came and stood by the bed for an hour with an expression of dumb grief on her face. And Dr. Khobotov visited him. He brought a bottle of bromine drops and ordered Nikita to fumigate the ward.

Toward evening Andrei Yefimych died of an apoplectic stroke. He first suffered violent chills and nausea; something loathsome seemed to permeate his entire body even to his finger tips; it rose from his stomach to his head and flooded his eyes and ears. Everything turned green before him. Andrei Yefimych realized that the end had come and remembered that Ivan Dmitrich, Mikhail Averyanych, and millions of others believed in immortality. And what if they were right? But he felt no desire for immortality, and gave it only a momentary thought. A herd of reindeer, about which he had been reading the day before, extraordinarily beautiful and graceful, ran by him; a peasant woman held out a registered letter to him. . . . Mikhail Averyanych said something. . . . Then all was gone, and Andrei Yefimych lost consciousness forever.

Attendants came, picked him up by the arms and legs, and carried him into the chapel. There he lay on a table, his eyes open, with the moon shining down on him through the night.

In the morning Sergei Sergeich came, and after piously praying before the crucifix, closed the eyes of his former chief.

Andrei Yefimych was buried the following day. Only Mikhail Averyanych and Daryushka were at the funeral.

Translated by Ann Dunnigan

Topics for Discussion and Writing

1. What specifically does Shakespeare's sonnet "My love is as a fever, longing still" have in common with D. H. Lawrence's "The Horse Dealer's Daughter," especially with the last passionate scenes of that story? Discuss.
2. What effects did the sedatives, tonics, and advice that Sir Augustus prescribed for Lord Mountdrago have? Why did Lord Mountdrago seek out Dr. Audlin? While the story outlines for the reader a case in which psychoanalysis helps clarify a patient's problem, why does Maugham conclude with two mysterious deaths and a doctor who admits "I'm not well"?
3. In James Dickey's "Diabetes," we find a physical disease with mental ramifications; in Maugham's "Lord Mountdrago," we find a mental disease with physical ramifications. Using these two literary texts—the

poem and the story—to help you make your points, come to some supportable conclusions about the relationship between the body and the mind. Summarize your argument in a short essay.

4. Explore in an original essay the concept of the "split self" in "Lord Mountdrago" and "Borges and Myself." You might review Nathaniel Hawthorne's humorous tale "The Haunted Quack" as well. How are conscience and nightmares especially important in the Maugham and Hawthorne stories? Modern psychiatric medicine attempts to do what with the split personality?

5. During her adult life, Anne Sexton was a suburban housewife, a poet, and a victim of mental illness. Do you see any way in which Borges' comment, "Which of us is writing this page I don't know," might serve as a gloss on the three Sexton poems? Are creativity and madness sometimes closely related?

6. Prepare a short oral report on the imagery in "You, Doctor Martin." One approach to this project might be to focus on references to the patient as child and to the doctor as father.

7. Point out in an original essay how "Said the Poet to the Analyst" reveals a hopeful process of communication between patient and physician that is essentially absent from Chekhov's "Ward Six."

8. The speaker in "Lullaby" mentions her surroundings as "the TV parlor / in the best ward at Bedlam." Look up the word "bedlam" in your dictionary. What are its meanings? Do you think that the "I" in "Lullaby" is facing anything like the brutality found in "Ward Six"?

9. Write an evaluative character sketch of Ivan Dmitrich. Why does Chekhov introduce this character early in "Ward Six"? Comment on the partly parallel fates of Ivan Dmitrich and his physician, Andrei Yefimych.

10. If Andrei Yefimych knows that his small town's "entire hospital system is based on theft, wrangling scandal-mongering, favoritism, and gross quackery, exactly as it was twenty years ago, and remains a vicious institution" (section VII), why does he do nothing to remedy the situation?

11. Chekhov's Dr. Yefimych knows about modern advances in medical science and in psychiatry, but he allows Ward Six to exist unchanged during his tenure. Yet, by the end of the novella, Chekhov makes us sympathize with such a physician. Does Yefimych change, grow, or attain any self-knowledge as the narrative progresses?

12. What picture do you get of health-care personnel (nurses and attendants, among others) in Sexton and Chekhov? Does this picture square with the American medical scene in the 1970s? Do you see any distortions? Why?

Part 4

Medicine and the Scientific Impulse

Our fourth medicine-in-literature topic, around which a considerable body of writing has developed, concerns the relationship (and often the conflict) between medical practice and medical science. In this connection it may be useful to remember the shocking discrepancy between Dr. Andrei Yefimych's actual practice in the town's inferior hospital and his knowledge of recent scientific developments in distant but more enlightened medical centers, detailed in section VII of Chekhov's "Ward Six."

In his acerbic 1911 "Preface on Doctors" (introducing his play *The Doctor's Dilemma*), Bernard Shaw posed the question, "Are Doctors Men of Science?" Shaw viewed "doctoring" as an art, "the art of curing illnesses," and not as a science. In Shaw's opinion, doctors were mostly interested in making a living at the expense of their patients; they had a vested interest in ill health and in selling cures. And Shaw considered licensed doctors no better than the quacks. He had "never been able to perceive any distinction between the science of the herbalist and that of the duly registered doctor."

The next three selections shed light on the medicine-and-science theme in surprisingly different ways. "Rappaccini's Daughter," Nathaniel Hawthorne's grimly ambiguous nineteenth-century allegorical tale about a physician who cares more for science than for mankind, tells the story of the man of science as cold experimenter. Here we see the scientific impulse run riot. People are not really important in Dr. Rappaccini's mysterious world. Healing is not this doctor's goal. On the other hand, in the legend of "The First Cure," from *Black Elk Speaks*, healing—specifically, saving the life of a little Indian boy— is the young Sioux medicine man's primary aim. An older and wiser Black Elk here reviews a dramatic scene from his youth in which both the spiritual (faith in divine powers) and the natural (use of special herbs) play a part in the healing ceremony. The story is told through author John G. Neihardt's vivid prose. The contrasts between Neihardt and Hawthorne are both striking and moving. "Of Medicine and Poetry," an autobiographical essay by William Carlos Williams, supplies ironical insight into the nature of modern cures through scientific advances: "It is noteworthy that the sulfonamids, penicillin, came in about simultaneously with Ted Williams, Ralph Kiner, and the rubber ball. We want home runs, antibiotics to 'cure' man with a single shot in the buttocks." Williams, a physician as well as a man of letters, downplays science and miracle drugs and instead emphasizes how treating man "as material for a work of [literary] art made him somehow come alive to me." In short, Williams finds it but "an indifferent matter" to treat man "as something to which surgery, drugs and hoodoo" apply.

The next selection, act one from Henrik Ibsen's late nineteenth-century play *An Enemy of the People,* reveals the doctor as a man of science who unfortunately discovers that the town's lucrative Baths are unsafe and that the whole water system will have to be relaid. Initially elated by his singular discovery, Dr. Thomas Stockmann soon finds that he is regarded as an enemy of the people for disturbing the status quo. The playwright closely scrutinizes a medical/political/ethical triangle; while act one sets up the problem and ends on a happy note, yet disaster for Dr. Stockmann and his family will inevitably follow such a prideful outburst as "Well, now I'll give them a real broadside. Of course, I've written a full report to the Baths Committee; it's been ready for a whole week, I've only been waiting to receive this. (*Shows the letter.*) But now I shall send it to them at once!" So even in act one there are foreshadowings of the doctor's greater interest in himself, his cause, and his own moral principles than in his plan for actually solving the health problem with and for the many people concerned.

Unlike Ibsen's rather stubborn Dr. Stockmann, Sinclair Lewis' Dr. Martin Arrowsmith much better represents devotion to pure scientific idealism. Martin's mentor, Dr. Max Gottlieb, carefully defines the religion of a scientist in our excerpt from the novel, *Arrowsmith.* Martin then says the prayer of the scientist, and when he at last returns to his hotel room and to Leora, his wife, he is so excited about the opportunity for research at the McGurk Institute that he has neglected to ask what his new salary will be. In contrast, money is quite important to gerontologist Dr. Raúl Narbondo in Jorge Luis Borges' "The Immortals." For the right price, Dr. Narbondo can keep a man alive forever as a furniturelike cube. Borges' science-fiction tale explores issues such as euthanasia, the man of science gone mad, medical ethics, the nature of immortality, and the mind-body relationship. In the end, the cost of immortality seems just too great—to become machinelike, a freak, and totally dependent on the doctor and his corporation for what little existence remains for a disembodied brain. The emphasis is on getting rid of, not curing, the body. Here we have science without humanity.

The last two selections, both written by physicians, help complete the somewhat complicated picture of medicine and the scientific impulse. Sir Arthur Conan Doyle's brilliant story "The Doctors of Hoyland" pits Dr. James Ripley against Dr. Verrinder Smith in a male-female struggle for dominance. Dr. Ripley admires, hates, needs, loves, then loses Dr. Smith, the pure scientist who also happens to be a woman. Doyle enmeshes his two main characters in various intricate interpersonal relationships and also raises the twin "problems" of women as doctors and of women (or men) as steadfastly devoted to science beyond regular medical practice. And finally, Oliver Wendell Holmes' poem "A Sentiment" serves to balance the warring elements in this part, for it brings into a kind of unity the body, emotion, and reason with the lines: "A TRIPLE health to Friendship, Science, Art, / From heads and hands that own a common heart!"

BERNARD SHAW

Are Doctors Men of Science?

I presume nobody will question the existence of a widely spread popular delusion that every doctor is a man of science. It is escaped only in the very small class which understands by science something more than conjuring with retorts and spirit lamps, magnets and microscopes, and discovering magical cures for disease. To a sufficiently ignorant man every captain of a trading schooner is a Galileo, every organ-grinder a Beethoven, every piano-tuner a Helmholtz, every Old Bailey barrister a Solon, every Seven Dials pigeon-dealer a Darwin, every scrivener a Shakespeare, every locomotive engine a miracle, and its driver no less wonderful than George Stephenson. As a matter of fact, the rank and file of doctors are no more scientific than their tailors; or, if you prefer to put it the reverse way, their tailors are no less scientific than they. Doctoring is an art, not a science: any layman who is interested in science sufficiently to take in one of the scientific journals and follow the literature of the scientific movement, knows more about it than those doctors (probably a large majority) who are not interested in it, and practise only to earn their bread. Doctoring is not even the art of keeping people in health (no doctor seems able to advise you what to eat any better than his grandmother or the nearest quack): it is the art of curing illnesses. It does happen exceptionally that a practising doctor makes a contribution to science (my play describes a very notable one); but it happens much oftener that he draws disastrous conclusions from his clinical experience because he has no conception of scientific method, and believes, like any rustic, that the handling of evidence and statistics needs no expertness. The distinction between a quack doctor and a qualified one is mainly that only the qualified one is authorized to sign death certificates, for which both sorts seem to have about equal occasion. Unqualified practitioners now make large incomes as hygienists, and are resorted to as frequently by cultivated amateur scientists who understand quite well what they are doing as by ignorant people who are simply dupes. Bone-setters make fortunes under the very noses of our greatest surgeons from educated and wealthy patients; and some of the most successful doctors on the register use quite heretical methods of treating disease, and have qualified themselves solely for convenience. Leaving out of account the village witches who prescribe spells and sell charms, the humblest professional healers in this country are the herbalists. These men wander through the fields on Sunday seeking for herbs with magic properties of curing disease, preventing childbirth, and the like. Each of them believes that he is on the verge of a great discovery, in which Virginia Snake Root will be an ingredient, heaven knows why! Virginia Snake Root fascinates the imagination of the herbalist as mercury used to fascinate the alchemists. On week days he keeps a shop in which he sells packets of penny-royal, dandelion, &c., labelled with little lists of the diseases they are supposed to cure, and apparently do cure to the satisfaction of the people who keep on buying them. I have never been able to perceive any distinction between the science of the herbalist and that of the duly registered doctor. A relative of mine recently consulted a doctor about some of the ordinary symptoms which indicate the need for a holiday and a change. The doctor satisfied himself that the patient's heart was a little depressed. Digitalis being a drug labelled as a heart specific by the profession, he promptly administered a stiff dose. Fortunately the patient was a hardy old lady who was not easily killed. She recovered with no worse result than her conversion to Christian Science, which owes its vogue quite as much to public despair of doctors as to superstition. I am not, observe, here concerned with the question as to whether the dose of digitalis was judicious or not: the point is, that a farm laborer consulting a herbalist would have been treated in exactly the same way.

NATHANIEL HAWTHORNE

Rappaccini's Daughter

A young man, named Giovanni Guasconti, came, very long ago, from the more southern region of Italy, to pursue his studies at the University of Padua. Giovanni, who had but a scanty supply of gold ducats in his pocket, took lodgings in a high and gloomy chamber of an old edifice which looked not unworthy to have been the palace of a Paduan noble, and which, in fact, exhibited over its entrance the armorial bearings of a family long since extinct. The young stranger, who was not unstudied in the great poem of his country, recollected that one of the ancestors of this family, and perhaps an occupant of this very mansion, had been pictured by Dante as a partaker of the immortal agonies of his Inferno. These reminiscences and associations, together

with the tendency to heartbreak natural to a young man for the first time
out of his native sphere, caused Giovanni to sigh heavily as he looked around
the desolate and ill-furnished apartment.

"Holy Virgin, signor!" cried old Dame Lisabetta, who, won by the youth's
remarkable beauty of person, was kindly endeavoring to give the chamber a
habitable air, "what a sigh was that to come out of a young man's heart! Do
you find this old mansion gloomy? For the love of Heaven, then, put your
head out of the window, and you will see as bright sunshine as you have left
in Naples."

Guasconti mechanically did as the old woman advised, but could not quite
agree with her that the Paduan sunshine was as cheerful as that of southern
Italy. Such as it was, however, it fell upon a garden beneath the window and
expended its fostering influences on a variety of plants, which seemed to have
been cultivated with exceeding care.

"Does this garden belong to the house?" asked Giovanni.

"Heaven forbid, signor, unless it were fruitful of better pot herbs than any
that grow there now," answered old Lisabetta. "No; that garden is cultivated
by the own hands of Signor Giacomo Rappaccini, the famous doctor, who, I
warrant him, has been heard of as far as Naples. It is said that he distils these
plants into medicines that are as potent as a charm. Oftentimes you may see
the signor doctor at work, and perchance the signora, his daughter, too, gathering the strange flowers that grow in the garden."

The old woman had now done what she could for the aspect of the chamber;
and, commending the young man to the protection of the saints, took her
departure.

Giovanni still found no better occupation than to look down into the garden beneath his window. From its appearance, he judged it to be one of
those botanic gardens which were of earlier date in Padua than elsewhere in
Italy or in the world. Or, not improbably, it might once have been the
pleasure-place of an opulent family; for there was the ruin of a marble
fountain in the centre, sculptured with rare art, but so wofully shattered that
it was impossible to trace the original design from the chaos of remaining
fragments. The water, however, continued to gush and sparkle into the sun-
beams as cheerfully as ever. A little gurgling sound ascended to the young
man's window, and made him feel as if the fountain were an immortal spirit
that sung its song unceasingly and without heeding the vicissitudes around it,
while one century imbodied it in marble and another scattered the perishable
garniture on the soil. All about the pool into which the water subsided grew
various plants, that seemed to require a plentiful supply of moisture for the
nourishment of gigantic leaves, and, in some instances, flowers gorgeously
magnificent. There was one shrub in particular, set in a marble vase in the
midst of the pool, that bore a profusion of purple blossoms, each of which
had the lustre and richness of a gem; and the whole together made a show
so resplendent that it seemed enough to illuminate the garden, even had

there been no sunshine. Every portion of the soil was peopled with plants and herbs, which, if less beautiful, still bore tokens of assiduous care, as if all had their individual virtues, known to the scientific mind that fostered them. Some were placed in urns, rich with old carving, and others in common garden pots; some crept serpent-like along the ground or climbed on high, using whatever means of ascent was offered them. One plant had wreathed itself round a statue of Vertumnus, which was thus quite veiled and shrouded in a drapery of hanging foliage, so happily arranged that it might have served a sculptor for a study.

While Giovanni stood at the window he heard a rustling behind a screen of leaves, and became aware that a person was at work in the garden. His figure soon emerged into view, and showed itself to be that of no common laborer, but a tall, emaciated, sallow, and sickly-looking man, dressed in a scholar's garb of black. He was beyond the middle term of life, with gray hair, a thin, gray beard, and a face singularly marked with intellect and cultivation, but which could never, even in his more youthful days, have expressed much warmth of heart.

Nothing could exceed the intentness with which this scientific gardener examined every shrub which grew in his path: it seemed as if he was looking into their inmost nature, making observations in regard to their creative essence, and discovering why one leaf grew in this shape and another in that, and wherefore such and such flowers differed among themselves in hue and perfume. Nevertheless, in spite of this deep intelligence on his part, there was no approach to intimacy between himself and these vegetable existences. On the contrary, he avoided their actual touch or the direct inhaling of their odors with a caution that impressed Giovanni most disagreeably; for the man's demeanor was that of one walking among malignant influences, such as savage beasts, or deadly snakes, or evil spirits, which, should he allow them one moment of license, would wreak upon him some terrible fatality. It was strangely frightful to the young man's imagination to see this air of insecurity in a person cultivating a garden, that most simple and innocent of human toils, and which had been alike the joy and labor of the unfallen parents of the race. Was this garden, then, the Eden of the present world? And this man, with such a perception of harm in what his own hands caused to grow,—was he the Adam?

The distrustful gardener, while plucking away the dead leaves or pruning the too luxuriant growth of the shrubs, defended his hands with a pair of thick gloves. Nor were these his only armor. When, in his walk through the garden, he came to the magnificent plant that hung its purple gems beside the marble fountain, he placed a kind of mask over his mouth and nostrils, as if all this beauty did but conceal a deadlier malice; but, finding his task still too dangerous, he drew back, removed the mask, and called loudly, but in the infirm voice of a person affected with inward disease,—

"Beatrice! Beatrice!"

"Here am I, my father. What would you?" cried a rich and youthful voice from the window of the opposite house—a voice as rich as a tropical sunset, and which made Giovanni, though he knew not why, think of deep hues of purple or crimson and of perfumes heavily delectable. "Are you in the garden?"

"Yes, Beatrice," answered the gardener, "and I need your help."

Soon there emerged from under a sculptured portal the figure of a young girl, arrayed with as much richness of taste as the most splendid of the flowers, beautiful as the day, and with a bloom so deep and vivid that one shade more would have been too much. She looked redundant with life, health, and energy; all of which attributes were bound down and compressed, as it were, and girdled tensely, in their luxuriance, by her virgin zone. Yet Giovanni's fancy must have grown morbid while he looked down into the garden, for the impression which the fair stranger made upon him was as if here were another flower, the human sister of those vegetable ones, as beautiful as they, more beautiful than the richest of them, but still to be touched only with a glove, nor to be approached without a mask. As Beatrice came down the garden path, it was observable that she handled and inhaled the odor of several of the plants which her father had most sedulously avoided.

"Here, Beatrice," said the latter, "see how many needful offices require to be done to our chief treasure. Yet, shattered as I am, my life might pay the penalty of approaching it so closely as circumstances demand. Henceforth, I fear, this plant must be consigned to your sole charge."

"And gladly will I undertake it," cried again the rich tones of the young lady, as she bent towards the magnificent plant and opened her arms as if to embrace it. "Yes, my sister, my splendor, it shall be Beatrice's task to nurse and serve thee; and thou shalt reward her with thy kisses and perfumed breath, which to her is as the breath of life."

Then, with all the tenderness in her manner that was so strikingly expressed in her words, she busied herself with such attentions as the plant seemed to require; and Giovanni, at his lofty window, rubbed his eyes and almost doubted whether it were a girl tending her favorite flower, or one sister performing the duties of affection to another. The scene soon terminated. Whether Dr. Rappaccini had finished his labors in the garden, or that his watchful eye had caught the stranger's face, he now took his daughter's arm and retired. Night was already closing in; oppressive exhalations seemed to proceed from the plants and steal upward past the open window; and Giovanni, closing the lattice, went to his couch and dreamed of a rich flower and beautiful girl. Flower and maiden were different, and yet the same, and fraught with some strange peril in either shape.

But there is an influence in the light of morning that tends to rectify whatever errors of fancy, or even of judgment, we may have incurred during the sun's decline, or among the shadows of the night, or in the less wholesome glow of moonshine. Giovanni's first movement, on starting from sleep, was to throw open the window and gaze down into the garden which his dreams had made so fertile of mysteries. He was surprised and a little ashamed to find how real and matter-of-fact an affair it proved to be, in the first rays of the sun which gilded the dew-drops that hung upon leaf and blossom, and, while giving a brighter beauty to each rare flower, brought everything within the limits of ordinary experience. The young man rejoiced that, in the heart of the barren city, he had the privilege of overlooking this spot of lovely and luxuriant vegetation. It would serve, he said to himself, as a symbolic language to keep him in communion with Nature. Neither the sickly and thoughtworn Dr. Giacomo Rappaccini, it is true, nor his brilliant daughter, were now visible; so that Giovanni could not determine how much of the singularity which he attributed to both was due to their own qualities and how much to his wonder-working fancy; but he was inclined to take a most rational view of the whole matter.

In the course of the day he paid his respects to Signor Pietro Baglioni, professor of medicine in the university, a physician of eminent repute, to whom Giovanni had brought a letter of introduction. The professor was an elderly personage, apparently of genial nature, and habits that might almost be called jovial. He kept the young man to dinner, and made himself very agreeable by the freedom and liveliness of his conversation, especially when warmed by a flask or two of Tuscan wine. Giovanni, conceiving that men of science, inhabitants of the same city, must needs be on familiar terms with one another, took an opportunity to mention the name of Dr. Rappaccini. But the professor did not respond with so much cordiality as he had anticipated.

"Ill would it become a teacher of the divine art of medicine," said Professor Pietro Baglioni, in answer to a question of Giovanni, "to withhold due and well-considered praise of a physician so eminently skilled as Rappaccini; but, on the other hand, I should answer it but scantily to my conscience were I to permit a worthy youth like yourself, Signor Giovanni, the son of an ancient friend, to imbibe erroneous ideas respecting a man who might here-after chance to hold your life and death in his hands. The truth is, our worshipful Dr. Rappaccini has as much science as any member of the faculty—with perhaps one single exception—in Padua, or all Italy; but there are certain grave objections to his professional character."

"And what are they?" asked the young man.

"Has my friend Giovanni any disease of body or heart, that he is so inquisitive about physicians?" said the professor, with a smile. "But as for Rappaccini, it is said of him—and I, who know the man well, can answer for its truth—that he cares infinitely more for science than for mankind. His patients are interesting to him only as subjects for some new experiment. He would sacrifice human life, his own among the rest, or whatever else was dearest to him, for the sake of adding so much as a grain of mustard seed to the great heap of his accumulated knowledge."

"Methinks he is an awful man indeed," remarked Guasconti, mentally recalling the cold and purely intellectual aspect of Rappaccini. "And yet, worshipful professor, is it not a noble spirit? Are there many men capable of so spiritual a love of science?"

"God forbid," answered the professor, somewhat testily; "at least, unless they take sounder views of the healing art than those adopted by Rappaccini. It is his theory that all medicinal virtues are comprised within those substances which we term vegetable poisons. These he cultivates with his own hands, and is said even to have produced new varieties of poison, more horribly deleterious than Nature, without the assistance of this learned person, would ever have plagued the world withal. That the signor doctor does less mischief than might be expected with such dangerous substances is undeniable. Now and then, it must be owned, he has effected, or seemed to effect, a marvellous cure; but, to tell you my private mind, Signor Giovanni, he should receive little credit for such instances of success,—they being probably the work of chance,—but should be held strictly accountable for his failures, which may justly be considered his own work."

The youth might have taken Baglioni's opinions with many grains of allowance had he known that there was a professional warfare of long continuance between him and Dr. Rappaccini, in which the latter was generally thought to have gained the advantage. If the reader be inclined to judge for himself, we refer him to certain black-letter tracts on both sides, preserved in the medical department of the University of Padua.

"I know not, most learned professor," returned Giovanni, after musing on what had been said of Rappaccini's exclusive zeal for science,—"I know not how dearly this physician may love his art; but surely there is one object more dear to him. He has a daughter."

"Aha!" cried the professor, with a laugh. "So now our friend Giovanni's secret is out. You have heard of this daughter, whom all the young men in Padua are wild about, though not half a dozen have ever had the good hap to see her face. I know little of the Signora Beatrice save that Rappaccini is said to have instructed her deeply in his science, and that, young and beautiful as fame reports her, she is already qualified to fill a professor's chair. Perchance her father destines her for mine! Other absurd rumors there be, not worth talking about or listening to. So now, Signor Giovanni, drink off your glass of lachryma."

Guasconti returned to his lodgings somewhat heated with the wine he had quaffed, and which caused his brain to swim with strange fantasies in reference to Dr. Rappaccini and the beautiful Beatrice. On his way, happening to pass by a florist's, he bought a fresh bouquet of flowers.

Ascending to his chamber, he seated himself near the window, but within the shadow thrown by the depth of the wall, so that he could look down into the garden with little risk of being discovered. All beneath his eye was a solitude. The strange plants were basking in the sunshine, and now and then nodding gently to one another, as if in acknowledgment of sympathy and kindred. In the midst, by the shattered fountain, grew the magnificent shrub, with its purple gems clustering all over it; they glowed in the air, and gleamed back again out of the depths of the pool, which thus seemed to overflow with colored radiance from the rich reflection that was steeped in it. At first, as we have said, the garden was a solitude. Soon, however,—as Giovanni had half hoped, half feared, would be the case,—a figure appeared beneath the antique sculptured portal, and came down between the rows of plants, inhaling their various perfumes as if she were one of those beings of old classic fable that lived upon sweet odors. On again beholding Beatrice, the young man was even startled to perceive how much her beauty exceeded his recollection of it; so brilliant, so vivid, was its character, that she glowed amid the sunlight, and, as Giovanni whispered to himself, positively illuminated the more shadowy intervals of the garden path. Her face being now more revealed than on the former occasion, he was struck by its expression of simplicity and sweetness,— qualities that had not entered into his idea of her character, and which made him ask anew what manner of mortal she might be. Nor did he fail again to observe, or imagine, an analogy between the beautiful girl and the gorgeous shrub that hung its gemlike flowers over the fountain,—a resemblance which Beatrice seemed to have indulged a fantastic humor in heightening, both by the arrangement of her dress and the selection of its hues.

Approaching the shrub, she threw open her arms, as with a passionate ardor, and drew its branches into an intimate embrace—so intimate that her features were hidden in its leafy bosom and her glistening ringlets all intermingled with the flowers.

"Give me thy breath, my sister," exclaimed Beatrice; "for I am faint with common air. And give me this flower of thine, which I separate with gentlest fingers from the stem and place it close beside my heart."

With these words the beautiful daughter of Rappaccini plucked one of the richest blossoms of the shrub, and was about to fasten it in her bosom. But now, unless Giovanni's draughts of wine had bewildered his senses, a singular incident occurred. A small orange-colored reptile, of the lizard or chameleon species, chanced to be creeping along the path, just at the feet of Beatrice. It appeared to Giovanni,—but, at the distance from which he gazed, he could scarcely have seen anything so minute,—it appeared to him, however, that a drop or two of moisture from the broken stem of the flower descended upon the lizard's head. For an instant the reptile contorted itself violently, and then lay motionless in the sunshine. Beatrice observed this remarkable phenomenon, and crossed herself, sadly, but without surprise; nor did she therefore hesitate to arrange the fatal flower in her bosom. There it blushed, and almost glimmered with the dazzling effect of a precious stone, adding to her dress and aspect the one appropriate charm which nothing else in the world could have supplied. But Giovanni, out of the shadow of his window, bent forward and shrank back, and murmured and trembled.

"Am I awake? Have I my senses?" said he to himself. "What is this being? Beautiful shall I call her, or inexpressibly terrible?"

Beatrice now strayed carelessly through the garden, approaching closer beneath Giovanni's window, so that he was compelled to thrust his head quite out of its concealment in order to gratify the intense and painful curiosity which she excited. At this moment there came a beautiful insect over the garden wall; it had, perhaps, wandered through the city, and found no flowers of verdue among those antique haunts of men until the heavy perfumes of Dr. Rappaccini's shrubs had lured it from afar. Without alighting on the flowers, this winged brightness seemed to be attracted by Beatrice, and lingered in the air and fluttered about her head. Now, here it could not be but that Giovanni Guasconti's eyes deceived him. Be that as it might, he fancied that, while Beatrice was gazing at the insect with childish delight, it grew faint and fell at her feet; its bright wings shivered; it was dead—from no cause that he could discern, unless it were the atmosphere of her breath. Again Beatrice crossed herself and sighed heavily as she bent over the dead insect.

An impulsive movement of Giovanni drew her eyes to the window. There she beheld the beautiful head of the young man—rather a Grecian than an Italian head, with fair, regular features, and a glistening of gold among his ringlets—gazing down upon her like a being that hovered in mid air. Scarcely knowing what he did, Giovanni threw down the bouquet which he had hitherto held in his hand.

"Signora," said he, "there are pure and healthful flowers. Wear them for the sake of Giovanni Guasconti."

"Thanks, signor," replied Beatrice, with her rich voice, that came forth as it were like a gush of music, and with a mirthful expression half childish and half woman-like. "I accept your gift, and would fain recompense it with this precious purple flower; but if I toss it into the air it will not reach you. So Signor Guasconti must even content himself with my thanks."

She lifted the bouquet from the ground, and then, as if inwardly ashamed at having stepped aside from her maidenly reserve to respond to a stranger's greeting, passed swiftly homeward through the garden. But few as the moments were, it seemed to Giovanni, when she was on the point of vanishing beneath the sculptured portal, that his beautiful bouquet was already beginning to wither in her grasp. It was an idle thought; there could be no possibility of distinguishing a faded flower from a fresh one at so great a distance.

For many days after this incident the young man avoided the window that looked into Dr. Rappaccini's garden, as if something ugly and monstrous would have blasted his eyesight had he been betrayed into a glance. He felt conscious of having put himself, to a certain extent, within the influence of an unintelligible power by the communication which he had opened with Beatrice. The wisest course would have been, if his heart were in any real danger, to quit his lodgings and Padua itself at once; the next wiser, to have accustomed himself, as far as possible, to the familiar and daylight view of Beatrice—thus bringing her rigidly and systematically within the limits of ordinary experience. Least of all, while avoiding her sight, ought Giovanni to have remained so near this extraordinary being that the proximity and possibility even of intercourse should give a kind of substance and reality to the wild vagaries which his imagination ran riot continually in producing. Guasconti had not a deep heart—or, at all events, its depths were not sounded now; but he had a quick fancy, and an ardent southern temperament, which rose every instant to a higher fever pitch. Whether or no Beatrice possessed those terrible attributes, that fatal breath, the affinity with those so beautiful and deadly flowers which were indicated by what Giovanni had witnessed, she had at least instilled a fierce and subtle poison into his system. It was not love, although her rich beauty was a madness to him; nor horror, even while he fancied her spirit to be imbued with the same baneful essence that seemed to pervade her physical frame; but a wild offspring of both love and horror that had each parent in it, and burned like one and shivered like the other. Giovanni knew not what to dread; still less did he know what to hope; yet hope and dread kept a continual warfare in his breast, alternately vanquishing one another and starting up afresh to renew the contest. Blessed are all simple emotions, be they dark or bright! It is the lurid intermixture of the two that produces the illuminating blaze of the infernal regions.

Sometimes he endeavored to assuage the fever of his spirit by a rapid walk through the streets of Padua or beyond its gates: his footsteps kept time with the throbbings of his brain, so that the walk was apt to accelerate itself to a race. One day he found himself arrested; his arm was seized by a portly personage, who had turned back on recognizing the young man and expended much breath in overtaking him.

"Signor Giovanni! Stay, my young friend!" cried he. "Have you forgotten me? That might well be the case if I were as much altered as yourself."

It was Baglioni, whom Giovanni had avoided ever since their first meeting, from a doubt that the professor's sagacity would look too deeply into his secrets. Endeavoring to recover himself, he stared forth wildly from his inner world into the outer one and spoke like a man in a dream.

"Yes; I am Giovanni Guasconti. You are Professor Pietro Baglioni. Now let me pass!"

"Not yet, not yet, Signor Giovanni Guasconti," said the professor, smiling, but at the same time scrutinizing the youth with an earnest glance. "What!" did I grow up side by side with your father? and shall his son pass me like a stranger in these old streets of Padua? Stand still, Signor Giovanni; for we must have a word or two before we part."

"Speedily, then, most worshipful professor, speedily," said Giovanni, with feverish impatience. "Does not your worship see that I am in haste?"

Now, while he was speaking there came a man in black along the street, stooping and moving feebly like a person in inferior health. His face was all overspread with a most sickly and sallow hue, but yet so pervaded with an expression of piercing and active intellect that an observer might easily have overlooked the merely physical attributes and have seen only this wonderful energy. As he passed, this person exchanged a cold and distant salutation with Baglioni, but fixed his eyes upon Giovanni with an intentness that seemed to bring out whatever was within him worthy of notice. Nevertheless, there was a peculiar quietness in the look, as if taking merely a speculative, not a human, interest in the young man.

"It is Dr. Rappaccini!" whispered the professor when the stranger had passed. "Has he ever seen your face before?"

"Not that I know," answered Giovanni, starting at the name.

"He *has* seen you! he must have seen you!" said Baglioni, hastily. "For some purpose or other, this man of science is making a study of you. I know that look of his! It is the same that coldly illuminates his face as he bends over a bird, a mouse, or a butterfly, which, in pursuance of some experiment, he has killed by the perfume of a flower; a look as deep as Nature itself, but without Nature's warmth of love. Signor Giovanni, I will stake my life upon it, you are the subject of one of Rappaccini's experiments!"

"Will you make a fool of me?" cried Giovanni, passionately. "*That,* signor professor, were an untoward experiment."

"Patience! patience!" replied the imperturbable professor. "I tell thee, my poor Giovanni, that Rappaccini has a scientific interest in thee. Thou hast fallen into fearful hands! And the Signora Beatrice,—what part does she act in this mystery?"

But Guasconti, finding Baglioni's pertinacity intolerable, here broke away, and was gone before the professor could again seize his arm. He looked after the young man intently and shook his head.

"This must not be," said Baglioni to himself. "The youth is the son of my old friend, and shall not come to any harm from which the arcana of medical science can preserve him. Besides, it is too insufferable an impertinence in Rappaccini, thus to snatch the lad out of my own hands, as I may say, and make use of him for his infernal experiments. This daughter of his! It shall be looked to. Perchance, most learned Rappaccini, I may foil you where you little dream of it!"

Meanwhile Giovanni had pursued a circuitous route, and at length found himself at the door of his lodgings. As he crossed the threshold he was met by old Lisabetta, who smirked and smiled, and was evidently desirous to attract his attention; vainly, however, as the ebullition of his feelings had momentarily subsided into a cold and dull vacuity. He turned his eyes full upon the withered face that was puckering itself into a smile, but seemed to behold it not. The old dame, therefore, laid her grasp upon his cloak.

"Signor! signor!" whispered she, still with a smile over the whole breadth of her visage, so that it looked not unlike a grotesque carving in wood, darkened by centuries. "Listen, signor! There is a private entrance into the garden!"

"What do you say?" exclaimed Giovanni, turning quickly about, as if an inanimate thing should start into feverish life. "A private entrance into Dr. Rappaccini's garden?"

"Hush! hush! not so loud!" whispered Lisabetta, putting her hand over his mouth. "Yes; into the worshipful doctor's garden, where you may see all his fine shrubbery. Many a young man in Padua would give gold to be admitted among those flowers."

Giovanni put a piece of gold into her hand.

"Show me the way," said he.

A surmise, probably excited by his conversation with Baglioni, crossed his mind, that this interposition of old Lisabetta might perchance be connected with the intrigue, whatever were its nature, in which the professor seemed to suppose that Dr. Rappaccini was involving him. But such a suspicion, though it disturbed Giovanni, was inadequate to restrain him. The instant that he was aware of the possibility of approaching Beatrice, it seemed an absolute necessity of his existence to do so. It mattered not whether she were angel or demon; he was irrevocably within her sphere, and must obey the law that whirled him onward, in ever-lessening circles, towards a result which he did not attempt to foreshadow; and yet, strange to say, there came across him a sudden doubt whether this intense interest on his part were not delusory; whether it were really of so deep and positive a nature as to justify him in now thrusting himself into an incalculable position; whether it were not merely the fantasy of a young man's brain, only slightly or not at all connected with his heart.

He paused, hesitated, turned half about, but again went on. His withered guide led him along several obscure passages, and finally undid a door, through which, as it was opened, there came the sight and sound of rustling leaves, with the broken sunshine glimmering among them. Giovanni stepped forth, and, forcing himself through the entanglement of a shrub that wreathed its tendrils over the hidden entrance, stood beneath his own window in the open area of Dr. Rappaccini's garden.

How often is it the case that, when impossibilities have come to pass and dreams have condensed their misty substance into tangible realities, we find ourselves calm, and even coldly self-possessed, amid circumstances which it would have been a delirium of joy or agony to anticipate! Fate delights to thwart us thus. Passion will choose his own time to rush upon the scene, and lingers sluggishly behind when an appropriate adjustment of events would seem to summon his appearance. So was it now with Giovanni. Day after day his pulse had throbbed with feverish blood at the improbable idea of an interview with Beatrice, and of standing with her, face to face, in this very garden, basking in the Oriental sunshine of her beauty, and snatching from her full gaze the mystery which he deemed the riddle of his own existence. But now there was a singular and untimely equanimity within his breast. He threw a glance around the garden to discover if Beatrice or her father were present, and, perceiving that he was alone, began a critical observation of the plants.

The aspect of one and all of them dissatisfied him; their gorgeousness seemed fierce, passionate, and even unnatural. There was hardly an individual shrub which a wanderer, straying by himself through a forest, would not have been startled to find growing wild, as if an unearthly face had glared at him out of the thicket. Several also would have shocked a delicate instinct by an appearance of artificialness indicating that there had been such commixture, and, as it were, adultery, of various vegetable species, that the production was no longer of God's making, but the monstrous offspring of man's depraved fancy, glowing with only an evil mockery of beauty. They were probably the result of experiment, which in one or two cases had succeeded in mingling plants individually lovely into a compound possessing the questionable and ominous character that distinguished the whole growth of the garden. In fine, Giovanni recognized but two or three plants in the collection, and those of a kind that he well knew to be poisonous. While busy with these contemplations he heard the rustling of a silken garment, and, turning, beheld Beatrice emerging from beneath the sculptured portal.

Giovanni had not considered with himself what should be his deportment; whether he should apologize for his intrusion into the garden, or assume that he was there with the privity at least, if not by the desire, of Dr. Rappaccini or his daughter; but Beatrice's manner placed him at his ease, though leaving him still in doubt by what agency he had gained admittance. She came lightly along the path and met him near the broken fountain. There was surprise in her face, but brightened by a simple and kind expression of pleasure.

"You are a connoisseur in flowers, signor," said Beatrice, with a smile, alluding to the bouquet which he had flung her from the window. "It is no marvel, therefore, if the sight of my father's rare collection has tempted you to take a nearer view. If he were here, he could tell you many strange and interesting facts as to the nature and habits of these shrubs; for he has spent a lifetime in such studies, and this garden is his world."

"And yourself, lady," observed Giovanni, "if fame says true,—you likewise are deeply skilled in the virtues indicated by these rich blossoms and these spicy perfumes. Would you deign to be my instructress, I should prove an apter scholar than if taught by Signor Rappaccini himself."

"Are there such idle rumors?" asked Beatrice, with the music of a pleasant laugh. "Do people say that I am skilled in my father's science of plants? What a jest is there! No; though I have grown up among these flowers, I know no more of them than their hues and perfume; and sometimes methinks I would fain rid myself of even that small knowledge. There are many

flowers here, and those not the least brilliant, that shock and offend me when
they meet my eye. But pray, signor, do not believe these stories about my
science. Believe nothing of me save what you see with your own eyes."

"And must I believe all that I have seen with my own eyes?" asked Giovanni, pointedly, while the recollection of former scenes made him shrink.
"No, signora; you demand too little of me. Bid me believe nothing save what
comes from your own lips."

It would appear that Beatrice understood him. There came a deep flush to
her cheek; but she looked full into Giovanni's eyes, and responded to his gaze
of uneasy suspicion with a queenlike haughtiness.

"I do so bid you, signor," she replied. "Forget whatever you may have
fancied in regard to me. If true to the outward senses, still it may be false
in its essence; but the words of Beatrice Rappaccini's lips are true from the
depths of the heart outward. Those you may believe."

A fervor glowed in her whole aspect and beamed upon Giovanni's consciousness like the light of truth itself; but while she spoke there was a fragrance in
the atmosphere around her, rich and delightful, though evanescent, yet which
the young man, from an indefinable reluctance, scarcely dared to draw into
his lungs. It might be the odor of the flowers. Could it be Beatrice's breath
which thus embalmed her words with a strange richness, as if by steeping
them in her heart? A faintness passed like a shadow over Giovanni and flitted
away; he seemed to gaze through the beautiful girl's eyes into her transparent
soul, and felt no more doubt or fear.

The tinge of passion that had colored Beatrice's manner vanished; she became gay, and appeared to derive a pure delight from her communion with
the youth not unlike what the maiden of a lonely island might have felt
conversing with a voyager from the civilized world. Evidently her experience
of life had been confined within the limits of that garden. She talked now
about matters as simple as the daylight or summer clouds, and now asked
questions in reference to the city, or Giovanni's distant home, his friends, his
mother, and his sisters—questions indicating such seclusion, and such lack of
familiarity with modes and forms, that Giovanni responded as if to an infant.
Her spirit gushed out before him like a fresh rill that was just catching its
first glimpse of the sunlight and wondering at the reflections of earth and sky
which were flung into its bosom. There came thoughts, too, from a deep
source, and fantasies of a gemlike brilliancy, as if diamonds and rubies
sparkled upward among the bubbles of the fountain. Ever and anon there
gleamed across the young man's mind a sense of wonder that he should be
walking side by side with the being who had so wrought upon his imagination,
whom he had idealized in such hues of terror, in whom he had positively
witnessed such manifestations of dreadful attributes,—that he should be conversing with Beatrice like a brother, and should find her so human and so
maidenlike. But such reflections were only momentary; the effect of her
character was too real not to make itself familiar at once.

In this free intercourse they had strayed through the garden, and now, after many turns among its avenues, were come to the shattered fountain, beside which grew the magnificent shrub, with its treasury of glowing blossoms. A fragrance was diffused from it which Giovanni recognized as identical with that which he had attributed to Beatrice's breath, but incomparably more powerful. As her eyes fell upon it, Giovanni beheld her press her hand to her bosom as if her heart were throbbing suddenly and painfully.

"For the first time in my life," murmured she, addressing the shrub, "I had forgotten thee."

"I remember, signora," said Giovanni, "that you once promised to reward me with one of these living gems for the bouquet which I had the happy boldness to fling to your feet. Permit me now to pluck it as a memorial of this interview."

He made a step toward the shrub with extended hand; but Beatrice darted forward, uttering a shriek that went through his heart like a dagger. She caught his hand and drew it back with the whole force of her slender figure. Giovanni felt her touch thrilling through his fibres.

"Touch it not!" exclaimed she, in a voice of agony. "Not for thy life! It is fatal!"

Then, hiding her face, she fled from him and vanished beneath the sculptured portal. As Giovanni followed her with his eyes, he beheld the emaciated figure and pale intelligence of Dr. Rappaccini, who had been watching the scene, he knew not how long, within the shadow of the entrance.

No sooner was Guasconti alone in his chamber than the image of Beatrice came back to his passionate musings, invested with all the witchery that had been gathering around it ever since his first glimpse of her, and now likewise imbued with a tender warmth of girlish womanhood. She was human; her nature was endowed with all gentle and feminine qualities; she was worthiest to be worshipped; she was capable, surely, on her part, of the height and heroism of love. Those tokens which he had hitherto considered as proofs of a frightful peculiarity in her physical and moral system were now either forgotten, or, by the subtle sophistry of passion transmitted into a golden crown of enchantment, rendering Beatrice the more admirable by so much as she was the more unique. Whatever had looked ugly was now beautiful; or, if incapable of such a change, it stole away and hid itself among those shapeless half ideas which throng the dim region beyond the daylight of our perfect consciousness. Thus did he spend the night, nor fell asleep until the dawn had begun to awake the slumbering flowers in Dr. Rappaccini's garden, whither Giovanni's dreams doubtless led him. Up rose the sun in his due season, and, flinging his beams upon the young man's eyelids, awoke him to a sense of pain. When thoroughly aroused, he became sensible of a burning and tingling agony in his hand—in his right hand—the very hand which Beatrice had grasped in her own when he was on the point of plucking one of the gemlike flowers. On the back of that hand there was now a purple print like that of four small fingers, and the likeness of a slender thumb upon his wrist.

Oh, how stubbornly does love,—or even that cunning semblance of love which flourishes in the imagination, but strikes no depth of root into the heart,—how stubbornly does it hold its faith until the moment comes when it is doomed to vanish into thin mist! Giovanni wrapped a handkerchief about his hand and wondered what evil thing had stung him, and soon forgot his pain in a reverie of Beatrice.

After the first interview, a second was in the inevitable course of what we call fate. A third; a fourth; and a meeting with Beatrice in the garden was no longer an incident in Giovanni's daily life, but the whole space in which he might be said to live; for the anticipation and memory of that ecstatic hour made up the remainder. Nor was it otherwise with the daughter of Rappaccini. She watched for the youth's appearance, and flew to his side with confidence as unreserved as if they had been playmates from early infancy—as if they were such playmates still. If, by any unwonted chance, he failed to come at the appointed moment, she stood beneath the window and sent up the rich sweetness of her tones to float around him in his chamber and echo and reverberate throughout his heart: "Giovanni! Giovanni! Why tarriest thou? Come down!" And down he hastened into that Eden of poisonous flowers.

But, with all this intimate familiarity, there was still a reserve in Beatrice's demeanor, so rigidly and invariably sustained that the idea of infringing it scarcely occurred to his imagination. By all applicable signs, they loved; they had looked love with eyes that conveyed the holy secret from the depths of one soul into the depths of the other, as if it were too sacred to be whispered by the way; they had even spoken love in those gushes of passion when their spirits darted forth in articulated breath like tongues of long-hidden flame; and yet there had been no seal of lips, no clasp of hands, nor any slightest caress such as love claims and hallows. He had never touched one of the gleaming ringlets of her hair; her garment—so marked was the physical barrier between them—had never been waved against him by a breeze. On the few occasions when Giovanni had seemed tempted to overstep the limit, Beatrice grew so sad, so stern, and withal wore such a look of desolate separation, shuddering at itself, that not a spoken word was requisite to repel him. At such times he was startled at the horrible suspicions that rose, monster-like, out of the caverns of his heart and stared him in the face; his love grew thin and faint as the morning mist, his doubts alone had substance. But, when Beatrice's face brightened again after the momentary shadow, she was transformed at once from the mysterious, questionable being whom he had watched with so much awe and horror; she was now the beautiful and unsophisticated girl whom he felt that his spirit knew with a certainty beyond all other knowledge.

A considerable time had now passed since Giovanni's last meeting with Baglioni. One morning, however, he was disagreeably surprised by a visit from the professor, whom he had scarcely thought of for whole weeks, and would willingly have forgotten still longer. Given up as he had long been to a pervading excitement, he could tolerate no companions except upon condition of their perfect sympathy with his present state of feeling. Such sympathy was not to be expected from Professor Baglioni.

The visitor chatted carelessly for a few moments about the gossip of the city and the university, and then took up another topic.

"I have been reading an old classic author lately," said he, "and met with a story that strangely interested me. Possibly you may remember it. It is of an Indian prince, who sent a beautiful woman as a present to Alexander the Great. She was as lovely as the dawn and gorgeous as the sunset; but what especially distinguished her was a certain rich perfume in her breath—richer than a garden of Persian roses. Alexander, as was natural to a youthful conqueror, fell in love at first sight with this magnificent stranger; but a certain sage physician, happening to be present, discovered a terrible secret in regard to her."

"And what was that?" asked Giovanni, turning his eyes downward to avoid those of the professor.

"That this lovely woman," continued Baglioni, with emphasis, "had been nourished with poisons from her birth upward, until her whole nature was so imbued with them that she herself had become the deadliest poison in existence. Poison was her element of life. With that rich perfume of her breath she blasted the very air. Her love would have been poison—her embrace death. Is not this a marvelous tale?"

"A childish fable," answered Giovanni, nervously starting from his chair. "I marvel how your worship finds time to read such nonsense among your graver studies."

"By the by," said the professor, looking uneasily about him, "what singular fragrance is this in your apartment? Is it the perfume of your gloves? It is faint, but delicious; and yet, after all, by no means agreeable. Were I to breathe it long, methinks it would make me ill. It is like the breath of a flower; but I see no flowers in the chamber."

"Nor are there any," replied Giovanni, who had turned pale as the professor spoke; "nor, I think, is there any fragrance except in your worship's imagination. Odors, being a sort of element combined of the sensual and the spiritual, are apt to deceive us in this manner. The recollection of a perfume, the bare idea of it, may easily be mistaken for a present reality."

"Aye; but my sober imagination does not often play such tricks," said Baglioni; "and, were I to fancy any kind of odor, it would be that of some vile apothecary drug, wherewith my fingers are likely enough to be imbued. Our worshipful friend Rappaccini, as I have heard, tinctures his medicaments with odors richer than those of Araby. Doubtless, likewise, the fair and learned Signora Beatrice would minister to her patients with draughts as sweet as a maiden's breath; but woe to him that sips them!"

Giovanni's face evinced many contending emotions. The tone in which the professor alluded to the pure and lovely daughter of Rappaccini was a torture to his soul; and yet the intimation of a view of her character, opposite to his own, gave instantaneous distinctness to a thousand dim suspicions, which now grinned at him like so many demons. But he strove hard to quell them and to respond to Baglioni with a true lover's perfect faith.

"Signor professor," said he, "you were my father's friend; perchance, too, it is your purpose to act a friendly part towards his son. I would fain feel nothing towards you save respect and deference; but I pray you to observe, signor, that there is one subject on which we must not speak. You know not the Signora Beatrice. You cannot, therefore, estimate the wrong—the blasphemy, I may even say—that is offered to her character by a light or injurious word."

"Giovanni! my poor Giovanni!" answered the professor, with a calm expression of pity, "I know this wretched girl far better than yourself. You shall hear the truth in respect to the poisoner Rappaccini and his poisonous daughter; yes, poisonous as she is beautiful. Listen; for, even should you do violence to my gray hairs, it shall not silence me. That old fable of the Indian woman has become a truth by the deep and deadly science of Rappaccini and in the person of the lovely Beatrice."

Giovanni groaned and hid his face.

"Her father," continued Baglioni, "was not restrained by natural affection from offering up his child in this horrible manner as the victim of his insane zeal for science; for, let us do him justice, he is as true a man of science as ever distilled his own heart in an alembic. What, then, will be your fate? Beyond a doubt you are selected as the material of some new experiment. Perhaps the result is to be death; perhaps a fate more awful still. Rappaccini, with what he calls the interest of science before his eyes, will hesitate at nothing."

"It is a dream," muttered Giovanni to himself; "surely it is a dream."

"But," resumed the professor, "be of good cheer, son of my friend. It is not yet too late for the rescue. Possibly we may even succeed in bringing back this miserable child within the limits of ordinary nature, from which her father's madness has estranged her. Behold this little silver vase! It was wrought by the hands of the renowned Benvenuto Cellini, and is well worthy to be a love gift to the fairest dame in Italy. But its contents are invaluable. One little sip of this antidote would have rendered the most virulent poisons of the Borgias innocuous. Doubt not that it will be as efficacious against those of Rappaccini. Bestow the vase, and the precious liquid within it, on your Beatrice, and hopefully await the result."

Baglioni laid a small, exquisitely wrought silver vial on the table and withdrew, leaving what he had said to produce its effect upon the young man's mind.

"We will thwart Rappaccini yet," thought he, chuckling to himself, as he descended the stairs; "but, let us confess the truth of him, he is a wonderful man—a wonderful man indeed; a vile empiric, however, in his practice, and therefore not to be tolerated by those who respect the good old rules of the medical profession."

Throughout Giovanni's whole acquaintance with Beatrice, he had occasionally, as we have said, been haunted by dark surmises as to her character; yet so thoroughly had she made herself felt by him as a simple, natural, most affectionate, and guileless creature, that the image now held up by Professor Baglioni looked as strange and incredible as if it were not in accordance with his own original conception. True, there were ugly recollections connected with his first glimpses of the beautiful girl; he could not quite forget the bouquet that withered in her grasp, and the insect that perished amid the sunny air, by no ostensible agency save the fragrance of her breath. These incidents, however, dissolving in the pure light of her character, had no longer the efficacy of facts, but were acknowledged as mistaken fantasies, by whatever testimony of the senses they might appear to be substantiated. There is something truer and more real than what we can see with the eyes and touch with the finger. On such better evidence had Giovanni founded his confidence in Beatrice, though rather by the necessary force of her high attributes than by any deep and generous faith on his part. But now his spirit was incapable of sustaining itself at the height to which the early enthusiasm of passion had exalted it; he fell down, grovelling among earthly doubts, and defiled therewith the pure whiteness of Beatrice's image. Not that he gave her up; he did but distrust. He resolved to institute some decisive test that should satisfy him, once for all, whether there were those dreadful peculiarities in her physical nature which could not be supposed to exist without some corresponding monstrosity of soul. His eyes, gazing down afar, might have deceived him as to the lizard, the insect, and the flowers; but if he could witness, at the distance of a few paces, the sudden blight of one fresh and healthful flower in Beatrice's hand, there would be room for no further question. With this idea he hastened to the florist's and purchased a bouquet that was still gemmed with the morning dew-drops.

It was now the customary hour of his daily interview with Beatrice. Before descending into the garden, Giovanni failed not to look at his figure in the mirror,—a vanity to be expected in a beautiful young man, yet, as displaying itself at that troubled and feverish moment, the token of a certain shallowness of feeling and insincerity of character. He did gaze, however, and said to himself that his features had never before possessed so rich a grace, nor his eyes such vivacity, nor his cheeks so warm a hue of superabundant life.

"At least," thought he, "her poison has not yet insinuated itself into my system. I am no flower to perish in her grasp."

With that thought he turned his eyes on the bouquet, which he had never once laid aside from his hand. A thrill of indefinable horror shot through his frame on perceiving that those dewy flowers were already beginning to droop; they wore the aspect of things that had been fresh and lovely yesterday. Gio-

vanni grew white as marble, and stood motionless before the mirror, staring
at his own reflection there as at the likeness of something frightful. He remembered Baglioni's remark about the fragrance that seemed to pervade the
chamber. It must have been the poison in his breath! Then he shuddered—
shuddered at himself. Recovering from his stupor, he began to watch with
curious eye a spider that was busily at work hanging its web from the antique
cornice of the apartment, crossing and recrossing the artful system of inter-
woven lines—as vigorous and active a spider as ever dangled from an old ceiling. Giovanni bent towards the insect, and emitted a deep, long breath. The
spider suddenly ceased its toil; the web vibrated with a tremor originating in
the body of the small artisan. Again Giovanni sent forth a breath, deeper,
longer, and imbued with a venomous feeling out of his heart: he knew not
whether he were wicked, or only desperate. The spider made a convulsive
gripe with his limbs and hung dead across the window.

"Accursed! accursed!" muttered Giovanni, addressing himself. "Hast thou
grown so poisonous that this deadly insect perishes by thy breath?"

At that moment a rich, sweet voice came floating up from the garden.

"Giovanni! Giovanni! It is past the hour! Why tarriest thou? Come down!"

"Yes," muttered Giovanni again. "She is the only being whom my breath
may not slay! Would that it might!"

He rushed down, and in an instant was standing before the bright and
loving eyes of Beatrice. A moment ago his wrath and despair had been so
fierce that he could have desired nothing so much as to wither her by a glance;
but with her actual presence there came influences which had too real an existence to be at once shaken off: recollections of the delicate and benign power
of her feminine nature, which had so often enveloped him in a religious calm;
recollections of many a holy and passionate outgush of her heart, when the
pure fountain had been unsealed from its depths and made visible in its trans-
parency to his mental eye; recollections which, had Giovanni known how to
estimate them, would have assured him that all this ugly mystery was but an
earthly illusion, and that, whatever mist of evil might seem to have gathered
over her, the real Beatrice was a heavenly angel. Incapable as he was of such
high faith, still her presence had not utterly lost its magic. Giovanni's rage
was quelled into an aspect of sullen insensibility. Beatrice, with a quick spiritual sense, immediately felt that there was a gulf of blackness between them
which neither he nor she could pass. They walked on together, sad and silent,
and came thus to the marble fountain and to its pool of water on the ground,
in the midst of which grew the shrub that bore gem-like blossoms. Giovanni
was affrighted at the eager enjoyment—the appetite, as it were—with which
he found himself inhaling the fragrance of the flowers.

"Beatrice," asked he, abruptly, "whence came this shrub?"

"My father created it," answered she, with simplicity.

"Created it! created it!" repeated Giovanni. "What mean you, Beatrice?"

"He is a man fearfully acquainted with the secrets of Nature," replied

Beatrice; "and, at the hour when I first drew breath, this plant sprang from the soil, the offspring of his science, of his intellect, while I was but his earthly child. Approach it not!" continued she, observing with terror that Giovanni was drawing nearer to the shrub. "It has qualities that you little dream of. But I, dearest Giovanni,—grew up and blossomed with the plant and was nourished with its breath. It was my sister, and I loved it with a human affection; for, alas!—hast thou not suspected it?—there was an awful doom."

Here Giovanni frowned so darkly upon her that Beatrice paused and trembled. But her faith in his tenderness reassured her, and made her blush that she had doubted for an instant.

"There was an awful doom," she continued, "the effect of my father's fatal love of science, which estranged me from all society of my kind. Until Heaven sent thee, dearest Giovanni, oh, how lonely was thy poor Beatrice!"

"Was it a hard doom?" asked Giovanni, fixing his eyes upon her.

"Only of late have I known how hard it was," answered she, tenderly. "Oh, yes; but my heart was torpid, and therefore quiet."

Giovanni's rage broke forth from his sullen gloom like a lightning flash out of a dark cloud.

"Accursed one!" cried he, with venomous scorn and anger. "And, finding thy solitude wearisome, thou hast severed me likewise from all the warmth of life and enticed me into thy region of unspeakable horror!"

"Giovanni!" exclaimed Beatrice, turning her large bright eyes upon his face. The force of his words had not found its way into her mind; she was merely thunderstruck.

"Yes, poisonous thing!" repeated Giovanni, beside himself with passion. "Thou hast done it! Thou hast blasted me! Thou hast filled my veins with poison! Thou hast made me as hateful, as ugly, as loathsome and deadly a creature as thyself—a world's wonder of hideous monstrosity! Now, if our breath be happily as fatal to ourselves as to all others, let us join our lips in one kiss of unutterable hatred, and so die!"

"What has befallen me?" murmured Beatrice, with a low moan out of her heart. "Holy Virgin, pity me, a poor heart-broken child!"

"Thou,—dost thou pray?" cried Giovanni, still with the same fiendish scorn. "Thy very prayers, as they come from thy lips, taint the atmosphere with death. Yes, yes; let us pray! Let us to church and dip our fingers in the holy water at the portal! They that come after us will perish as by a pestilence! Let us sign crosses in the air! It will be scattering curses abroad in the likeness of holy symbols!"

"Giovanni," said Beatrice, calmly, for her grief was beyond passion, "why dost thou join thyself with me thus in those terrible words? I, it is true, am the horrible thing thou namest me. But thou,—what hast thou to do, save with one other shudder at my hideous misery to go forth out of the garden and mingle with thy race, and forget that there ever crawled on earth such a monster as poor Beatrice?"

"Dost thou pretend ignorance?" asked Giovanni, scowling upon her. "Behold! this power have I gained from the pure daughter of Rappaccini."

There was a swarm of summer insects flitting through the air in search of the food promised by the flower odors of the fatal garden. They circled round Giovanni's head, and were evidently attracted towards him by the same influence which had drawn them for an instant within the sphere of several of the shrubs. He sent forth a breath among them, and smiled bitterly at Beatrice as at least a score of the insects fell dead upon the ground.

"I see it! I see it!" shrieked Beatrice. "It is my father's fatal science! No, no, Giovanni; it was not I! Never! never! I dreamed only to love thee and be with thee a little time, and so to let thee pass away, leaving but thine image in mine heart; for, Giovanni, believe it, though my body be nourished with poison, my spirit is God's creature, and craves love as its daily food. But my father,—he has united us in this fearful sympathy. Yes; spurn me, tread upon me, kill me! Oh, what is death after such words as thine? But it was not I. Not for a world of bliss would I have done it."

Giovanni's passion had exhausted itself in its outburst from his lips. There now came across him a sense, mournful, and not without tenderness, of the intimate and peculiar relationship between Beatrice and himself. They stood, as it were, in an utter solitude, which would be made none the less solitary by the densest throng of human life. Ought not, then, the desert of humanity around them to press this insulated pair closer together? If they should be cruel to one another, who was there to be kind to them? Besides, thought Giovanni, might there not still be a hope of his returning within the limits of ordinary nature, and leading Beatrice, the redeemed Beatrice, by the hand? O, weak, and selfish, and unworthy spirit, that could dream of an earthly union and earthly happiness as possible, after such deep love had been so bitterly wronged as was Beatrice's love by Giovanni's blighting words! No, no; there could be no such hope. She must pass heavily, with that broken heart, across the borders of Time—she must bathe her hurts in some fount of paradise, and forget her grief in the light of immortality, and *there* be well.

But Giovanni did not know it.

"Dear Beatrice," said he, approaching her, while she shrank away as always at his approach, but now with a different impulse, "dearest Beatrice, our fate is not yet so desperate. Behold! there is a medicine, potent, as a wise physician has assured me, and almost divine in its efficacy. It is composed of ingredients the most opposite to those by which thy awful father has brought this calamity upon thee and me. It is distilled of blessed herbs. Shall we not quaff it together, and thus be purified from evil?"

"Give it me!" said Beatrice, extending her hand to receive the little silver vial which Giovanni took from his bosom. She added, with a peculiar emphasis, "I will drink; but do thou await the result."

She put Baglioni's antidote to her lips; and at the same moment, the figure of Rappaccini emerged from the portal and came slowly towards the marble fountain. As he drew near, the pale man of science seemed to gaze with a triumphant expression at the beautiful youth and maiden, as might an artist who should spend his life in achieving a picture or a group of statuary and finally be satisfied with his success. He paused; his bent form grew erect with conscious power; he spread out his hands over them in the attitude of a father imploring a blessing upon his children; but those were the same hands that had thrown poison into the stream of their lives. Giovanni trembled. Beatrice shuddered nervously, and pressed her hand upon her heart.

"My daughter," said Rappaccini, "thou art no longer lonely in the world. Pluck one of those precious gems from thy sister shrub and bid thy bridegroom wear it in his bosom. It will not harm him now. My science and the sympathy between thee and him have so wrought within his system that he now stands apart from common men, as thou dost, daughter of my pride and triumph, from ordinary women. Pass on, then, through the world, most dear to one another and dreadful to all besides!"

"My father," said Beatrice, feebly,—and still as she spoke she kept her hand upon her heart,—"wherefore didst thou inflict this miserable doom upon thy child?"

"Miserable!" exclaimed Rappaccini. "What mean you, foolish girl? Dost thou deem it misery to be endowed with marvellous gifts against which no power nor strength could avail an enemy—misery, to be able to quell the mightiest with a breath—misery, to be as terrible as thou art beautiful? Wouldst thou, then, have preferred the condition of a weak woman, exposed to all evil and capable of none?"

"I would fain have been loved, not feared," murmured Beatrice, sinking down upon the ground. "But now it matters not. I am going, father, where the evil which thou hast striven to mingle with my being will pass away like a dream—like the fragrance of these poisonous flowers, which will no longer taint my breath among the flowers of Eden. Farewell, Giovanni! Thy words of hatred are like lead within my heart; but they, too, will fall away as I ascend. Oh, was there not, from the first, more poison in thy nature than in mine?"

To Beatrice,—so radically had her earthly part been wrought upon by Rappaccini's skill,—as poison had been life, so the powerful antidote was death; and thus the poor victim of man's ingenuity and of thwarted nature, and of the fatality that attends all such efforts of perverted wisdom, perished there, at the feet of her father and Giovanni. Just at that moment Professor Pietro Baglioni looked forth from the window, and called loudly, in a tone of triumph mixed with horror, to the thunderstricken man of science,—

"Rappaccini! Rappaccini! and is *this* the upshot of your experiment!"

JOHN G. NEIHARDT

The First Cure

After the heyoka ceremony, I came to live here where I am now between Wounded Knee Creek and Grass Creek. Others came too, and we made these little gray houses of logs that you see, and they are square. It is a bad way to live, for there can be no power in a square.

You have noticed that everything an Indian does is in a circle, and that is because the Power of the World always works in circles, and everything tries to be round. In the old days when we were a strong and happy people, all our power came to us from the sacred hoop of the nation, and so long as the hoop was unbroken, the people flourished. The flowering tree was the living center of the hoop, and the circle of the four quarters nourished it. The east gave peace and light, the south gave warmth, the west gave rain, and the north with its cold and mighty wind gave strength and endurance. This knowledge came to us from the outer world with our religion. Everything the Power of the World does is done in a circle. The sky is round, and I have heard that the earth is round like a ball, and so are all the stars. The wind, in its greatest power, whirls. Birds make their nests in circles, for theirs is the same religion as ours. The sun comes forth and goes down again in a circle. The moon does the same, and both are round. Even the seasons form a great circle in their changing, and always come back again to where they were. The life of a man is a circle from childhood to childhood, and so it is in everything where power moves. Our tepees were round like the nests of birds, and these were always set in a circle, the nation's hoop, a nest of many nests, where the Great Spirit meant for us to hatch our children.

But the Wasichus have put us in these square boxes. Our power is gone and we are dying, for the power is not in us any more. You can look at our boys and see how it is with us. When we were living by the power of the circle in the way we should, boys were men at twelve or thirteen years of age. But now it takes them very much longer to mature.

Well, it is as it is. We are prisoners of war while we are waiting here. But there is another world.

It was in the Moon of Shedding Ponies (May) when we had the heyoka ceremony. One day in the Moon of Fatness (June), when everything was blooming, I invited One Side to come over and eat with me. I had been thinking about the four-rayed herb that I had now seen twice—the first time in the great vision when I was nine years old, and the second time when I was lamenting on the hill. I knew that I must have this herb for curing, and thought I could recognize the place where I had seen it growing that night when I lamented.

After One Side and I had eaten, I told him there was a herb I must find, and I wanted him to help me hunt for it. Of course I did not tell him I had seen it in a vision. He was willing to help, so we got on our horses and rode over to Grass Creek. Nobody was living over there. We came to the top of a high hill above the creek, and there we got off our horses and sat down, for I felt that we were close to where I saw the herb growing in my vision of the dog.

We sat there awhile singing together some heyoka songs. Then I began to sing alone a song I had heard in my first great vision:

"In a sacred manner they are sending voices."

After I had sung this song, I looked down towards the west, and yonder at a certain spot beside the creek were crows and magpies, chicken hawks and spotted eagles circling around and around.

Then I knew, and I said to One Side: "Friend, right there is where the herb is growing." He said: "We will go forth and see." So we got on our horses and rode down Grass Creek until we came to a dry gulch, and this we followed up. As we neared the spot the birds all flew away, and it was a place where four or five dry gulches came together. There right on the side of the bank the herb was growing, and I knew it, although I had never seen one like it before, except in my vision.

It had a root about as long as to my elbow, and this was a little thicker than my thumb. It was flowering in four colors, blue, white, red, and yellow.

We got off our horses, and after I had offered red willow bark to the Six Powers, I made a prayer to the herb, and said to it: "Now we shall go forth to the two-leggeds, but only to the weakest ones, and there shall be happy days among the weak."

It was easy to dig the herb, because it was growing in the edge of the clay gulch. Then we started back with it. When we came to Grass Creek again, we wrapped it in some good sage that was growing there.

Something must have told me to find the herb just then, for the next evening I needed it and could have done nothing without it.

I was eating supper when a man by the name of Cuts-to-Pieces came in, and he was saying: "Hey, hey, hey!" for he was in trouble. I asked him what was the matter, and he said: "I have a boy of mine, and he is very sick and I am afraid he will die soon. He has been sick a long time. They say you have great power from the horse dance and the heyoka ceremony, so maybe you can save him for me. I think so much of him."

I told Cuts-to-Pieces that if he really wanted help, he should go home and bring me back a pipe with an eagle feather on it. While he was gone, I thought about what I had to do; and I was afraid, because I had never cured anybody yet with my power, and I was very sorry for Cuts-to-Pieces. I prayed hard for help. When Cuts-to-Pieces came back with the pipe, I told him to take it around to the left of me, leave it there, and pass out again to the right of me. When he had done this, I sent for One Side to come and help me. Then I took the pipe and went to where the sick little boy was. My father and my mother went with us, and my friend, Standing Bear, was already there.

I first offered the pipe to the Six Powers, then I passed it, and we all smoked. After that I began making a rumbling thunder sound on the drum. You know, when the power of the west comes to the two-leggeds, it comes with rumbling, and when it has passed, everything lifts up its head and is glad and there is greenness. So I made this rumbling sound. Also, the voice of the drum is an offering to the Spirit of the World. Its sound arouses the mind and makes men feel the mystery and power of things.

The sick little boy was on the northeast side of the tepee, and when we entered at the south, we went around from left to right, stopping on the west side when we had made the circle.

You want to know why we always go from left to right like that. I can tell you something of the reason, but not all. Think of this: Is not the south the source of life, and does not the flowering stick truly come from there? And does not man advance from there toward the setting sun of his life? Then does he not approach the colder north where the white hairs are? And does he not then arrive, if he lives, at the source of light and understanding, which is the east? Then does he not return to where he began, to his second childhood, there to give back his life to all life, and his flesh to the earth whence it came? The more you think about this, the more meaning you will see in it.

As I said, we went into the tepee from left to right, and sat ourselves down on the west side. The sick little boy was on the northeast side, and he looked as though he were only skin and bones. I had the pipe, the drum and the four-rayed herb already, so I asked for a wooden cup, full of water, and an eagle bone whistle, which was for the spotted eagle of my great vision. They placed the cup of water in front of me; and then I had to think awhile, because I had never done this before and I was in doubt.

I understood a little more now, so I gave the eagle bone whistle to One Side and told him how to use it in helping me. Then I filled the pipe with red willow bark, and gave it to the pretty young daughter of Cuts-to-Pieces, telling her to hold it, just as I had seen the virgin of the east holding it in my great vision.

Everything was ready now, so I made low thunder on the drum, keeping time as I sent forth a voice. Four times I cried "Hey-a-a-hey," drumming as I cried to the Spirit of the World, and while I was doing this I could feel the power coming through me from my feet up, and I knew that I could help the sick little boy.

I kept on sending a voice, while I made low thunder on the drum, saying: "My Grandfather, Great Spirit, you are the only one and to no other can any one send voices. You have made everything, they say, and you have made it good and beautiful. The four quarters and the two roads crossing each other, you have made. Also you have set a power where the sun goes down. The two-leggeds on earth are in despair. For them, my Grandfather, I send a voice to you. You have said this to me: The weak shall walk. In vision you have taken me to the center of the world and there you have shown me the power to make over. The water in the cup that you have given me, by its power shall the dying live. The herb that you have shown me, through its power shall the feeble walk upright. From where we are always facing (the south), behold, a virgin shall appear, walking the good red road, offering the pipe as she walks, and hers also is the power of the flowering tree. From where the Giant lives (the north), you have given me a sacred, cleasing wind, and where this wind passes the weak shall have strength. You have said this to me. To you and to all your powers and to Mother Earth I send a voice for help."

You see, I had never done this before, and I know now that only one power would have been enough. But I was so eager to help the sick little boy that I called on every power there is.

I had been facing the west, of course, while sending a voice. Now I walked to the north and to the east and to the south, stopping there where the source of all life is and where the good red road begins. Standing there, I sang thus:

> "In a sacred manner I have made them walk.
> A sacred nation lies low.
> In a sacred manner I have made them walk.
> A sacred two-legged, he lies low.
> In a sacred manner, he shall walk."

While I was singing this I could feel something queer all through my body, something that made me want to cry for all unhappy things, and there were tears on my face.

Now I walked to the quarter of the west, where I lit the pipe, offered it to the powers, and, after I had taken a whiff of smoke, I passed it around.

When I looked at the sick little boy again, he smiled at me, and I could feel that the power was getting stronger.

I next took the cup of water, drank a little of it, and went around to where the sick little boy was. Standing before him, I stamped the earth four times. Then, putting my mouth to the pit of his stomach, I drew through him the cleansing wind of the north. I next chewed some of the herb and put it in the water, afterward blowing some of it on the boy and to the four quarters. The cup with the rest of the water I gave to the virgin, who gave it to the sick little boy to drink. Then I told the virgin to help the boy stand up and to walk around the circle with him, beginning at the south, the source of life. He was very poor and weak, but with the virgin's help he did this.

Then I went away.

Next day Cuts-to-Pieces came and told me that his little boy was feeling better and was sitting up and could eat something again. In four days he could walk around. He got well and lived to be thirty years old.

Cuts-to-Pieces gave me a good horse for doing this; but of course I would have done it for nothing.

When the people heard about how the little boy was cured, many came to me for help, and I was busy most of the time.

This was in the summer of my nineteenth year (1882), in the Moon of Making Fat.

WILLIAM CARLOS WILLIAMS

Of Medicine and Poetry

When they ask me, as of late they frequently do, how I have for so many years continued an equal interest in medicine and the poem, I reply that they amount for me to nearly the same thing. Any worth-his-salt physician knows that no one is "cured." We recover from some somatic, some bodily "fever" where as observers we have seen various engagements between our battalions of cells playing at this or that lethal maneuver with other natural elements. It has been interesting. Various sewers or feed-mains have given way here or there under pressure: various new patterns have been thrown up for us upon the screen of our knowledge. But a cure is absurd, as absurd as calling these deployments "diseases." Sometimes the home team wins, sometimes the visitors. Great excitement. It is noteworthy that the sulfonamids, penicillin, came in about simultaneously with Ted Williams, Ralph Kiner and the rubber ball. We want home runs, antibiotics to "cure" man with a single shot in the buttocks.

But after you've knocked the ball into the center-field bleachers and won the game, you still have to go home to supper. So what? The ball park lies empty-eyed until the next game, the next season, the next bomb. Peanuts.

Medicine, as an art, never had much attraction for me, though it fascinated me, especially the physiology of the nervous system. That's something. Surgery always seemed to me particularly unsatisfying. What is there to cut off or out that will "cure" us? And to stand there for a lifetime sawing away! You'd better be a chef, if not a butcher. There is a joy in it, I realize, to know that you've really cut the cancer out and that the guy will come in to score, but I never wanted to be a surgeon. Marvelous men—I take my hat off to them. I knew one once who whenever he'd get into a malignant growth would take a hunk of it and rub it into his armpit afterward. Never knew why. It never hurt him, and he lived to a great old age. He had imagination, curiosity and a sense of humor, I suppose.

The cured man, I want to say, is no different from any other. It is a trivial business unless you add the zest, whatever that is, to the picture. That's how I came to find writing such a necessity, to relieve me from such a dilemma. I found by practice, by trial and error, that to treat a man as something to which surgery, drugs and hoodoo applied was an indifferent matter; to treat him as material for a work of art made him somehow come alive to me.

What I wanted to do with him (or her, or it) fascinated me. And it didn't make any difference, apparently, that he was in himself distinguished or otherwise. It wasn't that I wanted to save him because he was a good and useful member of society. Death had no respect for him for that reason, neither does the artist, neither did I. As far as I can tell that kind of "use" doesn't enter into it; I am myself curious as to what I do find. The attraction is bizarre.

Thus I have said "the mind." And the mind? I can't say that I have ever been interested in a completely mindless person. But I have known one or two that are close to mindless, certainly useless, even fatal to their families, or what remains of their families, whom yet I find far more interesting than plenty of others whom I serve.

These are the matters which obsess me so that I cannot stop writing. I can recall many from the past, boys and girls, bad pupils, renegades, dirty-minded and -fisted, that I miss keenly. When some old woman tells me of her daughter now happily married to a handicapper at the Garden City track, that she has two fine sons, I want to sing and dance. I am happy. I am stimulated. She is still alive. Why should I feel that way? She almost caused me to flunk out of grammar school. I almost ruined my young days over her.

But I didn't. I love her, ignorant, fulsome bit of flesh that she was, and some other really vicious bits of childhood who ruined the record of the whole class—dead of their excesses, most of them. They flatter my memory. The thing, the thing, of which I am in chase. The thing I cannot quite name was there then. My writing, the necessity for a continued assertion, the need for me to go on will not let me stop. To this day I am in pursuit of it, actually—not there, in the academies, nor in the pursuit of a remote and difficult knowledge or skill.

They had no knowledge and no skill at all. They flunked out, got jailed, got "Mamie" with child, and fell away, if they survived, from their perfections.

There again, a word: their perfections. They were perfect, they seem to have been born perfect, to need nothing else. They were there, living before me, and I lived beside them, associated with them. Their very presence denied the need of "study," that is study by degrees to elucidate them. They were, living, the theme that all my life I have labored to elucidate, and when I could not elucidate them I have tried to put them down, to lay them upon the paper to record them: for to do that is, after all, a sort of elucidation.

It isn't because they fascinated me by their evildoings that they were "bad" boys or girls. Not at all. It was because they were there full of a perfection of the longest leap, the most unmitigated daring, the longest chances.

This immediacy, the thing, as I went on writing, living as I could, thinking a secret life I wanted to tell openly—if only I could—how it lives, secretly about us as much now as ever. It is the history, the anatomy of this, not subject to surgery, plumbing or cures, that I wanted to tell. I don't know why. Why tell that which no one wants to hear? But I saw that when I was successful in portraying something, by accident, of that secret world of perfection, that they did want to listen. Definitely. And my "medicine" was the thing which gained me entrance to these secret gardens of the self. It lay there, another world, in the self. I was permitted by my medical badge to follow the poor, defeated body into those gulfs and grottos. And the astonishing thing is that at such times and in such places—foul as they may be with the stinking ischio-rectal abscesses of our comings and goings—just there, the thing, in all its greatest beauty, may for a moment be freed to fly for a moment guiltily about the room. In illness, in the permission I as a physician have had to be present at deaths and births, at the tormented battles between daughter and diabolic mother, shattered by a gone brain—just there—for a split second—from one side or the other, it has fluttered before me for a moment, a phrase which I quickly write down on anything at hand, any piece of paper I can grab.

It is an identifiable thing, and its characteristic, its chief character is that it is sure, all of a piece and, as I have said, instant and perfect: it comes, it is there, and it vanishes. But I have seen it, clearly. I have seen it. I know it because there it is. I have been possessed by it just as I was in the fifth grade —when she leaned over the back of the seat before me and greeted me with some obscene remarks—which I cannot repeat even if made by a child forty years ago, because no one would or could understand what I am saying that then, there, it had appeared.

The great world never much interested me (except at the back of my head) since its effects, from what I observed, were so disastrously trivial—other than in their bulk; smelled the same as most public places. As Bob McAlmon said after the well-dressed Spanish woman passed us in Juarez (I had said, Wow! there's perfume for you!):

"You mean that?" he said. "That's not perfume, I just call that whores."

HENRIK IBSEN

An Enemy of the People

CHARACTERS

DR. THOMAS STOCKMANN, medical officer at the Baths
MRS. STOCKMANN, his wife
PETRA, their daughter, a schoolteacher
EILIF
MORTEN } their sons, aged thirteen and ten
PETER STOCKMANN, the DOCTOR's elder brother, Mayor and
    Chief Constable, Chairman of the Baths Committee, etc.
MORTON KIIL, master tanner, foster father to MRS. STOCK-
    MANN
HOVSTAD, editor of the *People's Tribune*
BILLING, an employee on the newspaper
HORSTER, a sea captain
ASLAKSEN, a printer

People at a public meeting—men of all classes, a few women
and a bunch of schoolboys.

The action takes place in a coastal town in Southern Norway.

ACT I

Evening in DR. STOCKMANN's *living-room. It is humbly but neatly furnished
and decorated. In the wall to the right are two doors, of which the further
leads out to the hall and the nearer to the* DOCTOR's *study. In the opposite
wall, facing the hall door, is a door that leads to the other rooms occupied
by the family. In the middle of this wall stands a tiled stove; further downstage
is a sofa with a mirror above it. In front of the sofa is an oval table with a
cloth on it. Upon this table stands a lighted lamp with a shade. Upstage, an
open door to the dining-room, in which can be seen a table laid for the evening meal, with a lamp on it.*

At this table BILLING *is seated, a napkin tucked beneath his chin.* MRS. STOCK-
MANN *is standing by the table, offering him a plate with a large joint of beef*

on it. The other places around the table are empty, and the table is in the disorder of a meal that has been finished.

MRS. STOCKMANN: There, Mr. Billing! But if you will come an hour late, you'll have to put up with cold.

BILLING (*eating*):   Oh, but this is capital. Absolutely capital!

MRS. STOCKMANN: Well, you know how punctually my husband always likes to eat.

BILLING: It doesn't bother me. I enjoy eating alone, without having to talk to anyone.

MRS. STOCKMANN: Oh. Well, as long as you're *enjoying* it, that's— (*Listens towards the hall.*) Ah, this must be Mr. Hovstad.

BILLING: Very likely.

PETER STOCKMANN *enters wearing an overcoat and his mayoral hat, and carrying a stick.*

MAYOR: Good evening to you, my dear sister-in-law.

MRS. STOCKMANN (*goes into the living-room*):   Why, good evening! Fancy seeing you here! How nice of you to come and call on us!

MAYOR: I just happened to be passing, so— (*Glances towards the dining-room.*) But I hear you have company.

MRS. STOCKMANN (*a little embarrassed*):   Oh no, no, that's no one. (*Quickly.*) Won't you have something too?

MAYOR: I? No, thank you! A cooked meal at night! My digestion would never stand that!

MRS. STOCKMANN: Oh, but surely just for once—

MAYOR: No, no! It's very kind of you, but I'll stick to my tea and sandwiches. It's healthier in the long run; and a little less expensive.

MRS. STOCKMANN (*smiles*):   You speak as though Thomas and I were spendthrifts!

MAYOR: Not you, my dear sister-in-law. Such a thought was far from my mind. (*Points towards the* DOCTOR's *study.*) Isn't he at home?

MRS. STOCKMANN: No, he's gone for a little walk with the boys.

MAYOR: I wonder if that's wise so soon after a meal? (*Listens.*) Ah, this must be he.

MRS. STOCKMANN: No, I don't think it can be, yet. (*A knock on the door.*)
Come in!

HOVSTAD, *the editor of the local newspaper, enters from the hall.*

MRS. STOCKMANN: Oh—Mr. Hovstad—?

HOVSTAD: Yes. Please excuse me, I was detained down at the printer's. Good
evening, Your Worship.

MAYOR (*greets him somewhat stiffly*):   Good evening. I suppose you are here
on business?

HOVSTAD: Partly. About an article for my newspaper—

MAYOR: I guessed as much. I hear my brother is a regular contributor to the
People's Tribune.

HOVSTAD: Yes, he usually drops us a line when he thinks the truth needs to
be told about something.

MRS. STOCKMANN (*to* HOVSTAD, *pointing towards the dining-room*):   Er—
won't you—?

MAYOR: Great heavens, you mustn't think I blame him for writing for the
kind of public he's most likely to find sympathetic to his ideas. Besides, I
have no reason to bear your newspaper any ill will, Mr. Hovstad—

HOVSTAD: I should hope not.

MAYOR: On the whole I think I may say that an admirable spirit of tolerance
reigns in our town. A fine communal spirit! And the reason for this is that
we have this great common interest that binds us together—an interest
which is the close concern of every right-minded citizen—

HOVSTAD: You mean the Baths?

MAYOR: Exactly! Our magnificent new Baths! Mark my words, sir! These
Baths will prove the very heart and essence of our life! There can be no
doubt about it.

MRS. STOCKMANN: Yes, that's just what Thomas says.

MAYOR: It's really astounding the strides this place has made during the past
two or three years! The town is becoming prosperous. People are waking up
and beginning to live. Buildings and ground rents are increasing in value
every day.

HOVSTAD: And unemployment is going down.

MAYOR: Yes, there's that too. The burden upon the propertied classes of poor relief has been most gratifyingly reduced—and will be still more if only we have a really good summer this year, with plenty of visitors. What we want most is invalids. They'll give the Baths a good name.

HOVSTAD: And I hear the indications are promising.

MAYOR: They are indeed. Enquiries about accommodation are pouring in every day.

HOVSTAD: Well then, the Doctor's article will be most opportune.

MAYOR: Oh, has he written something new?

HOVSTAD: No, it's something he wrote last winter; a eulogy of the Baths and the excellent health facilities of the town. But I decided to hold it over.

MAYOR: Ah, there was a snag somewhere?

HOVSTAD: No, it wasn't that. I just thought it would be better to wait till the spring. Now people are thinking about where to spend their summer holidays—

MAYOR: Quite right! Quite right, Mr. Hovstad!

MRS. STOCKMANN: Thomas never stops thinking about those Baths.

MAYOR: Well, he is employed there.

HOVSTAD: Yes, and he was the one who really created it all, wasn't he?

MAYOR: Was he? Really? Yes, I have heard that certain people do hold that opinion. I must say I was labouring under the delusion that I had some modest share in promoting the enterprise.

MRS. STOCKMANN: That's what Thomas is always telling people.

HOVSTAD: No one denies that, Your Worship. You got it going and saw to all the practical details—we all know that. I only meant that the idea originated with the Doctor.

MAYOR: Yes, my brother's always been full of ideas—unfortunately. But when things have to be done, another kind of man is needed, Mr. Hovstad. And I should have thought that least of all in this house would—

MRS. STOCKMANN: But my dear brother-in-law—!

HOVSTAD: Surely Your Worship doesn't—?

MRS. STOCKMANN: Do go inside and get yourself something to eat, Mr. Hovstad. My husband will be here any moment.

HOVSTAD: Thank you—just a bite, perhaps. (*Goes into the dining-room.*)

MAYOR (*lowers his voice slightly*):   It's extraordinary about people of peasant stock. They never learn the meaning of tact.

MRS. STOCKMANN: But is it really anything to bother about? Can't you and Thomas share the honour as brothers?

MAYOR: Well, I should have thought so; but it seems not everyone is content to share.

MRS. STOCKMANN: Oh, nonsense! You and Thomas always get on so well together. Ah, this sounds like him.

Goes over and opens the door leading to the hall.

DR. STOCKMANN (*laughing and boisterous*):   Hullo, Catherine! I've another guest for you here! The more the merrier, what? Come in, Captain Horster! Hang your overcoat up there on the hook. No, of course, you don't wear an overcoat, do you? Fancy, Catherine, I bumped into him in the street! Had the devil of a job persuading him to come back with me!

CAPTAIN HORSTER *enters and shakes hands with* MRS. STOCKMANN.

DR. STOCKMANN (*in the doorway*):   Run along in now, lads. (*To* MRS. STOCKMANN.) They're hungry again already! This way Captain Horster, you're going to have the finest roast beef you ever—!

Drives HORSTER *into the dining-room.* EILIF *and* MORTEN *go in too.*

MRS. STOCKMANN: Thomas! Don't you see who's—?

DR. STOCKMANN (*turns in the doorway*):   Oh, hullo, Peter! (*Goes over and shakes his hand.*) Well, it's good to see you!

MAYOR: I'm afraid I can only spare a few minutes—

DR. STOCKMANN: Rubbish, we'll be having some hot toddy soon. You haven't forgotten the toddy, Catherine?

MRS. STOCKMANN: No, of course not. I've got the kettle on—(*Goes into the dining-room.*)

MAYOR: Hot toddy too—!

DR. STOCKMANN: Yes. Now sit down, and we'll have a good time.

MAYOR: Thank you. I never partake in drinking parties.

DR. STOCKMANN: But this isn't a party.

MAYOR: Well, but—! (*Glances towards the dining-room.*) It's really extraordinary the amount they eat!

DR. STOCKMANN (*rubs his hands*): Yes, there's nothing better than to see young people tuck in, is there? Always hungry! That's the way it should be! They've got to have food! Gives them strength! They're the ones who've got to ginger up the future, Peter.

MAYOR: May one ask what it is that needs to be "gingered up," as you put it?

DR. STOCKMANN: You must ask the young ones that—when the time comes. We can't see it, of course. Obviously—a couple of old fogeys like you and me—

MAYOR: Well, really! That's a most extraordinary way to describe us—

DR. STOCKMANN: Oh, you mustn't take me too seriously, Peter. I feel so happy and exhilarated, you see! It's so wonderful to be alive at a time like this, with everything germinating and bursting all around us! Oh, it's a glorious age we live in! It's as though a whole new world were coming to birth before our eyes!

MAYOR: Do you really feel that?

DR. STOCKMANN: Yes. Of course, you can't see it as clearly as I do. You've spent your life in this background, so it doesn't make the same impression on you as it does on me. But I've had to spend all these years sitting up there in that damned northern backwater, hardly ever seeing a new face that had a stimulating word to say to me. To me it's as though I had moved into the heart of some pulsing metropolis—

MAYOR: Hm; metropolis—!

DR. STOCKMANN: Oh, I know it must seem small in comparison with lots of other cities. But there's life here—promise—so many things to work and fight for! And that's what matters. (*Shouts.*) Catherine, hasn't the post come yet?

MRS. STOCKMANN (*from the dining-room*): No, not yet.

DR. STOCKMANN: And to be making a decent living, Peter! That's something one learns to appreciate when one's been living on the edge of starvation, as we have—

MAYOR: Oh, surely!

DR. STOCKMANN: Oh yes, I can tell you we were often pretty hard pressed up there. But now, we can live like lords! Today, for instance, we had roast beef for dinner; *and* there was enough left over for supper! Won't you have a bit? Let me show it to you anyway. Come on, have a look—

MAYOR: No, really—

DR. STOCKMANN: Well, look at this, then! Do you see? We've got a table-cloth!

MAYOR: Yes, I've noticed it.

DR. STOCKMANN: And a lampshade too! See? All from what Catherine's managed to save! It makes the room so cosy, don't you think? Come and stand here—no, no, no, not there! There, now! Look! See how the light sort of concentrates downwards? I really think it looks very elegant, don't you?

MAYOR: Well, if one can indulge in that kind of luxury—

DR. STOCKMANN: Oh, I think I can permit myself that now. Catherine says I earn almost as much as we spend.

MAYOR: Almost!

DR. STOCKMANN: Well, a man of science ought to live in a little style. I'm sure any magistrate spends far more in a year than I do.

MAYOR: Yes, I should think so! After all, a magistrate is an important public official—

DR. STOCKMANN: Well, a wholesale merchant, then. A man like that spends much more—

MAYOR: His circumstances are different.

DR. STOCKMANN: Oh, it isn't that I'm wasteful, Peter. I just can't deny my-self the pleasure of having people around me! I need that, you know. I've been living outside the world for so long, and for me it's a necessity to be with people who are young, bold, and cheerful, and have lively, liberal minds—and that's what they are, all the men who are sitting in there en-joying a good meal! I wish you knew Hovstad a little better—

MAYOR: That reminds me, Hovstad told me he's going to print another article by you.

DR. STOCKMANN: An article by me?

MAYOR: Yes, about the Baths. Something you wrote last winter.

DR. STOCKMANN: Oh, that. No, I don't want them to print that now.

MAYOR: No? But I should have thought now would be the most suitable time.

DR. STOCKMANN: I dare say it would under ordinary circumstances. (*Walks across the room.*)

MAYOR (*watches him*):   And what is extraordinary about the circumstances now?

DR. STOCKMANN (*stops*):   I'm sorry, Peter, I can't tell you that yet. Not this evening, anyway. There may be a great deal that's extraordinary; or there may be nothing at all. It may be my imagination—

MAYOR: I must say you're making it all sound very mysterious. Is there something the matter? Something I mustn't be told about? I should have thought that I, as Chairman of the Baths Committee—

DR. STOCKMANN: And I should have thought that I, as—well, let's not start flying off the handle.

MAYOR: Heaven forbid. I'm not in the habit of flying off the handle, as you phrase it. But I must absolutely insist that all arrangements be made and executed through the proper channels and through the authorities legally appointed for that purpose. I cannot permit any underhand or backdoor methods.

DR. STOCKMANN: Have I ever used underhand or backdoor methods?

MAYOR: You will always insist on going your own way. And that's almost equally inadmissible in a well-ordered community. The individual must learn to fall in line with the general will, or, to be more accurate, with that of the authorities whose business it is to watch over the common good.

DR. STOCKMANN: I dare say. But what the hell has that to do with me?

MAYOR: Because that, my dear Thomas, is what you seem never to be willing to learn. But take care. You'll pay for it some time. Well, I've warned you. Goodbye.

DR. STOCKMANN: Are you raving mad? You're barking completely up the wrong tree—

MAYOR: I'm not in the habit of doing that. Well, if you'll excuse me— (*Bows towards the dining-room.*) Goodbye, sister-in-law. Good day, gentlemen. (*Goes.*)

MRS. STOCKMANN (*comes back into the living-room*):   Has he gone?

DR. STOCKMANN: Yes, Catherine, and in a damned bad temper.

MRS. STOCKMANN: Oh, Thomas, what have you done to him now?

DR. STOCKMANN: Absolutely nothing. He can't expect me to account to him until the time comes.

MRS. STOCKMANN: Account to him? For what?

DR. STOCKMANN: Hm; never mind, Catherine. Why the devil doesn't the post come?

HOVSTAD, BILLING, *and* HORSTER *have got up from the dining table and come into the living-room.* EILIF *and* MORTEN *follow a few moments later.*

BILLING (*stretches his arms*):   Ah, a meal like that makes one feel like a new man! By jingo, yes!

HOVSTAD: His Worship wasn't in a very cheerful mood tonight.

DR. STOCKMANN: Oh, that's his stomach. He's got a bad digestion.

HOVSTAD: I expect we radical journalists stuck in his gullet.

MRS. STOCKMANN: I thought you were getting on rather well with him.

HOVSTAD: Oh, it's only an armistice.

BILLING: That's it! The word epitomises the situation in a nutshell.

DR. STOCKMANN: Peter's a lonely man, poor fellow; we must remember that. He has no home where he can relax; only business, business. And all that damned tea he pours into himself! Well, lads, pull up your chairs! Catherine, where's that toddy?

MRS. STOCKMANN (*goes into the dining-room*):   It's just coming.

DR. STOCKMANN: You sit down here on the sofa with me, Captain Horster. You're too rare a guest in this house! Sit, sit, gentlemen!

The GENTLEMEN *sit at the table.* MRS. STOCKMANN *brings a tray with a kettle, decanters, glasses, etc.*

MRS. STOCKMANN: Here you are. This is arrack, and this is rum; and there's the brandy. Now everyone must help himself.

DR. STOCKMANN (*takes a glass*):   Don't you worry about that! (*As the toddy is mixed.*) But where are the cigars? Eilif, you know where the box is. Morten, you can bring me my pipe. (*The* BOYS *go into the room on the right.*) I've a suspicion Eilif pinches a cigar once in a while, but I pretend I don't know! (*Shouts.*) And my smoking cap, Morten! Catherine, can't you tell him where I've put it? Oh, good, he's found it. (*The* BOYS *return with the things he asked for.*) Help yourself, my friends! I stick to my pipe, you know; this old friend's been my companion on many a stormy round up there in the north. (*Clinks his glass with theirs.*) Skol! Ah, I must say it's better to be sitting here, warm and relaxed!

MRS. STOCKMANN (*who is sitting, knitting*):   Will you be sailing soon, Captain Horster?

HORSTER: I expect to be off next week.

MRS. STOCKMANN: It's America this time, isn't it?

HORSTER: That's the idea.

BILLING: But then you won't be able to vote in the next council elections!

HORSTER: Is there going to be a new election?

BILLING: Didn't you know?

HORSTER: No, such things don't interest me.

BILLING: But you must care about public affairs?

HORSTER: No, I don't understand these matters.

BILLING: All the same, one ought at least to vote.

HORSTER: Even if one doesn't understand what it's about?

BILLING: Understand? What's that got to do with it? Society's like a ship; everyone's got to lend a hand at the rudder.

HORSTER: Not in my ship!

HOVSTAD: It's curious how little sailors bother about what goes on in their own country.

BILLING: Most abnormal.

DR. STOCKMANN: Sailors are like birds of passage; wherever they happen to be, they regard that as home. Which means the rest of us must be all the more active, Mr. Hovstad. Have you anything salutary to offer us in the *People's Tribune* tomorrow?

HOVSTAD: Nothing of local interest. But the day after, I thought of printing your article—

DR. STOCKMANN: Oh God, yes, that article! No, look, you'll have to sit on that.

HOVSTAD: Oh? We've plenty of space just now; and I thought this would be the most suitable time—

DR. STOCKMANN: Yes, yes, I dare say you're right, but you'll have to wait all the same. I'll explain later—

PETRA, *in hat and cloak, with a pile of exercise books under her arm, enters from the hall.*

PETRA: Good evening.

DR. STOCKMANN: Hullo, Petra, is that you?

The others greet her, and she them. She puts down her cloak, hat and books on a chair by the door.

PETRA: And you're all sitting here having a party while I've been out working!

DR. STOCKMANN: Well, come and have a party too.

BILLING: May I mix you a tiny glass?

PETRA (*comes over to the table*): Thanks, I'll do it myself; you always make it too strong. Oh, by the way, Father, I've a letter for you.

Goes over to the chair on which her things are lying.

DR. STOCKMANN: A letter? Who from?

PETRA (*looks in her coat pocket*): The postman gave it to me just as I was going out—

DR. STOCKMANN (*gets up and goes over to her*): Why on earth didn't you let me have it before?

PETRA: I really didn't have time to run up again. Here it is.

DR. STOCKMANN (*seizes the letter*): Let me see it, child, let me see it! (*Looks at the envelope.*) Yes, this is it!

MRS. STOCKMANN: Is this what you've been waiting for so anxiously, Thomas?

DR. STOCKMANN: It is indeed. I must go and read it at once. Where can I find a light, Catherine? Is there no lamp in my room again?

MRS. STOCKMANN: Yes, there's one burning on your desk.

DR. STOCKMANN: Good, good. Excuse me a moment—

Goes into the room on the right.

PETRA: What on earth can that be. Mother?

MRS. STOCKMANN: I don't know. These last few days he's done nothing but ask about the post.

BILLING: Probably some patient out of town—

PETRA: Poor Father! He'll soon find he's bitten off more than he can chew. (*Mixes herself a glass.*) Ah, that tastes good!

HOVSTAD: Have you been at evening classes tonight, too?

PETRA (*sips her drink*):   Two hours.

BILLING: And four hours this morning at the technical college—

PETRA (*sits at the table*):   Five hours.

MRS. STOCKMANN: And you've got exercises to correct tonight, I see.

PETRA: Yes, lots.

HORSTER: You seem to have bitten off more than you can chew too, by the sound of it.

PETRA: Yes, but I like it. One feels so wonderfully tired afterwards.

BILLING: Wonderfully?

PETRA: Yes. One sleeps so soundly, afterwards.

MORTEN: You must be very wicked, Petra.

PETRA: Wicked?

MORTEN: Yes, if you work so much. Dr. Roerlund says work is a punishment for our sins.

EILIF (*sniffs*):   Silly! Fancy believing stuff like that!

MRS. STOCKMANN: Now, now, Eilif!

BILLING (*laughs*):   Ha! Very good!

HOVSTAD: Don't you want to work hard too, Morten?

MORTEN: No! Not me!

HOVSTAD: But surely you want to become something?

MORTEN: I want to be a Viking!

EILIF: But then you'll have to be a heathen.

MORTEN: All right, I'll be a heathen!

BILLING: I'm with you there, Morten! That's just the way I feel!

MRS. STOCKMANN (*makes a sign*):   I'm sure you don't really, Mr. Billing.

BILLING: By jingo, I do! I *am* a heathen, and I'm proud of it! Before long we'll all be heathens. Just you wait and see.

MORTEN: Shall we be able to do anything we like then?

BILLING: Yes, Morten! You see—!

MRS. STOCKMANN: Hurry off now, boys. I'm sure you've some homework to do.

EILIF: I can stay a few minutes longer—

MRS. STOCKMANN: No, you can't. Be off, the pair of you!

The BOYS *say good night and go into the room on the left.*

HOVSTAD: Do you really think it can do the boys any harm to hear this kind of thing?

MRS. STOCKMANN: Well, I don't know. I just don't like it.

PETRA: Oh, really, Mother! I think you're being very stupid.

MRS. STOCKMANN: Perhaps I am; but I don't like it. Not here in the home.

PETRA: Oh, there's so much fear of the truth everywhere! At home and at school. Here we've got to keep our mouths shut, and at school we have to stand up and tell lies to the children.

HORSTER: Lie to them?

PETRA: Yes, surely you realise we have to teach them all kinds of things we don't believe in ourselves.

BILLING: I fear that is all too true!

PETRA: If only I had money, I'd start a school of my own. And there things would be different.

BILLING: Ah! Money!

HORSTER: If you mean that seriously, Miss Stockmann, I could gladly let you have a room at my place. My father's old house is almost empty; there's a great big dining-room downstairs—

PETRA (*laughs*):   Thank you! But I don't suppose it'll ever come to anything.

HOVSTAD: No, I think Miss Petra will probably turn to journalism. By the way, have you found time to look at that English novel you promised to translate for us?

PETRA: Not yet. But I'll see you get it in time.

DR. STOCKMANN *enters from his room with the letter open in his hand.*

DR. STOCKMANN (*waves the letter*):   Here's news that's going to set this town by the ears, believe you me!

BILLING: News?

MRS. STOCKMANN: Why, what's happened?

DR. STOCKMANN: A great discovery has been made, Catherine!

HOVSTAD: Really?

MRS. STOCKMANN: By you?

DR. STOCKMANN: Precisely! By me! (*Walks up and down.*) Now let them come as usual and say it's all madman's talk and I'm imagining things! But they'll have to watch their step this time! (*Laughs.*) Yes, I fancy they'll have to watch their step!

PETRA: Father, for Heaven's sake tell us what it is!

DR. STOCKMANN: Yes, yes, just give me time and you'll hear everything. Oh, if only I had Peter here now! Well, it only goes to show how blindly we mortals can form our judgments—

HOVSTAD: What do you mean by that, Doctor?

DR. STOCKMANN (*stops by the table*):   Is it not popularly supposed that our town is a healthy place?

HOVSTAD: Yes, of course.

DR. STOCKMANN: A quite unusually healthy place? A place which deserves to be recommended in the warmest possible terms both for the sick and for their more fortunate brethren?

MRS. STOCKMANN: Yes, but my dear Thomas—!

DR. STOCKMANN: And we ourselves have praised and recommended it, have we not? I have written thousands of words of eulogy both in the *People's Tribune,* and in pamphlets—

HOVSTAD: Yes, well, what of it?

DR. STOCKMANN: These Baths, which have been called the artery of the town, and its central nerve and—and God knows what else—

BILLING: "The pulsing heart of our city" is a phrase I once, in a festive moment, ventured to—

DR. STOCKMANN: No doubt. But do you know what they really are, these beloved Baths of ours which have been so puffed up and which have cost so much money? Do you know what they are?

HOVSTAD: No, what are they?

DR. STOCKMANN: Nothing but a damned cesspit!

PETRA: The Baths, Father?

MRS. STOCKMANN (*simultaneously*):   Our Baths!

HOVSTAD (*simultaneously*):   But, Doctor—!

BILLING: Absolutely incredible!

DR. STOCKMANN: These Baths are a whited sepulchre—and a poisoned one at that. Dangerous to health in the highest degree! All that filth up at Moellerdal—you know, that stinking refuse from the tanneries—has infected the water in the pipes that feed the Pump Room. And that's not all. This damnable muck has even seeped out onto the beach—

HORSTER: Where the sea baths are?

DR. STOCKMANN: Exactly!

HOVSTAD: But how can you be so sure about all this, Doctor?

DR. STOCKMANN: I've investigated the whole thing most thoroughly. Oh, I've long suspected something of the kind. Last year there were a lot of curious complaints among visitors who'd come for the bathing—typhoid, and gastric troubles—

MRS. STOCKMANN: Yes, so there were.

DR. STOCKMANN: At the time we thought these people had brought the disease with them. But later, during the winter, I began to have other thoughts. So I set to work to analyse the water as closely as I was able.

MRS. STOCKMANN: So that's what you've been toiling so hard at!

DR. STOCKMANN: Yes, you may well say I have toiled, Catherine. But of course I lacked the proper scientific facilities. So I sent specimens of both the drinking water and the sea water to the University to have them analysed by a chemist.

HOVSTAD: And now you have that analysis?

DR. STOCKMANN (*shows the letter*):   Here it is! It establishes conclusively that the water here contains putrid organic matter—millions of bacteria! It is definitely noxious to the health even for external use.

MRS. STOCKMANN: What a miracle you found this out in time!

DR. STOCKMANN: You may well say that, Catherine.

HOVSTAD: And what do you intend to do now, Doctor?

DR. STOCKMANN: Put the matter right, of course.

HOVSTAD: Can that be done?

DR. STOCKMANN: It must be done! Otherwise the Baths are unusable—and all our work has been wasted. But don't worry. I'm pretty sure I know what needs to be done.

MRS. STOCKMANN: But, my dear Thomas, why have you kept all this so secret?

DR. STOCKMANN: Did you expect me to go round the town talking about it before I was certain? No, thank you, I'm not that mad.

PETRA: You might have told us—

DR. STOCKMANN: I wasn't going to tell anyone. But tomorrow you can run along to the Badger and—

MRS. STOCKMANN: Thomas, really!

DR. STOCKMANN: Sorry; I mean your grandfather. It'll shock the old boy out of his skin. He thinks I'm a bit gone in the head anyway—oh, and there are plenty of others who think the same! I know! But now these good people shall see! Now they shall see! (*Walks around and rubs his hands.*) There's going to be such a to-do in this town, Catherine! You've no idea! The whole water system will have to be relaid.

HOVSTAD (*gets up*):   The whole of the water system—?

DR. STOCKMANN: Of course. The intake is too low. It'll have to be raised much higher up.

PETRA: Then you were right after all!

DR. STOCKMANN: Yes, Petra, do you remember? I wrote protesting against the plans when they were about to start laying it. But no one would listen to me then. Well, now I'll give them a real broadside. Of course, I've written a full report to the Baths Committee; it's been ready for a whole week, I've only been waiting to receive this. (*Shows the letter.*) But now I shall send it to them at once! (*Goes into his room and returns with a sheaf of papers.*) Look at this! Ten foolscap pages—closely written! I'm sending the analysis with it. A newspaper, Catherine! Get me something to wrap these up in. Good! There, now! Give it to—to—! (*Stamps his foot.*) What the devil's her name? You know, the maid! Tell her to take it straight down to the Mayor.

MRS. STOCKMANN *goes out through the dining-room with the parcel.*

PETRA: What do you think Uncle Peter will say, Father?

DR. STOCKMANN: What can he say? He must be grateful that so important a fact has been brought to light.

HOVSTAD: May I have your permission to print a short piece about your discovery in the *People's Tribune?*

DR. STOCKMANN: I'd be very grateful if you would.

HOVSTAD: I think it's desirable that the community should be informed as quickly as possible.

DR. STOCKMANN: Yes, yes, of course.

MRS. STOCKMANN (*comes back*): She's gone with it now.

BILLING: You'll be the first citizen in the town, Doctor, by jingo, you will!

DR. STOCKMANN (*walks round contentedly*): Oh, nonsense. I've really done nothing except my duty. I dug for treasure and struck lucky, that's all. All the same—!

BILLING: Hovstad, don't you think the town ought to organize a torchlight procession in honour of Dr. Stockmann?

HOVSTAD: I'll suggest it, certainly.

BILLING: And I'll have a word with Aslaksen.

DR. STOCKMANN: No, my dear friends, please don't bother with that nonsense. I don't want any fuss made. And if the Baths Committee should decide to raise my salary, I won't accept it! It's no good, Catherine, I won't accept it!

MRS. STOCKMANN: Quite right, Thomas.

PETRA (*raises her glass*): Skol, Father!

HOVSTAD
BILLING } (*together*): Skol, skol, Doctor!

HORSTER (*clinks his glass with the* DOCTOR's): Here's hoping your discovery will bring you nothing but joy!

DR. STOCKMANN: Thank you, my dear friends, thank you! I'm so deeply happy! Oh, it's good to know that one has the respect of one's fellow-citizens! Hurrah, Catherine!

Seizes her round the neck with both hands and whirls round with her. MRS. STOCKMANN *screams and struggles. Laughter, applause, and cheers for the* DOCTOR. *The* BOYS *stick their heads in through the door.*

Translated by Michael Meyer

SINCLAIR LEWIS

The Religion of a Scientist

I

The McGurk Building. A sheer wall, thirty blank stories of glass and lime-stone, down in the pinched triangle whence New York rules a quarter of the world.

Martin was not overwhelmed by his first hint of New York; after a year in the Chicago Loop, Manhattan seemed leisurely. But when from the elevated railroad he beheld the Woolworth Tower, he was exalted. To him architec-ture had never existed; buildings were larger or smaller bulks containing more or less interesting objects. His most impassioned architectural comment had been, "There's a cute bungalow; be nice place to live." Now he pondered, "Like to see that tower every day—clouds and storms behind it and every-thing—so sort of satisfying."

He came along Cedar Street, among thunderous trucks portly with wares from all the world; came to the bronze doors of the McGurk Building and a corridor of intemperately colored terra-cotta, with murals of Andean Indians, pirates booming up the Spanish Main, guarded gold-trains, and the stout walls of Cartagena. At the Cedar Street end of the corridor, a private street, one block long, was the Bank of the Andes and Antilles (Ross McGurk chairman of the board), in whose gold-crusted sanctity red-headed Yankee exporters drew drafts on Quito, and clerks hurled breathless Spanish at bulky women. A sign indicated, at the Liberty Street end, "Passenger Offices, McGurk Line, weekly sailings for the West Indies and South America."

Born to the prairies, never far from the sight of the cornfields, Martin was conveyed to blazing lands and portentous enterprises.

One of the row of bronze-barred elevators was labeled "Express to McGurk Institute." He entered it proudly, feeling himself already a part of the godly association. They rose swiftly, and he had but half-second glimpses of ground glass doors with the signs of mining companies, lumber companies, Central American railroad companies.

The McGurk Institute is probably the only organization for scientific re-search in the world which is housed in an office building. It has the twenty-ninth and thirtieth stories of the McGurk Building, and the roof is devoted to its animal house and to tiled walks along which (above a world of stenog-raphers and bookkeepers and earnest gentlemen who desire to sell Better-bilt Garments to the golden dons of the Argentine) saunter rapt scientists dream-ing of osmosis in Spirogyra.

Later, Martin was to note that the reception-room of the Institute was smaller, yet more forbiddingly polite, in its white paneling and Chippendale chairs, than the lobby of the Rouncefield Clinic, but now he was unconscious of the room, of the staccato girl attendant, of everything except that he was about to see Max Gottlieb, for the first time in five years.

At the door of the laboratory he stared hungrily.

Gottlieb was thin-cheeked and dark as ever, his hawk nose bony, his fierce eyes demanding, but his hair had gone gray, the flesh round his mouth was sunken, and Martin could have wept at the feebleness with which he rose. The old man peered down at him, his hand on Martin's shoulder, but he said only:

"Ah! Dis is good. . . . Your laboratory is three doors down the hall. . . . But I object to one thing in the good paper you send me. You say, 'The regularity of the rate at which the streptolysin disappears suggests that an equation may be found—' "

"But it can, sir!"

"Then why did you not make the equation?"

"Well— I don't know. I wasn't enough of a mathematician."

"Then you should not have published till you knew your math!"

"I— Look, Dr. Gottlieb, do you really think I know enough to work here? I want terribly to succeed."

"Succeed? I have heard that word. It is English? Oh, yes, it is a word that liddle schoolboys use at the University of Winnemac. It means passing examinations. But there are no examinations to pass here. . . . Martin, let us be clear. You know something of laboratory technique; you have heard about dese bacilli; you are not a good chemist, and mathematics—pfui!—most terrible! But you have curiosity and you are stubborn. You do not accept rules. Therefore I t'ink you will either make a very good scientist or a very bad one, and if you are bad enough, you will be popular with the rich ladies who rule this city, New York, and you can gif lectures for a living or even become, if you get to be plausible enough, a college president. So anyvay, it will be interesting."

Half an hour later they were arguing ferociously, Martin asserting that the whole world ought to stop warring and trading and writing and get straightway into laboratories to observe new phenomena; Gottlieb insisting that there were already too many facile scientists, that the one thing necessary was the mathematical analysis (and often the destruction) of phenomena already observed.

It sounded bellicose, and all the while Martin was blissful with the certainty that he had come home.

The laboratory in which they talked (Gottlieb pacing the floor, his long arms fantastically knotted behind his thin back; Martin leaping on and off tall stools) was not in the least remarkable—a sink, a bench with racks of numbered test-tubes, a microscope, a few note-books and hydrogen-ion charts, a grotesque series of bottles connected by glass and rubber tubes on an ordinary kitchen table at the end of the room—yet now and then during his tirades Martin looked about reverently.

Gottlieb interrupted their debate: "What work do you want to do here?"

"Why, sir, I'd like to help you, if I can. I suppose you're cleaning up some things on the synthesis of antibodies."

"Yes, I t'ink I can bring immunity reactions under the mass action law. But you are not to help me. You are to do your own work. What do you want to do? This is not a clinic, wit' patients going through so neat in a row!"

"I want to find a hemolysin for which there's an antibody. There isn't any for streptolysin. I'd like to work with staphylolysin. Would you mind?"

"I do not care what you do—if you just do not steal my staph cultures out of the ice-box, and if you will look mysterious all the time, so Dr. Tubbs, our Director, will t'ink you are up to something big. So! I haf only one suggestion: when you get stuck in a problem, I have a fine collection of detective stories in my office. But no. Should I be serious—this once, when you are just come?

"Perhaps I am a crank, Martin. There are many who hate me. There are plots against me—oh, you t'ink I imagine it, but you shall see! I make many mistakes. But one thing I keep always pure: the religion of a scientist.

"To be a scientist—it is not just a different job, so that a man should choose between being a scientist and being an explorer or a bond-salesman or a physician or a king or a farmer. It is a tangle of ver-y obscure emotions, like mysticism, or wanting to write poetry; it makes its victim all different from the good normal man. The normal man, he does not care much what he does except that he should eat and sleep and make love. But the scientist is intensely religious—he is so religious that he will not accept quarter-truths, because they are an insult to his faith.

"He wants that everything should be subject to inexorable laws. He is equal opposed to the capitalists who t'ink their silly money-grabbing is a system, and to liberals who t'ink man is not a fighting animal; he takes both the American booster and the European aristocrat, and he ignores all their blithering. Ignores it! All of it! He hates the preachers who talk their fables, but he iss not too kindly to the anthropologists and historians who can only make guesses, yet they have the nerf to call themselves scientists! Oh, yes, he is a man that all nice good-natured people should naturally hate!

"He speaks no meaner of the ridiculous faith-healers and chiropractors than he does of the doctors that want to snatch our science before it is tested and rush around hoping they heal people, and spoiling all the clues with their footsteps; and worse than the men like hogs, worse than the imbeciles who have not even heard of science, he hates pseudo-scientists, guess-scientists—like these psycho-analysts; and worse than those comic dream-scientists he hates the men that are allowed in a clean kingdom like biology but know only one text-book and how to lecture to nincompoops all so popular! He is the only real revolutionary, the authentic scientist, because he alone knows how liddle he knows.

"He must be heartless. He lives in a cold, clear light. Yet dis is a funny t'ing: really, in private, he is not cold nor heartless—so much less cold than the Professional Optimists. The world has always been ruled by the Philanthropists: by the doctors that want to use therapeutic methods they do not understand, by the soldiers that want something to defend their country against, by the preachers that yearn to make everybody listen to them, by the kind manufacturers that love their workers, by the eloquent statesmen and soft-hearted authors—and see once what a fine mess of hell they haf made of the world! Maybe now it is time for the scientist, who works and searches and never goes around howling how he loves everybody!

"But once again always remember that not all the men who work at science are scientists. So few! The rest—secretaries, press-agents, camp-followers! To be a scientist is like being a Goethe: it is born in you. Sometimes I t'ink you have a liddle of it born in you. If you haf, there is only one t'ing—no, there is two t'ings you must do: work twice as hard as you can, and keep people from using you. I will try to protect you from Success. It is all I can do. So. . . . I should wish, Martin, that you will be very happy here. May Koch bless you!"

II

Five rapt minutes Martin spent in the laboratory which was to be his—smallish but efficient, the bench exactly the right height, a proper sink with pedal taps. When he had closed the door and let his spirit flow out and fill that minute apartment with his own essence, he felt secure.

No Pickerbaugh or Rouncefield could burst in here and drag him away to be explanatory and plausible and public; he would be free to work, instead of being summoned to the package-wrapping and dictation of breezy letters which men call work.

He looked out of the broad window above his bench and saw that he did have the coveted Woolworth Tower, to keep and gloat on. Shut in to a joy of precision, he would nevertheless not be walled out from flowing life. He had, to the north, not the Woolworth Tower alone but the Singer Building, the arrogant magnificence of the City Investing Building. To the west, tall ships were riding, tugs were bustling, all the world went by. Below his cliff, the streets were feverish. Suddenly he loved humanity as he loved the decent, clean rows of test-tubes, and he prayed then the prayer of the scientist:

"God give me unclouded eyes and freedom from haste. God give me a quiet and relentless anger against all pretense and all pretentious work and all work left slack and unfinished. God give me a restlessness whereby I may neither sleep nor accept praise till my observed results equal my calculated results or in pious glee I discover and assault my error. God give me strength not to trust to God!"

<h2 style="text-align:center">III</h2>

He walked all the way up to their inconsiderable hotel in the Thirties, and all the way the crowds stared at him—this slim, pale, black-eyed, beaming young man who thrust among them, half-running, seeing nothing yet in a blur seeing everything: gallant buildings, filthy streets, relentless traffic, soldiers of fortune, fools, pretty women, frivolous shops, windy sky. His feet raced to the tune of "I've found my work, I've found my work, I've found my work!"

Leora was awaiting him—Leora whose fate it was ever to wait for him in creaky rocking-chairs in cheapish rooms. As he galloped in she smiled, and all her thin, sweet body was illumined. Before he spoke she cried:

"Oh, Sandy, I'm so glad!"

She interrupted his room-striding panegyrics on Max Gottlieb, on the McGurk Institute, on New York, on the charms of staphylolysin, by a meek "Dear, how much are they going to pay you?"

He stopped with a bump. "Gosh! I forgot to ask!"

"Oh!"

"Now you look here! This isn't a Rouncefield Clinic! I hate these buzzards that can't see anything but making money—"

"I know, Sandy. Honestly, I don't care. I was just wondering what kind of a flat we'll be able to afford, so I can begin looking for it. Go on. Dr. Gottlieb said—"

It was three hours after, at eight, when they went to dinner.

JORGE LUIS BORGES

The Immortals

And see, no longer blinded by our eyes.
RUPERT BROOKE

Whoever could have foreseen, way back in that innocent summer of 1923, that the novelette *The Chosen One* by Camilo N. Huergo, presented to me by the author with his personal inscription on the flyleaf (which I had the decorum to tear out before offering the volume for sale to successive men of the book trade), hid under the thin varnish of fiction a prophetic truth. Huergo's photograph, in an oval frame, adorns the cover. Each time I look at it, I have the impression that the snapshot is about to cough, a victim of that lung disease which nipped in the bud a promising career. Tuberculosis, in short, denied him the happiness of acknowledging the letter I wrote him in one of my characteristic outbursts of generosity.

The epigraph prefixed to this thoughtful essay has been taken from the aforementioned novelette; I requested Dr. Montenegro, of the Academy, to render it into Spanish, but the results were negative. To give the unprepared reader the gist of the matter, I shall now sketch, in condensed form, an out-line of Huergo's narrative, as follows:

The storyteller pays a visit, far to the south in Chubut, to the English rancher don Guillermo Blake, who devotes his energies not only to the breed-ing of sheep but also to the ramblings of the world-famous Plato and to the latest and more freakish experiments in the field of surgical medicine. On the basis of his reading, don Guillermo concludes that the five senses obstruct or deform the apprehension of reality and that, could we free ourselves of them, we would see the world as it is—endless and timeless. He comes to think that the eternal models of things lie in the depths of the soul and that the organs of perception with which the Creator has endowed us are, *grosso modo,* hindrances. They are no better than dark spectacles that blind us to what exists outside, diverting our attention at the same time from the splendor we carry within us.

Blake begets a son by one of the farm girls so that the boy may one day become acquainted with reality. To anesthetize him for life, to make him blind and deaf and dumb, to emancipate him from the senses of smell and taste, were the father's first concerns. He took, in the same way, all possible measures to make the chosen one unaware of his own body. As to the rest, this was arranged with contrivances designed to take over respiration, circula-tion, nourishment, digestion, and elimination. It was a pity that the boy, fully liberated, was cut off from all human contact.

Owing to the press of practical matters, the narrator goes away. After ten years, he returns. Don Guillermo has died; his son goes on living after his fashion, with natural breathing, heart regular, in a dusty shack cluttered with mechanical devices. The narrator, about to leave for good, drops a cigarette butt that sets fire to the shack and he never quite knows whether this act was done on purpose or by pure chance. So ends Huergo's story, strange enough. for its time but now, of course, more than outstripped by the rockets and astronauts of our men of science.

Having dashed off this disinterested compendium of the tale of a now dead and forgotten author—from whom I have nothing to gain—I steer back to the heart of the matter. Memory restores to me a Saturday morning in 1964 when I had an appointment with the eminent gerontologist Dr. Raúl Nar-bondo. The sad truth is that we young bloods of yesteryear are getting on; the thick mop begins to thin, one or another ear stops up, the wrinkles collect grime, molars grow hollow, a cough takes root, the backbone hunches up, the foot trips on a pebble, and, to put it plainly, the paterfamilias falters and withers. There was no doubt about it, the moment had come to see Dr. Narbondo for a general checkup, particularly considering the fact that he specialized in the replacement of malfunctioning organs.

Sick at heart because that afternoon the Palermo Juniors and the Spanish Sports were playing a return match and maybe I could not occupy my place in the front row to bolster my team, I betook myself to the clinic on Corrientes Avenue near Pasteur. The clinic, as its fame betrays, occupies the fifteenth floor of the Adamant Building. I went up by elevator (manufactured by the Electra Company). Eye to eye with Narbondo's brass shingle, I pressed the bell, and at long last, taking my courage in both hands, I slipped through the partly open door and entered into the waiting room proper. There, alone with the latest issues of *Ladies' Companion* and *Jumbo,* I whiled away the passing hours until a cuckoo clock struck twelve and sent me leaping from my armchair. At once, I asked myself, What happened? Planning my every move now like a sleuth, I took a step or two toward the next room, peeped in, ready, admittedly, to fly the coop at the slightest sound. From the streets far below came the noise of horns and traffic, the cry of a newspaper hawker, the squeal of brakes sparing some pedestrian, but, all around me, a reign of silence. I crossed a kind of laboratory, or pharmaceutical back room, furnished with instruments and flasks of all sorts. Stimulated by the aim of reaching the men's room, I pushed open a door at the far end of the lab.

Inside, I saw something that my eyes did not understand. The small enclosure was circular, painted white, with a low ceiling and neon lighting, and without a single window to relieve the sense of claustrophobia. The room was inhabited by four personages, or pieces of furniture. Their color was the same as the walls, their material wood, their form cubic. On each cube was another small cube with a latticed opening and below it a slot as in a mailbox. Carefully scrutinizing the grilled opening, you noted with alarm that from the interior you were being watched by something like eyes. The slots emitted, from time to time, a chorus of sighs or whisperings that the good Lord himself could not have made head or tail of. The placement of these cubes was such that they faced each other in the form of a square, composing a kind of conclave. I don't know how many minutes lapsed. At this point, the doctor came in and said to me, "My pardon, Bustos, for having kept you waiting. I was just out getting myself an advance ticket for today's match between the Palermo Juniors and the Spanish Sports." He went on, indicating the cubes, "Let me introduce you to Santiago Silberman, to retired clerk-of-court Ludueña, to Aquiles Molinari, and to Miss Bugard."

Out of the furniture came faint rumbling sounds. I quickly reached out a hand and, without the pleasure of shaking theirs, withdrew in good order, a frozen smile on my lips. Reaching the vestibule as best I could, I managed to stammer, "A drink. A stiff drink."

Narbondo came out of the lab with a graduated beaker filled with water and dissolved some effervescent drops into it. Blessed concoction—the wretched taste brought me to my senses. Then, the door to the small room closed and locked tight, came the explanation:

"I'm glad to see, my dear Bustos, that my immortals have made quite an impact on you. Whoever would have thought that *Homo sapiens,* Darwin's barely human ape, could achieve such perfection? This, my house, I assure you, is the only one in all Indo-America where Dr. Eric Stapledon's methodology has been fully applied. You recall, no doubt, the consternation that the death of the late lamented doctor, which took place in New Zealand, occasioned in scientific circles. I flatter myself, furthermore, for having implemented his precursory labors with a few Argentinean touches. In itself, the thesis—Newton's apple all over again—is fairly simple. The death of the body is a result, always, of the failure of some organ or other, call it the kidney, lungs, heart, or what you like. With the replacement of the organism's various components, in themselves perishable, with other corresponding stainless or polyethylene parts, there is no earthly reason whatever why the soul, why you yourself—Bustos Domecq—should not be immortal. None of your philosophical niceties here; the body can be vulcanized and from time to time recaulked, and so the mind keeps going. Surgery brings immortality to mankind. Life's essential aim has been attained—the mind lives on without fear of cessation. Each of our immortals is comforted by the certainty, backed by our firm's guarantee, of being a witness *in aeternum.* The brain, refreshed night and day by a system of electrical charges, is the last organic bulwark in which ball bearings and cells collaborate. The rest is Formica, steel, plastics. Respiration, alimentation, generation, mobility—elimination itself!—belong to the past. Our immortal is real estate. One or two minor touches are still missing, it's true. Oral articulation, dialogue, may still be improved. As for the costs, you need not worry yourself. By means of a procedure that circumvents legal red tape, the candidate transfers his property to us, and the Narbondo Company, Inc.—I, my son, his descendants—guarantees your upkeep, *in statu quo,* to the end of time. And, I might add, a moneyback guarantee."

It was then that he laid a friendly hand on my shoulder. I felt his will taking power over me. "Ha-ha! I see I've whetted your appetite, I've tempted you, dear Bustos. You'll need a couple of months or so to get your affairs in order and to have your stock portfolio signed over to us. As far as the operation goes, naturally, as a friend, I want to save you a little something. Instead of our usual fee of ten thousand dollars, for you, ninety-five hundred—in cash, of course. The rest is yours. It goes to pay your lodging, care, and service. The medical procedure in itself is painless. No more than a question of amputation and replacement. Nothing to worry about. On the eve, just keep yourself calm, untroubled. Avoid heavy meals, tobacco, and alcohol, apart from your accustomed and imported, I hope, Scotch or two. Above all, refrain from impatience."

"Why two months?" I asked him. "One's enough, and then some. I come out of the anesthesia and I'm one more of your cubes. You have my address and phone number. We'll keep in touch. I'll be back next Friday at the latest."

At the escape hatch he handed me the card of Nemirovski, Nemirovski, & Nemirovski, Counsellors at Law, who would put themselves at my disposal for all the details of drawing up the will. With perfect composure I walked to the subway entrance, then took the stairs at a run. I lost no time. That same night, without leaving the slightest trace behind, I moved to the New Impartial, in whose register I figure under the assumed name of Aquiles Silberman. Here, in my bedroom at the far rear of this modest hotel, wearing a false beard and dark spectacles, I am setting down this account of the facts.

Translated by Norman Thomas di Giovanni

SIR ARTHUR CONAN DOYLE

The Doctors of Hoyland

Dr. James Ripley was always looked upon as an exceedingly lucky dog by all of the profession who knew him. His father had preceded him in a practice in the village of Hoyland, in the north of Hampshire, and all was ready for him on the very first day that the law allowed him to put his name at the foot of a prescription. In a few years the old gentleman retired, and settled on the South Coast, leaving his son in undisputed possession of the whole countryside. Save for Dr. Horton, near Basingstoke, the young surgeon had a clear run of six miles in every direction, and took his fifteen hundred pounds a year, though, as is usual in country practices, the stable swallowed up most of what the consulting-room earned.

Dr. James Ripley was two-and-thirty years of age, reserved, learned, unmarried, with set, rather stern features, and a thinning of the dark hair upon the top of his head, which was worth quite a hundred a year to him. He was particularly happy in his management of ladies. He had caught the tone of bland sternness and decisive suavity which dominates without offending. Ladies, however, were not equally happy in their management of him. Professionally, he was always at their service. Socially, he was a drop of quicksilver. In vain the country mammas spread out their simple lures in front of him. Dances and picnics were not to his taste, and he preferred during his scanty leisure to shut himself up in his study, and to bury himself in Virchow's *Archives* and the professional journals.

Study was a passion with him, and he would have none of the rust which often gathers round a country practitioner. It was his ambition to keep his knowledge as fresh and bright as at the moment when he had stepped out of the examination hall. He prided himself on being able at a moment's notice to rattle off the seven ramifications of some obscure artery, or to give the exact percentage of any physiological compound. After a long day's work he would sit up half the night performing iridectomies and extractions upon the sheep's eyes sent in by the village butcher, to the horror of his housekeeper, who had to remove the *débris* next morning. His love for his work was the one fanaticism which found a place in his dry, precise nature.

It was the more to his credit that he should keep up to date in his knowledge, since he had no competition to force him to exertion. In the seven years during which he had practiced in Hoyland three rivals had pitted themselves against him, two in the village itself and one in the neighbouring hamlet of Lower Hoyland. Of these one had sickened and wasted, being, as it was said, himself the only patient whom he had treated during his eighteen months of ruralising. A second had bought a fourth share of a Basingstoke practice, and had departed honourably, while a third had vanished one September night, leaving a gutted house and an unpaid drug bill behind him. Since then the district had become a monopoly, and no one had dared to measure himself against the established fame of the Hoyland doctor.

It was, then, with a feeling of some surprise and considerable curiosity that on driving through Lower Hoyland one morning he perceived that the new house at the end of the village was occupied, and that a virgin brass plate glistened upon the swinging gate which faced the high road. He pulled up his fifty guinea chestnut mare and took a good look at it. "Verrinder Smith, M.D.," was printed across it in very neat, small lettering. The last man had had letters half a foot long, with a lamp like a fire-station. Dr. James Ripley noted the difference, and deduced from it that the newcomer might possibly prove a more formidable opponent. He was convinced of it that evening when he came to consult the current medical directory. By it he learned that Dr. Verrinder Smith was the holder of superb degrees, that he had studied with distinction at Edinburg, Paris, Berlin, and Vienna, and finally that he had been awarded a gold medal and the Lee Hopkins scholarship for original research, in recognition of an exhaustive inquiry into the functions of the anterior spinal nerve roots. Dr. Ripley passed his fingers through his thin hair in bewilderment as he read his rival's record. What on earth could so brilliant a man mean by putting up his plate in a little Hampshire hamlet.

But Dr. Ripley furnished himself with an explanation to the riddle. No doubt Dr. Verrinder Smith had simply come down there in order to pursue some scientific research in peace and quiet. The plate was up as an address rather than as an invitation to patients. Of course, that must be the true explanation. In that case the presence of this brilliant neighbour would be a splendid thing for his own studies. He had often longed for some kindred mind, some steel on which he might strike his flint. Chance had brought it to him, and he rejoiced exceedingly.

And this joy it was which led him to take a step which was quite at variance with his usual habits. It is the custom for a newcomer among medical men to call first upon the older, and the etiquette upon the subject is strict. Dr. Ripley was pedantically exact on such points, and yet he deliberately drove over next day and called upon Dr. Verrinder Smith. Such a waiving of ceremony was, he felt, a gracious act upon his part, and a fit prelude to the intimate relations which he hoped to establish with his neighbour.

The house was neat and well appointed, and Dr. Ripley was shown by a smart maid into a dapper little consulting-room. As he passed in he noticed two or three parasols and a lady's sun-bonnet hanging in the hall. It was a pity that his colleague should be a married man. It would put them upon a different footing, and interfere with those long evenings of high scientific talk which he had pictured to himself. On the other hand, there was much in the consulting-room to please him. Elaborate instruments, seen more often in hospitals than in the houses of private practitioners, were scattered about. A sphygmograph stood upon the table and a gasometer-like engine, which was new to Dr. Ripley, in the corner. A book-case full of ponderous volumes in French and German, paper-covered for the most part, and varying in tint from the shell to the yolk of a duck's egg, caught his wandering eyes, and he was deeply absorbed in their titles when the door opened suddenly behind him. Turning round, he found himself facing a little woman, whose plain, palish face was remarkable only for a pair of shrewd, humorous eyes of a blue which had two shades too much green in it. She held a *pince-nez* in her left hand, and the doctor's card in her right.

"How do you do, Doctor Ripley?" said she.

"How do you do, madam?" returned the visitor. "Your husband is perhaps out?"

"I am not married," said she simply.

"Oh, I beg your pardon! I meant the doctor—Doctor Verrinder Smith."

"I am Doctor Verrinder Smith."

Dr. Ripley was so surprised that he dropped his hat and forgot to pick it up again.

"What!" he gasped, "the Lee Hopkins prizeman! You!"

He had never seen a woman doctor before, and his whole conservative soul rose up in revolt at the idea. He could not recall any Biblical injunction that the man should remain ever the doctor and the woman the nurse, and yet he felt as if a blasphemy had been committed. His face betrayed his feelings only too clearly.

"I am sorry to disappoint you," said the lady drily.

"You certainly have surprised me," he answered, picking up his hat.

"You are not among our champions, then?"

"I cannot say that the movement has my approval."

"And why?"

"I should much prefer not to discuss it."

"But I am sure you will answer a lady's question."

"Ladies are in danger of losing their privileges when they usurp the place of the other sex. They cannot claim both."

"Why should a woman not earn her bread by her brains?"

Dr. Ripley felt irritated by the quiet manner in which the lady cross-questioned him.

"I should much prefer not to be led into a discussion, Miss Smith."

"Doctor Smith," she interrupted.

"Well, Doctor Smith! But if you insist upon an answer, I must say that I do not think medicine a suitable profession for women and that I have a personal objection to masculine ladies."

It was an exceedingly rude speech, and he was ashamed of it, the instant after he had made it. The lady however, simply raised her eyebrows and smiled.

"It seems to me that you are begging the question," said she. "Of course, if it makes women masculine that *would* be a considerable deterioration."

It was a neat little counter, and Dr. Ripley, like a pinked fencer, bowed his acknowledgment.

"I must go," said he.

"I am sorry that we cannot come to some more friendly conclusion since we are to be neighbours," she remarked.

He bowed again, and took a step towards the door.

"It was a singular coincidence," she continued, "that at the instant that you called I was reading your paper on 'Locomotor Ataxia,' in the *Lancet*."

"Indeed," said he drily.

"I thought it was a very able monograph."

"You are very good."

"But the views which you attribute to Professor Pitres, of Bordeaux, have been repudiated by him."

"I have his pamphlet of 1890," said Dr. Ripley angrily.

"Here is his pamphlet of 1891." She picked it from among a litter of periodicals. "If you have time to glance your eye down this passage—"

Dr. Ripley took it from her and shot rapidly through the paragraph which she indicated. There was no denying that it completely knocked the bottom out of his own article. He threw it down, and with another frigid bow he made for the door. As he took the reins from the groom he glanced round and saw that the lady was standing at her window, and it seemed to him that she was laughing heartily.

All day the memory of this interview haunted him. He felt that he had come very badly out of it. She had showed herself to be his superior on his own pet

subject. She had been courteous while he had been rude, self-possessed when
he had been angry. And then, above all, there was her presence, her monstrous
intrusion to rankle in his mind. A woman doctor had been an abstract thing
before, repugnant but distant. Now she was there in actual practice, with a
brass plate up just like his own, competing for the same patients. Not that he
feared competition, but he objected to this lowering of his ideal of womanhood. She could not be more than thirty, and had a bright, mobile face, too.
He thought of her humorous eyes, and of her strong, well-turned chin. It revolted him the more to recall the details of her education. A man, of course,
could come through such an ordeal with all his purity, but it was nothing
short of shameless in a woman.

But it was not long before he learned that even her competition was a
thing to be feared. The novelty of her presence had brought a few curious
invalids into her consulting-rooms, and, once there, they had been so impressed by the firmness of her manner and by the singular, new-fashioned instruments with which she tapped, and peered, and sounded, that it formed
the core of their conversation for weeks afterwards. And soon there were
tangible proofs of her powers upon the country-side. Farmer Eyton, whose
callous ulcer had been quietly spreading over his shin for years back under
a gentle régime of zinc ointment, was painted round with blistering fluid, and
found, after three blasphemous nights, that his sore was stimulated into healing. Mrs. Crowder, who had always regarded the birthmark upon her second
daughter Eliza as a sign of the indignation of the Creator at a third helping
of raspberry tart which she had partaken of during a critical period, learned
that, with the help of two galvanic needles, the mischief was not irreparable.
In a month Dr. Verrinder Smith was known, and in two she was famous.

Occasionally, Dr. Ripley met her as he drove upon his rounds. She had
started a high dog-cart, taking the reins herself, with a little tiger behind. When
they met he invariably raised his hat with punctilious politeness, but the grim
severity of his face showed how formal was the courtesy. In fact, his dislike
was rapidly deepening into absolute detestation. "The unsexed woman," was
the description of her which he permitted himself to give to those of his patients who still remained staunch. But, indeed, they were a rapidly-decreasing
body, and every day his pride was galled by the news of some fresh defection.
The lady had somehow impressed the country-folk with almost superstitious
belief in her power, and from far and near they flocked to her consulting-
room.

But what galled him most of all was, when she did something which he had
pronounced to be impracticable. For all his knowledge he lacked nerve as an
operator, and usually sent his worst cases up to London. The lady, however,
had no weakness of the sort, and took everything that came in her way. It was
agony to him to hear that she was about to straighten little Alec Turner's
club-foot, and right at the fringe of the rumour came a note from his mother,
the rector's wife, asking him if he would be so good as to act as chloroformist.

It would be inhumanity to refuse, as there was no other who could take the place, but it was gall and wormwood to his sensitive nature. Yet, in spite of his vexation, he could not but admire the dexterity with which the thing was done. She handled the little wax-like foot so gently, and held the tiny tenotomy knife as an artist holds his pencil. One straight insertion, one snick of a tendon, and it was all over without a stain upon the white towel which lay beneath. He had never seen anything more masterly, and he had the honesty to say so, though her skill increased his dislike of her. The operation spread her fame still further at his expense, and self-preservation was added to his other grounds for detesting her. And this very detestation it was which brought matters to a curious climax.

One winter's night, just as he was rising from his lonely dinner, a groom came riding down from Squire Faircastle's, the richest man in the district, to say that his daughter had scalded her hand, and that medical help was needed on the instant. The coachman had ridden for the lady doctor, for it mattered nothing to the Squire who came as long as it were speedily. Dr. Ripley rushed from his surgery with the determination that she should not effect an entrance into this stronghold of his if hard driving on his part could prevent it. He did not even wait to light his lamps, but sprang into his gig and flew off as fast as hoof could rattle. He lived rather nearer to the Squire's than she did, and was convinced that he could get there well before her.

And so he would but for that whimsical element of chance, which will for ever muddle up the affairs of this world and dumbfound the prophets. Whether it came from the want of his lights, or from his mind being full of the thoughts of his rival, he allowed too little by half a foot in taking the sharp turn upon the Basingstoke road. The empty trap and the frightened horse clattered away into the darkness, while the Squire's groom crawled out of the ditch into which he had been shot. He struck a match, looked down at his groaning companion, and then, after the fashion of rough, strong men when they see what they have not seen before, he was very sick.

The doctor raised himself a little on his elbow in the glint of the match. He caught a glimpse of something white and sharp bristling through his trouser-leg half-way down the shin.

"Compound!" he groaned. "A three months' job," and fainted.

When he came to himself the groom was gone, for he had scudded off to the Squire's house for help, but a small page was holding a gig-lamp in front of his injured leg, and a woman, with an open case of polished instruments gleaming in the yellow light, was deftly slitting up his trouser with a crooked pair of scissors.

"It's all right, doctor," said she soothingly. "I am so sorry about it. You can have Doctor Horton tomorrow, but I am sure you will allow me to help you tonight. I could hardly believe my eyes when I saw you by the roadside."

"The groom has gone for help," groaned the sufferer.

"When it comes we can move you into the gig. A little more light, John!

So! Ah, dear, dear, we shall have laceration unless we reduce this before we move you. Allow me to give you a whiff of chloroform, and I have no doubt that I can secure it sufficiently to—"

Dr. Ripley never heard the end of that sentence. He tried to raise a hand and to murmur something in protest, but a sweet smell was in his nostrils, and a sense of rich peace and lethargy stole over his jangled nerves. Down he sank, through clear, cool water, ever down and down into the green shadows beneath, gently, without effort, while the pleasant chiming of a great belfry rose and fell in his ears. Then he rose again, up and up, and ever up, with a terrible tightness about his temples, until at last he shot out of those green shadows and was in the light once more. Two bright, shining, golden spots gleamed before his dazed eyes. He blinked and blinked before he could give a name to them. They were only the two brass balls at the end posts of his bed, and he was lying in his own little room, with a head like a cannon ball, and a leg like an iron bar. Turning his eyes, he saw the calm face of Dr. Verrinder Smith looking down at him.

"Ah, at last!" said she. "I kept you under all the way home, for I knew how painful the jolting would be. It is in good position now with a strong side splint. I have ordered a morphia draught for you. Shall I tell your groom to ride for Doctor Horton in the morning?"

"I should prefer that you continue the case," said Dr. Ripley feebly, and then, with a half-hysterical laugh—"You have all the rest of the parish as patients, you know, so you may as well make the thing complete by having me also."

It was not a very gracious speech, but it was a look of pity and not of anger which shone in her eyes as she turned away from his bedside.

Dr. Ripley had a brother, William, who was assistant surgeon at a London hospital, and who was down in Hampshire within a few hours of his hearing of the accident. He raised his brows when he heard the details.

"What! You are pestered with one of those!" he cried.

"I don't know what I should have done without her."

"I've no doubt she's an excellent nurse."

"She knows her work as well as you or I."

"Speak for yourself, James," said the London man with a sniff. "But apart from that, you know that the principle of the thing is all wrong."

"You think there is nothing to be said on the other side?"

"Good heavens! do you?"

"Well, I don't know. It struck me during the night that we may have been a little narrow in our views."

"Nonsense, James. It's all very fine for women to win prizes in the lecture-room, but you know as well as I do that they are no use in an emergency. Now I warrant that this woman was all nerves when she was setting your leg. That reminds me that I had better just take a look at it and see that it is all right."

"I would rather that you did not undo it," said the patient. "I have her assurance that it is all right."

Brother William was deeply shocked.

"Of course, if a woman's assurance is of more value than the opinion of the assistant surgeon of a London hospital, there is nothing more to be said," he remarked.

"I should prefer that you did not touch it," said the patient firmly, and Dr. William went back to London that evening in a huff.

The lady, who had heard of his coming, was much surprised on learning of his departure.

"We had a difference upon a point of professional etiquette," said Dr. James, and it was all the explanation he would vouchsafe.

For two long months Dr. Ripley was brought in contact with his rival every day, and he learned many things which he had not known before. She was a charming companion, as well as a most assiduous doctor. Her short presence during the long, weary day was like a flower in a sand waste. What interested him was precisely what interested her, and she could meet him at every point upon equal terms. And yet under all her learning and her firmness ran a sweet, womanly nature, peeping out in her talk, shining in her greenish eyes, showing itself in a thousand subtle ways which the dullest of men could read. And he, though a bit of a prig and a pedant, was by no means dull, and had honesty enough to confess when he was in the wrong.

"I don't know how to apologise to you," he said in his shame-faced fashion one day, when he had progressed so far as to be able to sit in an arm-chair with his leg upon another one; "I feel that I have been quite in the wrong."

"Why, then?"

"Over this woman question. I used to think that a woman must inevitably lose something of her charm if she took up such studies."

"Oh, you don't think they are necessarily unsexed, then?" she cried, with a mischievous smile.

"Please don't recall my idiotic expression."

"I feel so pleased that I should have helped in changing your views. I think that it is the most sincere compliment that I have ever had paid me."

"At any rate, it is the truth," said he, and was happy all night at the remembrance of the flush of pleasure which made her pale face look quite comely for the instant.

For, indeed, he was already far past the stage when he would acknowledge her as the equal of any other woman. Already he could not disguise from himself that she had become the one woman. Her dainty skill, her gentle touch, her sweet presence, the community of their tastes, had all united to hopelessly upset his previous opinions. It was a dark day for him now when his convalescence allowed her to miss a visit, and darker still that other one which he saw approaching when all occasion for her visits would be at an end. It came round at last, however, and he felt that his whole life's fortune would hang upon the issue of that final interview. He was a direct man by nature, so he laid his hand upon hers as it felt for his pulse, and he asked her if she would be his wife.

"What, and unite the practices?" said she.

He started in pain and anger.

"Surely you do not attribute any such base motive to me!" he cried. "I love you as unselfishly as ever a woman was loved."

"No, I was wrong. It was a foolish speech," said she, moving her chair a little back, and tapping her stethoscope upon her knee. "Forget that I ever said it. I am so sorry to cause you any disappointment, and I appreciate most highly the honour which you do me, but what you ask is quite impossible."

With another woman he might have urged the point, but his instincts told him that it was quite useless with this one. Her tone of voice was conclusive. He said nothing, but leaned back in his chair a stricken man.

"I am so sorry," she said again. "If I had known what was passing in your mind I should have told you earlier that I intend to devote my life entirely to science. There are many women with a capacity for marriage, but few with a taste for biology. I will remain true to my own line, then. I came down here while waiting for an opening in the Paris Physiological Laboratory. I have just heard that there is a vacancy for me there, and so you will be troubled no more by my intrusion upon your practice. I have done you an injustice just as you did me one. I thought you narrow and pedantic, with no good quality. I have learned during your illness to appreciate you better, and the recollection of our friendship will always be a very pleasant one to me."

And so it came about that in a very few weeks there was only one doctor in Hoyland. But folks noticed that the one had aged many years in a few months, that a weary sadness lurked always in the depths of his blue eyes, and that he was less concerned than ever with the eligible young ladies whom chance, or their careful country mammas, placed in his way.

OLIVER WENDELL HOLMES

A Sentiment

[Distributed among the members gathered at the meeting of the American Medical Association, in Philadelphia, May 1, 1855.]

A TRIPLE health to Friendship, Science, Art,
From heads and hands that own a common
    heart!
Each in its turn the others' willing slave,
Each in its season strong to heal and save.

Friendship's blind service, in the hour of need,
Wipes the pale face, and lets the victim
  bleed.
Science must stop to reason and explain;
ART claps his finger on the streaming vein.

But Art's brief memory fails the hand at
  last;
Then SCIENCE lifts the flambeau of the past.
When both their equal impotence deplore,
When Learning sighs, and Skill can do no
  more,
The tear of FRIENDSHIP pours its heavenly
  balm,
And soothes the pang no anodyne may
  calm!

Topics for Discussion and Writing

1. In "Are Doctors Men of Science?" Shaw holds that "Doctoring is an art, not a science...." Explain his point by following the steps of his argument. Do you agree or disagree with Shaw? Have modern medical developments made some of his 1911 comments obsolete?

2. Read your library's copy of *The Doctor's Dilemma* (1906) in order to discover Shaw's fuller dramatic statement on medicine and science. In addition, review his "Preface on Doctors," which was printed with his play in 1911. Then prepare (1) a five-minute oral report of your findings for the class, and (2) a short written report for your instructor.

3. Who is the other doctor in "Rappaccini's Daughter"? How does he function in Hawthorne's story? Is he any more humane than Dr. Rappaccini? What is the meaning of the story's last two paragraphs? Is there irony? Explain.

4. Write an evaluative character sketch of Hawthorne's Beatrice. Quote from the text to support the main points of your original essay.

5. How exactly is the young Sioux medicine man, Black Elk, actually a better physician than the learned Dr. Giacomo Rappaccini?

6. In addition to the significant material on what the 1950s generation wanted from its superstars and miracle drugs, Williams' "Of Medicine and Poetry" is also interesting because of the doctor-author's opening

lines about how, for him, medicine and poetry are "nearly the same thing." Review Williams' "The Use of Force" (part 1) in light of this autobiographical essay. Does the essay illuminate that story? How?

7. From your reading of act one of Ibsen's *An Enemy of the People,* do you detect any elements of the "mad scientist" in Dr. Stockmann? Does Dr. Stockmann seek renown and status? Why? What backs up his claim that "the water here contains putrid organic matter—millions of bacteria"?

8. Read your library's copy of the last four acts of *An Enemy of the People.* Prepare a concisely written plot summary for the members of your discussion group. Are you satisfied with the play's ending?

9. What does the line "It was three hours after, at eight, when they went to dinner" indicate about Dr. Martin Arrowsmith's priorities? What is Leora's "place" in Martin's world of pure scientific research?

10. The narrator of "The Immortals," Bustos Domecq, feigns agreement with Dr. Narbondo. But after he leaves the doctor's office, what does Bustos proceed to do?

11. Picture yourself confronted with Dr. Narbondo's offer. Would you accept? Would you react as Bustos did? Explain your decision in an essay that weighs the science-versus-humanity issue. Should the mind and body ever be capable of a separation in which the mind could live on alone—would such a state of affairs be desirable?

12. What do you think Doyle is aiming at in having Dr. James Ripley say: " 'I should much prefer not to be led into a discussion, *Miss* Smith,' " only to be quickly corrected: " '*Doctor* Smith,' she interrupted" (italics added)?

13. What is the significance of Dr. Smith's concluding words—". . . I intend to devote my life entirely to science. There are many women with a capacity for marriage, but few with a taste for biology. I will remain true to my own line, then"—for "The Doctors of Hoyland" as a whole?

14. In a carefully planned essay, use Holmes' "A Sentiment" *and* your own powers of reasoning to help bring into clearer focus the diverse selections on the medicine-and-science theme in this part.

Part 5

*Medicine and
the Nurse*

The teacher of a course on medicine in literature can choose from scores of poems, stories, plays, and even novels that are doctor-oriented. But for reasons that might be profitably enumerated and discussed, very little creative literature on men and women in the allied health occupations seems to be available. What works we can discover focus primarily on nurses and their role in medicine, yet all too frequently the picture is either stereotyped or distorted. This part brings the nurse and other medical personnel to center stage.

Louisa May Alcott's "A Night" is one of the moving *Hospital Sketches* (1863) based on her brief experience in Washington as a volunteer Civil War nurse. Because Alcott was not specifically trained as a nurse, her night-shift duties consisted of showing "a motherly affection" for the Union men on Ward No. 1 and of "reading aloud, writing letters, waiting on and amusing the men, going the rounds with Dr. P., as he made his second daily survey, dressing my dozen wounds afresh, giving last doses, and making them cozy for the long hours to come. . . ." She tells of the three separate rooms on her ward, of her ward assistants, and of how she ministered to men in great pain or about to die. Dr. P. treated the soldiers but left it to a woman —Alcott—to break the sad news of impending death to those concerned. Even in the 1970s, it is difficult for the modern nurse to dissociate herself from the stereotype that appears in "A Night." To be sure, compassion and tenderness should continue as highly prized nursing qualities, but today's registered nurse should now be recognized as a fully trained professional and as a key member of the health-care team—a team that includes doctors, registered nurses, licensed practical nurses, orderlies, surgical technicians, and x-ray technicians, among many others.

In "The Wound-Dresser," Walt Whitman realistically describes some of his hospital activities during the time he, too, spent in Washington hospitals as a volunteer Civil War nurse. Whitman may be seen as the male counterpart of Alcott, for both worked under great pressure to ease the pain of the war-wounded. Fortunately, medicine has progressed much since the 1860s, and there is considerably more to nursing today than dressing wounds and giving comfort to those apparently fated to die. Moreover, many men

have decided to take up professional nursing as a career and to make significant contributions as nursing practitioners. What Alcott and Whitman described, therefore, was just a beginning for nursing.

But even William Carlos Williams' "Jean Beicke," a story set in the
Great Depression, presents the nurse somewhat ambivalently as both the
professional care-giver and the often emotional female. The doctor-narrator takes us onto a pediatrics ward where doctors and nurses "try to make
something out of" poor children who are very young, unwanted, dirty, and
diseased. The case of Jean Beicke, who is eleven months old and who suffers
from a mysterious illness, occupies most of this autobiographical tale. Jean
steals the hearts of those who labor to help her survive. Even the hard-
boiled doctor who claims not to care is touched by Jean's eventual death.
This story is especially rich in passages that reveal the feelings of nurses when
working with children as patients. The point seems to be that emotion plays
a necessary part for both the nurse *and* the doctor in the health-care system,
no matter how modern or scientifically advanced that system may be.

"The Big Nurse," a selection from Ken Kesey's popular novel *One Flew
Over the Cuckoo's Nest,* shows (1) how Miss Ratched, her staff nurses, her
attendants, and her technicians dominate the doctors and the patients, and
(2) how Miss Ratched in turn dominates *all* these. Obviously this sketch of
a contemporary nurse in charge of a psychiatric ward is a distortion of the
ideal as well as the real. The inmate-narrator, Chief Bromden, catalogues
the Big Nurse's strictly patterned routine so that we wonder just who is and
who is not insane in this mental institution. It is true that we have, in Kesey's
fiction, one of the few portraits of a nurse in a dominant literary role, but
we still have yet to see represented a fully modern, balanced, and professional nurse. Alcott's naiveté sharply contrasts with Miss Ratched's acerbic
cleverness, yet neither is an adequate portrayal of what a nurse is or should be.
In another pairing, the sympathetic nurses in "Jean Beicke" contrast with the
cold Miss Ratched and her crew, but here, too, neither case tells the whole story.

In an interview from his book *Working* with a devoted and sensitive West
Indian practical nurse in an old people's home, Studs Terkel lets the story
of Carmelita Lester dramatically unfold. Her moving nursing-home experiences, her positive and professional attitude toward the work, and her concluding suggestions about quality health care for our senior citizens—all these
points make Carmelita Lester a special health-care professional, indeed. The
negative stereotypes of the nurse as a plaything for medical men and as an
inferior care-giver are finally dying.

"Not Cancer at All," the opening section of Aleksandr Solzhenitsyn's
novel *The Cancer Ward,* sheds possibly more light on the contemporary
nurse's actual problems and responsibilities than do the other selections in
this part. Rusanov sadly enters the unlucky Ward No. 13, the cancer ward.
After bidding farewell to his wife and son, he experiences the inferior conditions of this public hospital and is shocked. The overworked nurses can

barely keep up with their excessive patient load and their paperwork; Rusanov soon realizes that they will not be able to give him any special attention. Solzhenitsyn exposes crowded hospital conditions as he also depicts the nurses' long hours, short staffing, and concern for patients, as well as their duty to keep moving and to concentrate on serious cases first. Here is a portrait that closely resembles today's American staff nurse—ethical, knowledgeable, hardworking, and often overtaxed. It is noteworthy that the senior nurse, Mita, refuses the bribe: " 'No, no!' the nurse said, her voice cold. 'We don't do these things.' " Is it the nurse's ethics or the Soviet Union's tight security regulations that make her refuse? Perhaps it is both.

LOUISA MAY ALCOTT

A Night

Being fond of the night side of nature, I was soon promoted to the post of night nurse, with every facility for indulging in my favorite pastime of "owling." My colleague, a black-eyed widow, relieved me at dawn, we two taking care of the ward, between us, like the immortal Sairy and Betsey,[1] "turn and turn about." I usually found my boys in the jolliest state of mind their condition allowed; for it was a known fact that Nurse Periwinkle objected to blue devils, and entertained a belief that he who laughed most was surest of recovery. At the beginning of my reign, dumps and dismals prevailed; the nurses looked anxious and tired, the men gloomy or sad; and a general "Hark!-from-the-tombs-a-doleful-sound" style of conversation seemed to be the fashion: a state of things which caused one coming from a merry, social New England town, to feel as if she had got into an exhausted receiver; and the instinct of self-preservation, to say nothing of a philanthropic desire to serve the race, caused a speedy change in Ward No. 1.

More flattering than the most gracefully turned compliment, more grateful than the most admiring glance, was the sight of those rows of faces, all strange to me a little while ago, now lighting up with smiles of welcome, as I came among them, enjoying that moment heartily, with a womanly pride in their regard, a motherly affection for them all. The evenings were spent in reading aloud, writing letters, waiting on and amusing the men, going the rounds with Dr. P., as he made his second daily survey, dressing my dozen

---

1. Sairy Gamp, in Charles Dickens' *Martin Chuzzlewit,* was one of Miss Alcott's favorite comic characters, with whom she often humorously identified herself. Her companion is Betsey Prig.

wounds afresh, giving last doses, and making them cozy for the long hours to come, till the nine o'clock bell rang, the gas was turned down, the day nurses went off duty, the night watch came on, and my nocturnal adventure began.

My ward was now divided into three rooms; and, under favor of the matron, I had managed to sort out the patients in such a way that I had what I called, "my duty room," my "pleasure room," and my "pathetic room," and worked for each in a different way. One I visited, armed with a dressing tray, full of rollers, plasters, and pins; another, with books, flowers, games, and gossip; a third, with teapots, lullabies, consolation, and, sometimes a shroud.

Wherever the sickest or most helpless man chanced to be, there I held my watch, often visiting the other rooms, to see that the general watchman of the ward did his duty by the fires and the wounds, the latter needing constant wetting. Not only on this account did I meander, but also to get fresher air than the close rooms afforded; for, owing to the stupidity of that mysterious "somebody" who does all the damage in the world the windows had been carefully nailed down above, and the lower sashes could only be raised in the mildest weather, for the men lay just below. I had suggested a summary smashing of a few panes here and there, when frequent appeals to headquarters had proved unavailing, and daily orders to lazy attendants had come to nothing. No one seconded the motion, however, and the nails were far beyond my reach; for, though, belonging to the sisterhood of "ministering angels," I had no wings, and might as well have asked for Jacob's ladder, as a pair of steps, in that charitable chaos.

One of the harmless ghosts who bore me company during the haunted hours, was Dan, the watchman, whom I regarded with a certain awe; for, though so much together, I never fairly saw his face, and, but for his legs, should never have recognized him, as we seldom met by day. These legs were remarkable, as was his whole figure, for his body was short, rotund, and done up in a big jacket, and muffler; his beard hid the lower part of his face, his hat-brim the upper; and all I ever discovered was a pair of sleepy eyes, and a very mild voice. But the legs!—very long, very thin, very crooked and feeble, looking like grey sausages in their tight coverings, without a ray of pegtopishness about them, and finished off with a pair of expansive, green cloth shoes, very like Chinese junks, with the sails down. This figure, gliding noiselessly about the dimly lighted rooms, was strongly suggestive of the spirit of a beer barrel mounted on cork-screws, haunting the old hotel in search of its lost mates, emptied and staved in long ago.

Another goblin who frequently appeared to me, was the attendant of the pathetic room, who, being a faithful soul, was often up to tend two or three men, weak and wandering as babies, after the fever had gone. The amiable creature beguiled the watches of the night by brewing jorums of a fearful beverage, which he called coffee, and insisted on sharing with me; coming in with a great bowl of something like mud soup, scalding hot, guiltless of cream, rich in an all-pervading flavor of molasses, scorch and tin pot. Such an amount of good will and neighborly kindness also went into the mess, that I never could find the heart to refuse, but always received it with thanks, sipped it with hypocritical relish while he remained, and whipped it into the slop-jar the instant he departed, thereby gratifying him, securing one rousing laugh in the doziest hour of the night, and no one was the worse for the transaction but the pigs. Whether they were "cut off untimely in their sins," or not, I carefully abstained from inquiring.

It was a strange life—asleep half the day, exploring Washington the other half, and all night hovering, like a massive cherubim, in a red rigolette,[2] over the slumbering sons of man. I liked it, and found many things to amuse, instruct, and interest me. The snores alone were quite a study, varying from the mild sniff to the stentorian snort, which startled the echoes and hoisted the performer erect to accuse his neighbor of the deed, magnanimously forgive him, and, wrapping the drapery of his couch about him, lie down to vocal slumber. After listening for a week to this band of wind instruments, I indulged in the belief that I could recognize each by the snore alone, and was tempted to join the chorus by breaking out with John Brown's favorite hymn:

"Blow ye the trumpet, blow!"

I would have given much to have possessed the art of sketching, for many of the faces became wonderfully interesting when unconscious. Some grew stern and grim, the men evidently dreaming of war, as they gave orders, groaned over their wounds, or damned the rebels vigorously; some grew sad and infinitely pathetic, as if the pain borne silently all day, revenged itself by now betraying what the man's pride had concealed so well. Often the roughest grew young and pleasant when sleep smoothed the hard lines away, letting the real nature assert itself; many almost seemed to speak, and I learned to know these men better by night than through any intercourse by day. Sometimes they disappointed me, for faces that looked merry and good in the light, grew bad and sly when the shadows came; and though they made no confidences in words, I read their lives, leaving them to wonder at the change of manner this midnight magic wrought in their nurse. A few talked busily; one drummer boy sang sweetly, though no persuasions could win a note from him by day; and several depended on being told what they had talked of in the morning. Even my constitutionals in the chilly halls, possessed a certain charm, for the house was never still. Sentinels tramped round it all night long, their muskets glittering in the wintry moonlight as they walked, or stood before the doors, straight and silent, as figures of stone,

2. A kind of wool scarf worn as a head covering.

causing one to conjure up romantic visions of guarded forts, sudden surprises, and daring deeds; for in these war times the hum drum life of Yankeedom has vanished, and the most prosaic feel some thrill of that excitement which stirs the nation's heart, and makes its capital a camp of hospitals. Wandering up and down these lower halls, I often heard cries from above, steps hurrying to and fro, saw surgeons passing up, or men coming down carrying a stretcher, where lay a long white figure, whose face was shrouded and whose fight was done. Sometimes I stopped to watch the passers in the street, the moonlight shining on the spire opposite, or the gleam of some vessel floating, like a white-winged sea-gull, down the broad Potomac, whose fullest flow can never wash away the red stain of the land.

The night whose events I have a fancy to record, opened with a little comedy, and closed with a great tragedy; for a virtuous and useful life untimely ended is always tragical to those who see not as God sees. My headquarters were beside the bed of a New Jersey boy, crazed by the horrors of that dreadful Saturday. A slight wound in the knee brought him there; but his mind had suffered more than his body; some string of that delicate machine was over strained, and, for days, he had been reliving, in imagination, the scenes he could not forget, till his distress broke out in incoherent ravings, pitiful to hear. As I sat by him, endeavoring to soothe his poor distracted brain by the constant touch of wet hands over his hot forehead, he lay cheering his comrades on, hurrying them back, then counting them as they fell around him, often clutching my arm, to drag me from the vicinity of a bursting shell, or covering up his head to screen himself from a shower of shot; his face brilliant with fever; his eyes restless; his head never still; every muscle strained and rigid; while an incessant stream of defiant shouts, whispered warnings, and broken laments, poured from his lips with that forceful bewilderment which makes such wanderings so hard to overhear.

It was past eleven, and my patient was slowly wearying himself into fitful intervals of quietude, when, in one of these pauses, a curious sound arrested my attention. Looking over my shoulder, I saw a one-legged phantom hopping nimbly down the room; and, going to meet it, recognized a certain Pennsylvania gentleman, whose wound-fever had taken a turn for the worse, and, depriving him of the few wits a drunken campaign had left him, set him literally tripping on the light, fantastic toe "toward home," as he blandly informed me, touching the military cap which formed a striking contrast to the severe simplicity of the rest of his decidedly *undress* uniform. When sane, the least movement produced a roar of pain or a volley of oaths; but the departure of reason seemed to have wrought an agreeable change, both in the man and his manners; for, balancing himself on one leg, like a meditative stork, he plunged into an animated discussion of the war, the President, lager beer, and Enfield rifles, regardless of any suggestions of mine as to the propriety of returning to bed, lest he be court-martialed for desertion.

Anything more supremely ridiculous can hardly be imagined than this figure, scantily draped in white, its one foot covered with a big blue sock, a dingy cap set rakingly askew on its shaven head, and placid satisfaction beaming in its broad red face, as it flourished a mug in one hand, an old boot in the other, calling them canteen and knapsack, while it skipped and fluttered in the most unearthly fashion. What to do with the creature I didn't know; Dan was absent, and if I went to find him, the perambulator might festoon himself out of the window, set his toga on fire, or do some of his neighbors a mischief. The attendant of the room was sleeping like a near relative of the celebrated Seven,[3] and nothing short of pins would rouse him; for he had been out that day, and whiskey asserted its supremacy in balmy whiffs. Still declaiming, in a fine flow of eloquence, the demented gentleman hopped on, blind and deaf to my graspings and entreaties; and I was about to slam the door in his face, and run for help, when a second and saner phantom, "all in white," came to the rescue, in the likeness of a big Prussian, who spoke no English, but divined the crisis, and put an end to it, by bundling the lively monoped into his bed, like a baby, with an authoritative command to "stay put," which received added weight from being delivered in an odd conglomeration of French and German, accompanied by warning wags of a head decorated with a yellow cotton night cap, rendered most imposing by a tassel like a bell-pull. Rather exhausted by his excursion, the member from Pennsylvania subsided; and, after an irrepressible laugh together, my Prussian ally and myself were returning to our places, when the echo of a sob caused us to glance along the beds. It came from one in the corner—such a little bed!—and such a tearful little face looked up at us, as we stopped beside it! The twelve years old drummer boy was not singing now, but sobbing, with a manly effort all the while to stifle the distressful sounds that would break out.

"What is it, Teddy?" I asked, as he rubbed the tears away, and checked himself in the middle of a great sob to answer plaintively:

"I've got a chill, ma'am, but I aint cryin' for that, 'cause I'm used to it. I dreamed Kit was here, and when I waked up he wasn't, and I couldn't help it, then."

The boy came in with the rest, and the man who was taken dead from the ambulance was the Kit he mourned. Well he might; for, when the wounded were brought from Fredericksburg, the child lay in one of the camps thereabout, and this good friend, though sorely hurt himself, would not leave him to the exposure and neglect of such a time and place; but, wrapping him in his own blanket, carried him in his arms to the transport, tended him during the passage, and only yielded up his charge when Death met him at the door of the hospital which promised care and comfort for the boy. For ten days,

3. The Seven Sleepers, in Christian tradition, were seven noble youths of Ephesus who fled during the persecution of Christians (A.D. 249–51), and slept in a cave for several hundred years until Christianity had become the accepted religion of the empire.

Teddy had shivered or burned with fever and ague, pining the while for Kit, and refusing to be comforted, because he had not been able to thank him for the generous protection, which, perhaps, had cost the giver's life. The vivid dream had wrung the childish heart with a fresh pang, and when I tried the solace fitted for his years, the remorseful fear that haunted him found vent in a fresh burst of tears, as he looked at the wasted hands I was endeavoring to warm:

"Oh! if I'd only been as thin when Kit carried me as I am now, maybe he wouldn't have died; but I was heavy, he was hurt worser than we knew, and so it killed him; and I didn't see him, to say good bye."

This thought had troubled him in secret; and my assurances that his friend would probably have died at all events, hardly assuaged the bitterness of his regretful grief.

At this juncture, the delirious man began to shout; the one-legged rose up in his bed, as if preparing for another dart; Teddy bewailed himself more piteously than before: and if ever a woman was at her wit's end, that distracted female was Nurse Periwinkle, during the space of two or three minutes, as she vibrated between the three beds, like an agitated pendulum. Like a most opportune reinforcement, Dan, the bandy, appeared, and devoted himself to the lively party, leaving me free to return to my post; for the Prussian, with a nod and a smile, took the lad away to his own bed, and lulled him to sleep with a soothing murmur, like a mammoth humble bee. I liked that in Fritz, and if he ever wondered afterward at the dainties which sometimes found their way into his rations, or the extra comforts of his bed, he might have found a solution of the mystery in sundry persons' knowledge of the fatherly action of that night.

Hardly was I settled again, when the inevitable bowl appeared, and its bearer delivered a message I had expected, yet dreaded to receive:

"John is going, ma'am, and wants to see you, if you can come."

"The moment this boy is asleep; tell him so, and let me know if I am in danger of being too late."

My Ganymede[4] departed, and while I quieted poor Shaw, I thought of John. He came in a day or two after the others; and, one evening, when I entered my "pathetic room," I found a lately emptied bed occupied by a large, fair man, with a fine face, and the serenest eyes I ever met. One of the earlier comers had often spoken of a friend, who had remained behind, that those apparently worse wounded than himself might reach a shelter first. It seemed a David and Jonathan sort of friendship. The man fretted for his mate, and was never tired of praising John—his courage, sobriety, self-denial, and unfailing kindliness of heart; always winding up with: "He's an out an' out fine feller, ma'am; you see if he aint."

4. Cupbearer to the gods.

I had some curiosity to behold this piece of excellence, and when he came, watched him for a night or two, before I made friends with him; for, to tell the truth, I was a little afraid of the stately looking man, whose bed had to be lengthened to accommodate his commanding stature; who seldom spoke, uttered no complaint, asked no sympathy, but tranquilly observed what went on about him; and, as he lay high upon his pillows, no picture of dying statesman or warrior was ever fuller of real dignity than this Virginia blacksmith. A most attractive face he had, framed in brown hair and beard, comely featured and full of vigor, as yet unsubdued by pain; thoughtful and often beautifully mild while watching the afflictions of others, as if entirely forgetful of his own. His mouth was grave and firm, with plenty of will and courage in its lines, but a smile could make it as sweet as any woman's; and his eyes were child's eyes, looking one fairly in the face, with a clear, straightforward glance, which promised well for such as placed their faith in him. He seemed to cling to life, as if it were rich in duties and delights, and he had learned the secret of content. The only time I saw his composure disturbed, was when my surgeon brought another to examine John, who scrutinized their faces with an anxious look, asking of the elder: "Do you think I shall pull through, sir?" "I hope so, my man." And, as the two passed on, John's eye still followed them, with an intentness which would have won a clearer answer from them, had they seen it. A momentary shadow flitted over his face; then came the usual serenity, as if, in that brief eclipse, he had acknowledged the existence of some hard possibility, and, asking nothing yet hoping all things, left the issue in God's hands, with that submission which is true piety.

The next night, as I went my rounds with Dr. P., I happened to ask which man in the room probably suffered most; and, to my great surprise, he glanced at John:

"Every breath he draws is like a stab; for the ball pierced the left lung, broke a rib, and did no end of damage here and there; so the poor lad can find neither forgetfulness nor ease, because he must lie on his wounded back or suffocate. It will be a hard struggle, and a long one, for he possesses great vitality; but even his temperate life can't save him; I wish it could."

"You don't mean he must die, Doctor?"

"Bless you, there's not the slightest hope for him; and you'd better tell him so before long; women have a way of doing such things comfortably, so I leave it to you. He won't last more than a day or two, at furthest."

I could have sat down on the spot and cried heartily, if I had not learned the wisdom of bottling up one's tears for leisure moments. Such an end seemed very hard for such a man, when half a dozen worn out, worthless bodies round him, were gathering up the remnants of wasted lives, to linger on for years perhaps, burdens to others, daily reproaches to themselves. The army needed men like John, earnest, brave, and faithful; fighting for liberty and justice with both heart and hand, true soldiers of the Lord. I could not give him up so soon, or think with any patience of so excellent a nature robbed of its fulfilment, and blundered into eternity by the rashness or stupidity of those at whose hands so many lives may be required. It was an easy thing for Dr. P. to say: "Tell him he must die," but a cruelly hard thing to do, and by no means as "comfortable" as he politely suggested. I had not the heart to do it then, and privately indulged the hope that some change for the better might take place, in spite of gloomy prophesies; so, rendering my task unnecessary. A few minutes later, as I came in again, with fresh rollers, I saw John sitting erect, with no one to support him, while the surgeon dressed his back. I had never hitherto seen it done; for, having simpler wounds to attend to, and knowing the fidelity of the attendant, I had left John to him, thinking it might be more agreeable and safe; for both strength and experience were needed in his case. I had forgotten that the strong man might long for the gentler tendance of a woman's hands, the sympathetic magnetism of a woman's presence, as well as the feebler souls about him. The Doctor's words caused me to reproach myself with neglect, not of any real duty perhaps, but of those little cares and kindnesses that solace homesick spirits, and make the heavy hours pass easier. John looked lonely and forsaken just then, as he sat with bent head, hands folded on his knee, and no outward sign of suffering, till, looking nearer, I saw great tears roll down and drop upon the floor. It was a new sight there; for, though I had seen many suffer, some swore, some groaned, most endured silently, but none wept. Yet it did not seem weak, only very touching, and straightway my fear vanished, my heart opened wide and took him in, as, gathering the bent head in my arms, as freely as if he had been a little child, I said, "Let me help you bear it, John."

Never, on any human countenance, have I seen so swift and beautiful a look of gratitude, surprise and comfort, as that which answered me more eloquently than the whispered—

"Thank you, ma'am, this is right good! this is what I wanted!"

"Then why not ask for it before?"

"I didn't like to be a trouble; you seemed so busy, and I could manage to get on alone."

"You shall not want it any more, John."

Nor did he; for now I understood the wistful look that sometimes followed me, as I went out, after a brief pause beside his bed, or merely a passing nod, while busied with those who seemed to need me more than he, because more urgent in their demands; now I knew that to him, as to so many, I was the poor substitute for mother, wife, or sister, and in his eyes no stranger, but a friend who hitherto had seemed neglectful; for, in his modesty, he had never guessed the truth. This was changed now; and, through the tedious operation of probing, bathing, and dressing his wounds, he leaned against me, holding my hand fast, and, if pain wrung further tears from him, no one saw them fall but me. When he was laid down again, I hovered about him, in a remorseful state of mind that would not let me rest, till I had bathed his face, brushed his "bonny brown hair," set all things smooth about him, and laid a knot of heath and heliotrope on his clean pillow. While doing this, he watched me with the satisfied expression I so liked to see; and when I offered the little nosegay, held it carefully in his great hand, smoothed a ruffled leaf or two, surveyed and smelt it with an air of genuine delight, and lay contentedly regarding the glimmer of the sunshine on the green. Although the manliest man among my forty, he said, "Yes, ma'am," like a little boy; received suggestions for his comfort with the quick smile that brightened his whole face; and now and then, as I stood tidying the table by his bed, I felt him softly touch my gown, as if to assure himself that I was there. Anything more natural and frank I never saw, and found this brave John as bashful as brave, yet full of excellencies and fine aspirations, which, having no power to express themselves in words, seemed to have bloomed into his character and made him what he was.

After that night, an hour of each evening that remained to him was devoted to his ease or pleasure. He could not talk much, for breath was precious, and he spoke in whispers; but from occasional conversations, I gleaned scraps of private history which only added to the affection and respect I felt for him. Once he asked me to write a letter, and as I settled pen and paper, I said, with an irrepressible glimmer of feminine curiosity, "Shall it be addressed to wife, or mother, John?"

"Neither, ma'am; I've got no wife, and will write to mother myself when I get better. Did you think I was married because of this?" he asked, touching a plain ring he wore, and often turned thoughtfully on his finger when he lay alone.

"Partly that, but more from a settled sort of look you have, a look which young men seldom get until they marry."

"I don't know that; but I'm not so very young, ma'am, thirty in May, and have been what you might call settled this ten years; for mother's a widow, I'm the oldest child she has, and it wouldn't do for me to marry until Lizzy has a home of her own, and Laurie's learned his trade; for we're not rich, and I must be father to the children and husband to the dear old woman, if I can."

"No doubt but you are both, John; yet how came you to go to war, if you felt so? Wasn't enlisting as bad as marrying?"

"No, ma'am, not as I see it, for one is helping my neighbor, the other pleasing myself. I went because I couldn't help it. I didn't want the glory or the pay; I wanted the right thing done, and people kept saying the men who were in earnest ought to fight. I was in earnest, the Lord knows! but I held off as long as I could, not knowing which was my duty; mother saw the case, gave me her ring to keep me steady, and said 'Go': so I went."

A short story and a simple one, but the man and the mother were portrayed better than pages of fine writing could have done it.

"Do you ever regret that you came, when you lie here suffering so much?"

"Never, ma'am; I haven't helped a great deal, but I've shown I was willing to give my life, and perhaps I've got to; but I don't blame anybody, and if it was to do over again, I'd do it. I'm a little sorry I wasn't wounded in front; it looks cowardly to be hit in the back, but I obeyed orders, and it don't matter in the end, I know."

Poor John! it did not matter now, except that a shot in front might have spared the long agony in store for him. He seemed to read the thought that troubled me, as he spoke so hopefully when there was no hope, for he suddenly added:

"This is my first battle; do they think it's going to be my last?"

"I'm afraid they do, John."

It was the hardest question I had ever been called upon to answer; doubly hard with those clear eyes fixed on mine, forcing a truthful answer by their own truth. He seemed a little startled at first, pondered over the fateful fact a moment then shook his head, with a glance at the broad chest and muscular limbs stretched out before him:

"I'm not afraid, but it's difficult to believe all at once. I'm so strong it don't seem possible for such a little wound to kill me."

Merry Mercutio's dying words glanced through my memory as he spoke: " 'Tis not so deep as a well, nor so wide as a church door, but 'tis enough." And John would have said the same could he have seen the ominous black holes between his shoulders, he never had; and, seeing the ghastly sights about him, could not believe his own wound more fatal than these, for all the suffering it caused him.

"Shall I write to your mother, now?" I asked, thinking that these sudden tidings might change all plans and purposes; but they did not; for the man received the order of the Divine Commander to march with the same unquestioning obedience with which the soldier had received that of the human one, doubtless remembering that the first led him to life, and the last to death.

"No, ma'am; to Laurie just the same; he'll break it to her best, and I'll add a line to her myself when you get done."

So I wrote the letter which he dictated, finding it better than any I had sent; for, though here and there a little ungrammatical or inelegant, each sentence came to me briefly worded, but most expressive; full of excellent counsel to the boy, tenderly bequeathing "mother and Lizzie" to his care, and bidding him good bye in words the sadder for their simplicity. He added a few lines, with steady hand, and, as I sealed it, said, with a patient sort of sigh, "I hope the answer will come in time for me to see it;" then turning away his face laid the flowers against his lips, as if to hide some quiver of emotion at the thought of such sudden sundering of all the dear home ties.

These things had happened two days before; now John was dying, and the letter had not come. I had been summoned to many death beds in my life, but to none that made my heart ache as it did then, since my mother called me to watch the departure of a spirit akin to this in its gentleness and patient strength. As I went in, John stretched out both hands:

"I knew you'd come! I guess I'm moving on, ma'am."

He was; and so rapidly that, even while he spoke, over his face I saw the grey veil falling that no human hand can lift. I sat down by him, wiped the drops from his forehead, stirred the air about him with the slow wave of a fan, and waited to help him die. He stood in sore need of help—and I could do so little; for, as the doctor had foretold, the strong body rebelled against death, and fought every inch of the way, forcing him to draw each breath with a spasm, and clench his hands with an imploring look, as if he asked, "How long must I endure this, and be still!" For hours he suffered dumbly, without a moment's respite, or a moment's murmuring; his limbs grew cold, his face damp, his lips white, and, again and again, he tore the covering off his breast, as if the lightest weight added to his agony; yet through it all, his eyes never lost their perfect serenity, and the man's soul seemed to sit therein, undaunted by the ills that vexed his flesh.

One by one, the men woke, and round the room appeared a circle of pale faces and watchful eyes, full of awe and pity; for, though a stranger, John was beloved by all. Each man there had wondered at his patience, respected his piety, admired his fortitude, and now lamented his hard death; for the influence of an upright nature had made itself deeply felt, even in one little week. Presently, the Jonathan who so loved this comely David, came creeping from his bed for a last look and word. The kind soul was full of trouble, as the choke in his voice, the grasp of his hand, betrayed; but there were no tears, and the farewell of the friends was the more touching for its brevity.

"Old boy, how are you?" faltered the one.

"Most through, thank heaven!" whispered the other.

"Can I say or do anything for you anywheres?"

"Take my things home, and tell them that I did my best."

"I will! I will!"

"Good bye, Ned."

"Good bye, John, good bye!"

They kissed eact other, tenderly as women, and so parted, for poor Ned could not stay to see his comrade die. For a little while, there was no sound in the room but the drip of water, from a stump or two, and John's distressful gasps, as he slowly breathed his life away. I thought him nearly gone, and had just laid down the fan, believing its help to be no longer needed, when suddenly he rose up in his bed, and cried out with a bitter cry that broke the silence, sharply startling every one with its agonized appeal:

"For God's sake, give me air!"

It was the only cry pain or death had wrung from him, the only boon he had asked; and none of us could grant it, for all the airs that blew were useless now. Dan flung up the window. The first red streak of dawn was warming the grey east, a herald of the coming sun; John saw it, and with the love of light which lingers in us to the end, seemed to read in it a sign of hope of help, for, over his whole face there broke that mysterious expression, brighter than any smile, which often comes to eyes that look their last. He laid himself gently down; and, stretching out his strong right arm, as if to grasp and bring the blessed air to his lips in a fuller flow, lapsed into a merciful unconsciousness, which assured us that for him suffering was forever past. He died then; for, though the heavy breaths still tore their way up for a little longer, they were but the waves of an ebbing tide that beat unfelt against the wreck, which an immortal voyager had deserted with a smile. He never spoke again, but to the end held my hand close, so close that when he was asleep at last, I could not draw it away. Dan helped me, warning me as he did so that it was unsafe for dead and living flesh to lie so long together; but though my hand was strangely cold and stiff, and four white marks remained across its back, even when warmth and color had returned elsewhere, I could not but be glad that, through its touch, the presence of human sympathy, perhaps, had lightened that hard hour.

When they had made him ready for the grave, John lay in state for half an hour, a thing which seldom happened in that busy place; but a universal sentiment of reverence and affection seemed to fill the hearts of all who had known or heard of him; and when the rumor of his death went through the house, always astir, many came to see him, and I felt a tender sort of pride in my lost patient; for he looked a most heroic figure, lying there stately and still as the statue of some young knight asleep upon his tomb. The lovely expression which so often beautifies dead faces, soon replaced the marks of pain, and I longed for those who loved him best to see him when half an hour's acquaintance with Death had made them friends. As we stood looking at him, the ward master handed me a letter, saying it had been forgotten the night before. It was John's letter, come just an hour too late to gladden the eyes that had longed and looked for it so eagerly: yet he had it; for, after I had cut some brown locks for his mother, and taken off the ring to send her, telling how well the talisman had done its work, I kissed this good son for her sake, and laid the letter in his hand, still folded as when I drew my own away, feeling that its place was there, and making myself happy with the thought, that, even in his solitary place in the "Government Lot," he would not be without some token of the love which makes life beautiful and outlives death. Then I left him, glad to have known so genuine a man, and carrying with me an enduring memory of the brave Virginia blacksmith, as he lay serenely waiting for the dawn of that long day which knows no night.

WALT WHITMAN

The Wound-Dresser

1

An old man bending I come among new faces,
Years looking backward resuming in answer to children,
Come tell us old man, as from young men and maidens that love
    me,
(Arous'd and angry, I'd thought to beat the alarum, and urge
    relentless war,
But soon my fingers fail'd me, my face droop'd and I resign'd
    myself,
To sit by the wounded and soothe them, or silently watch the
    dead;)
Years hence of these scenes, of these furious passions, these
    chances,
Of unsurpass'd heroes, (was one side so brave? the other was equally
    brave;)
Now be witness again, paint the mightiest armies of earth,
Of those armies so rapid so wondrous what saw you to tell us?
What stays with you latest and deepest? of curious panics,
Of hard-fought engagements or sieges tremendous what deepest
    remains?

2

O maidens and young men I love and that love me,
What you ask of my days those the strangest and sudden your
    talking recalls,
Soldier alert I arrive after a long march cover'd with sweat and dust,
In the nick of time I come, plunge in the fight, loudly shout in
    the rush of successful charge,
Enter the captur'd works—yet lo, like a swift-running river they
    fade,
Pass and are gone they fade—I dwell not on soldiers' perils or
    soldiers' joys,
(Both I remember well—many the hardships, few the joys, yet I
    was content.)

But in silence, in dreams' projections,
While the world of gain and appearance and mirth goes on,
So soon what is over forgotten, and waves wash the imprints off
    the sand,

With hinged knees returning I enter the doors, (while for you
    up there,
Whoever you are, follow without noise and be of strong heart.)

Bearing the bandages, water and sponge,
Straight and swift to my wounded I go,
Where they lie on the ground after the battle brought in,
Where their priceless blood reddens the grass the ground,
Or to the rows of the hospital tent, or under the roof'd hospital,
To the long rows of cots up and down each side I return,
To each and all one after another I draw near, not one do I miss,
An attendant follows holding a tray, he carries a refuse pail,
Soon to be fill'd with clotted rags and blood, emptied, and fill'd
    again.

I onward go, I stop,
With hinged knees and steady hand to dress wounds,
I am firm with each, the pangs are sharp yet unavoidable,
One turns to me his appealing eyes—poor boy! I never knew you,
Yet I think I could not refuse this moment to die for you, if that
    would save you.

3

On, on I go, (open doors of time! open hospital doors!)
The crush'd head I dress, (poor crazed hand tear not the bandage
    away,)
The neck of the cavalry-man with the bullet through and through
    I examine,
Hard the breathing rattles, quite glazed already the eye, yet life
    struggles hard,
(Come sweet death! be persuaded O beautiful death!
In mercy come quickly.)

From the stump of the arm, the amputated hand,
I undo the clotted lint, remove the slough, wash off the matter
    and blood,
Back on his pillow the soldier bends with curv'd neck and side-
    falling head,
His eyes are closed, his face is pale, he dares not look on the
    bloody stump,
And has not yet look'd on it.

I dress a wound in the side, deep, deep,
But a day or two more, for see the frame all wasted and sinking,
And the yellow-blue countenance see.

I dress the perforated shoulder, the foot with the bullet-wound,
Cleanse the one with a gnawing and putrid gangrene, so sickening,
    so offensive,
While the attendant stands behind aside me holding the tray and
    pail.

I am faithful, I do not give out,
The fractur'd thigh, the knee, the wound in the abdomen,
These and more I dress with impassive hand, (yet deep in my
    breast a fire, a burning flame.)

4

Thus in silence in dreams' projections,
Returning, resuming, I thread my way through the hospitals,
The hurt and wounded I pacify with soothing hand,
I sit by the restless all the dark night, some are so young,
Some suffer so much, I recall the experience sweet and sad,
(Many a soldier's loving arms about this neck have cross'd and
    rested,
Many a soldier's kiss dwells on these bearded lips.)

WILLIAM CARLOS WILLIAMS

Jean Beicke

During a time like this, they kid a lot among the doctors and nurses on the obstetrical floor because of the rushing business in new babies that's pretty nearly always going on up there. It's the Depression, they say, nobody has any money so they stay home nights. But one bad result of this is that in the children's ward, another floor up, you see a lot of unwanted children.

The parents get them into the place under all sorts of pretexts. For instance, we have two premature brats, Navarro and Cryschka, one a boy and one a girl; the mother died when Cryschka was born, I think. We got them within a few days of each other, one weighing four pounds and one a few ounces more. They dropped down below four pounds before we got them going but there they are; we had a lot of fun betting on their daily gains in weight but we still have them. They're in pretty good shape though now. Most of the kids that are left that way get along swell. The nurses grow attached to them and get a real thrill when they begin to pick up. It's great to see. And the parents sometimes don't even come to visit them, afraid we'll grab them and make them take the kids out, I suppose.

A funny one is a little Hungarian Gypsy girl that's been up there for the past month. She was about eight weeks old maybe when they brought her in with something on her lower lip that looked like a chancre. Everyone was interested but the Wassermann was negative. It turned out finally to be nothing but a peculiarly situated birthmark. But that kid is still there too. Nobody can find the parents. Maybe they'll turn up some day.

Even when we do get rid of them, they often come back in a week or so— sometimes in terrible condition, full of impetigo, down in weight—everything we'd done for them to do over again. I think it's deliberate neglect in most cases. That's what happened to this little Gypsy. The nurse was funny after the mother had left the second time. I couldn't speak to her, she said. I just couldn't say a word I was so mad. I wanted to slap her.

We had a couple of Irish girls a while back named Cowley. One was a red head with beautiful wavy hair and the other a straight haired blonde. They really were good looking and not infants at all. I should say they must have been two and three years old approximately. I can't imagine how the parents could have abandoned them. But they did. I think they were habitual drunkards and may have had to beat it besides on short notice. No fault of theirs maybe.

But all these are, after all, not the kind of kids I have in mind. The ones I mean are those they bring in stinking dirty, and I mean stinking. The poor brats are almost dead sometimes, just living skeletons, almost, wrapped in rags, their heads caked with dirt, their eyes stuck together with pus and their legs all excoriated from the dirty diapers no one has had the interest to take off them regularly. One poor little pot we have now with a thin purplish skin and big veins standing out all over its head had a big sore place in the fold of its neck under the chin. The nurse told me that when she started to undress it it had on a shirt with a neckband that rubbed right into that place. Just dirt. The mother gave a story of having had it in some sort of home in Paterson. We couldn't get it straight. We never try. What the hell? We take 'em and try to make something out of them.

Sometimes, you'd be surprised, some doctor has given the parents a ride before they bring the child to the clinic. You wouldn't believe it. They clean 'em out, maybe for twenty-five dollars—they maybe had to borrow—and then tell 'em to move on. It happens. Men we all know too. Pretty bad. But what can you do?

And sometimes the kids are not only dirty and neglected but sick, ready to die. You ought to see those nurses work. You'd think it was the brat of their best friend. They handle those kids as if they were worth a million dollars. Not that some nurses aren't better than others but in general they break their hearts over those kids, many times, when I, for one, wish they'd never get well.

I often kid the girls. Why not? I look at some miserable specimens they've dolled up for me when I make the rounds in the morning and I tell them: Give it an enema, maybe it will get well and grow up into a cheap prostitute or something. The country needs you, brat. I once proposed that we have a mock wedding between a born garbage hustler we'd saved and a little female with a fresh mug on her that would make anybody smile.

Poor kids! You really wonder sometimes if medicine isn't all wrong to try to do anything for them at all. You actually want to see them pass out, especially when they're deformed or—they're awful sometimes. Every one has rickets in an advanced form, scurvy too, flat chests, spindly arms and legs. They come in with pneumonia, a temperature of a hundred and six, maybe, and before you can do a thing, they're dead.

This little Jean Beicke was like that. She was about the worst you'd expect to find anywhere. Eleven months old. Lying on the examining table with a blanket half way up her body, stripped, lying there, you'd think it a five months baby, just about that long. But when the nurse took the blanket away, her legs kept on going for a good eight inches longer. I couldn't get used to it. I covered her up and asked two of the men to guess how long she was. Both guessed at least half a foot too short. One thing that helped the illusion besides her small face was her arms. They came about to her hips. I don't know what made that. They should come down to her thighs, you know.

She was just skin and bones but her eyes were good and she looked straight at you. Only if you touched her anywhere, she started to whine and then cry with a shrieking, distressing sort of cry that no one wanted to hear. We handled her as gently as we knew how but she had to cry just the same.

She was one of the damnedest looking kids I've ever seen. Her head was all up in front and flat behind, I suppose from lying on the back of her head so long the weight of it and the softness of the bones from the rickets had just flattened it out and pushed it up forward. And her legs and arms seemed loose on her like the arms and legs of some cheap dolls. You could bend her feet up on her shins absolutely flat—but there was no real deformity, just all loosened up. Nobody was with her when I saw her though her mother had brought her in.

It was about ten in the evening, the interne had asked me to see her because she had a stiff neck, and how! and there was some thought of meningitis—perhaps infantile paralysis. Anyhow, they didn't want her to go through the night without at least a lumbar puncture if she needed it. She had a fierce cough and a fairly high fever. I made it out to be a case of broncho-pneumonia with meningismus but no true involvement of the central nervous system. Besides she had inflamed ear drums.

I wanted to incise the drums, especially the left, and would have done it only the night superintendent came along just then and made me call the ear man on service. You know. She also looked to see if we had an operative release from the parents. There was. So I went home, the ear man came in a while later and opened the ears—a little bloody stream from both sides and that was that.

Next day we did a lumbar puncture, tapped the spine that is, and found clear fluid with a few lymphocytes in it, nothing diagnostic. The X-ray of the chest clinched the diagnosis of broncho-pneumonia, there was an extensive involvement. She was pretty sick. We all expected her to die from exhaustion before she'd gone very far.

I had to laugh every time I looked at the brat after that, she was such a funny looking one but one thing that kept her from being a total loss was that she did eat. Boy! how that kid could eat! As sick as she was she took her grub right on time every three hours, a big eight ounce bottle of whole milk and digested it perfectly. In this depression you got to be such a hungry baby, I heard the nurse say to her once. It's a sign of intelligence, I told her. But anyway, we all got to be crazy about Jean. She'd just lie there and eat and sleep. Or she'd lie and look straight in front of her by the hour. Her eyes were blue, a pale sort of blue. But if you went to touch her, she'd begin to scream. We just didn't, that's all, unless we absolutely had to. And she began to gain in weight. Can you imagine that? I suppose she had been so terribly run down that food, real food, was an entirely new experience to her. Anyway she took her food and gained on it though her temperature continued to run steadily around between a hundred and three and a hundred and four for the first eight or ten days. We were surprised.

When we were expecting her to begin to show improvement, however, she didn't. We did another lumbar puncture and found fewer cells. That was fine and the second X-ray of the chest showed it somewhat improved also. That wasn't so good though, because the temperature still kept up and we had no way to account for it. I looked at the ears again and thought they ought to be opened once more. The ear man disagreed but I kept after him and next day he did it to please me. He didn't get anything but a drop of serum on either side.

Well, Jean didn't get well. We did everything we knew how to do except the right thing. She carried on for another two—no I think it was three—weeks longer. A couple times her temperature shot up to a hundred and eight. Of course we knew then it was the end. We went over her six or eight times, three or four of us, one after the other, and nobody thought to take an X-ray of the mastoid regions. It was dumb, if you want to say it, but there wasn't a sign of anything but the history of the case to point to it. The ears had been opened early, they had been watched carefully, there was no discharge to speak of at any time and from the external examination, the mastoid processes showed no change from the normal. But that's what she died of, acute purulent mastoiditis of the left side, going on to involvement of the left lateral sinus and finally the meninges. We might, however, have taken a culture of the pus when the ear was first opened and I shall always, after this, in suspicious cases. I have been told since that if you get a virulent bug like the streptococcus mucosus capsulatus it's wise at least to go in behind the ear for drainage if the temperature keeps up. Anyhow she died.

I went in when she was just lying there gasping. Somehow or other, I hated to see that kid go. Everybody felt rotten. She was such a scrawny, misshapen, worthless piece of humanity that I had said many times that somebody ought to chuck her in the garbage chute—but after a month watching her suck up her milk and thrive on it—and to see those alert blue eyes in that face—well, it wasn't pleasant. Her mother was sitting by the bed crying quietly when I came in, the morning of the last day. She was a young woman, didn't look more than a girl, she just sat there looking at the child and crying without a sound.

I expected her to begin to ask me questions with that look on her face all doctors hate—but she didn't. I put my hand on her shoulder and told her we had done everything we knew how to do for Jean but that we really didn't know what, finally, was killing her. The woman didn't make any sign of hearing me. Just sat there looking in between the bars of the crib. So after a moment watching the poor kid beside her, I turned to the infant in the next crib to go on with my rounds. There was an older woman there looking in at that baby also—no better off than Jean, surely. I spoke to her, thinking she was the mother of this one, but she wasn't.

Before I could say anything, she told me she was the older sister of Jean's mother and that she knew that Jean was dying and that it was a good thing. That gave me an idea—I hated to talk to Jean's mother herself—so I beckoned the woman to come out in the hall with me.

I'm glad she's going to die, she said. She's got two others home, older, and her husband has run off with another woman. It's better off dead—never was any good anyway. You know her husband came down from Canada about a year and a half ago. She seen him and asked him to come back and live with her and the children. He come back just long enough to get her pregnant with this one then he left her again and went back to the other woman. And I suppose knowing she was pregnant, and suffering, and having no money and nowhere to get it, she was worrying and this one never was formed right. I seen it as soon as it was born. I guess the condition she was in was the cause. She's got enough to worry about now without this one. The husband's gone to Canada again and we can't get a thing out of him. I been keeping them, but we can't do much more. She'd work if she could find anything but what can you do with three kids in times like this? She's got a boy nine years old but her mother-in-law sneaked it away from her and now he's with his father in Canada. She worries about him too, but that don't do no good.

Listen, I said, I want to ask you something. Do you think she'd let us do an autopsy on Jean if she dies? I hate to speak to her of such a thing now but to tell you the truth, we've worked hard on that poor child and we don't exactly know what is the trouble. We know that she's had pneumonia but that's been getting well. Would you take it up with her for me, if—of course—she dies.

Oh, she's gonna die all right, said the woman. Sure, I will. If you can learn anything, it's only right. I'll see that you get the chance. She won't make any kick, I'll tell her.

Thanks, I said.

The infant died about five in the afternoon. The pathologist was dog-tired from a lot of extra work he'd had to do due to the absence of his assistant on her vacation so he put off the autopsy till next morning. They packed the body in ice in one of the service hoppers. It worked perfectly.

Next morning they did the postmortem. I couldn't get the nurse to go down to it. I may be a sap, she said, but I can't do it, that's all. I can't. Not when I've taken care of them. I feel as if they're my own.

I was amazed to see how completely the lungs had cleared up. They were almost normal except for a very small patch of residual pneumonia here and there which really amounted to nothing. Chest and abdomen were in excellent shape, otherwise, throughout—not a thing aside from the negligible pneumonia. Then he opened the head.

It seemed to me the poor kid's convolutions were unusually well developed. I kept thinking it's incredible that that complicated mechanism of the brain has come into being just for this. I never can quite get used to an autopsy.

The first evidence of the real trouble—for there had been no gross evidence of meningitis—was when the pathologist took the brain in his hand and made the long steady cut which opened up the left lateral ventricle. There was just a faint color of pus on the bulb of the choroid plexus there. Then the diagnosis all cleared up quickly. The left lateral sinus was completely thrombosed and on going into the left temporal bone from the inside the mastoid process was all broken down.

I called up the ear man and he came down at once. A clear miss, he said. I think if we'd gone in there earlier, we'd have saved her.

For what? said I. Vote the straight Communist ticket.

Would it make us any dumber? said the ear man.

KEN KESEY

The Big Nurse

In the glass Station the Big Nurse has opened a package from a foreign address and is sucking into hypodermic needles the grass-and-milk liquid that came in vials in the package. One of the little nurses, a girl with one wandering eye that always keeps looking worried over her shoulder while the other one goes about its usual business, picks up the little tray of filled needles but doesn't carry them away just yet.

"What, Miss Ratched, is your opinion of this new patient? I mean, gee, he's good-looking and friendly and everything, but in my humble opinion he certainly takes *over*."

The Big Nurse tests a needle against her fingertip. "I'm afraid"—she stabs the needle down in the rubber-capped vial and lifts the plunger—"that is exactly what the new patient is planning: to take over. He is what we call a 'manipulator,' Miss Flinn, a man who will use everyone and everything to his own ends."

"Oh. But. I mean, in a mental hospital? What could his ends be?"

"Any number of things." She's calm, smiling, lost in the work of loading the needles. "Comfort and an easy life, for instance; the feeling of power and respect, perhaps; monetary gain—perhaps all of these things. Sometimes a manipulator's own ends are simply the actual *disruption* of the ward for the sake of disruption. There are such people in our society. A manipulator can influence the other patients and disrupt them to such an extent that it may take months to get everything running smooth once more. With the present permissive philosophy in mental hospitals, it's easy for them to get away with it. Some years back it was quite different. I recall some years back we had a man, a Mr. Taber, on the ward, and he was an *intolerable* Ward Manipulator. For a while." She looks up from her work, needle half filled in front of her face like a little wand. Her eyes get far-off and pleased with the memory. "Mis-tur Tay-bur," she says.

"But, gee," the other nurse says, "what on earth would *make* a man want to do something like disrupt the ward for, Miss Ratched? What possible motive . . . ?"

She cuts the little nurse off by jabbing the needle back into the vial's rubber top, fills it, jerks it out, and lays it on the tray. I watch her hand reach for another empty needle, watch it dart out, hinge over it, drop.

"You seem to forget, *Miss* Flinn, that this is an institution for the insane."

The Big Nurse tends to get real put out if something keeps her outfit from running like a smooth, accurate, precision-made machine. The slightest thing messy or out of kilter or in the way ties her into a little white knot of tight-smiled fury. She walks around with that same doll smile crimped between her chin and her nose and that same calm whir coming from her eyes, but down inside of her she's tense as steel. I know, I can feel it. And she don't relax a hair till she gets the nuisance attended to—what she calls "adjusted to surroundings."

Under her rule the ward Inside is almost completely adjusted to surroundings. But the thing is she can't be on the ward all the time. She's got to spend some time Outside. So she works with an eye to adjusting the Outside world too. Working alongside others like her who I call the "Combine," which is a huge organization that aims to adjust the Outside as well as she has the Inside, has made her a real veteran at adjusting things. She was already the Big Nurse

in the old place when I came in from the Outside so long back, and she'd
been dedicating herself to adjustment for God knows how long.

And I've watched her get more and more skillful over the years. Practice
has steadied and strengthened her until now she wields a sure power that ex-
tends in all directions on hairlike wires too small for anybody's eye but
mine; I see her sit in the center of this web of wires like a watchful robot,
tend her network with mechanical insect skill, know every second which wire
runs where and just what current to send up to get the results she wants. I
was an electrician's assistant in training camp before the Army shipped me to
Germany and I had some electronics in my year in college is how I learned
about the way these things can be rigged.

What she dreams of there in the center of those wires is a world of precision
efficiency and tidiness like a pocket watch with a glass back, a place where
the schedule is unbreakable and all the patients who aren't Outside, obedient
under her beam, are wheelchair Chronics with catheter tubes run direct from
every pantleg to the sewer under the floor. Year by year she accumulates her
ideal staff: doctors, all ages and types, come and rise up in front of her with
ideas of their own about the way a ward should be run, some with backbone
enough to stand behind their ideas, and she fixes these doctors with dry-ice
eyes day in, day out, until they retreat with unnatural chills. "I tell you I don't
know *what* it is," they tell the guy in charge of personnel. "Since I started
on that ward with that woman I feel like my veins are running ammonia. I
shiver all the time, my kids won't sit in my lap, my wife won't sleep with me.
I *insist* on a transfer—neurology bin, the alky tank, pediatrics, I just don't
care!"

She keeps this up for years. The doctors last three weeks, three months.
Until she finally settles for a little man with a big wide forehead and wide
jowly cheeks and squeezed narrow across his tiny eyes like he once wore
glasses that were way too small, wore them for so long they crimped his face
in the middle, so now he has glasses on a string to his collar button; they
teeter on the purple bridge of his little nose and they are always slipping one
side or the other so he'll tip his head when he talks just to keep his glasses
level. That's the doctor.

Her three daytime black boys she acquires after more years of testing and
rejecting thousands. They come at her in a long black row of sulky, big-nosed
masks, hating her and her chalk doll whiteness from the first look they get.
She appraises them and their hate for a month or so, then lets them go because
they don't hate enough. When she finally gets the three she wants—gets them
one at a time over a number of years, weaving them into her plan and her
network—she's damn positive they hate enough to be capable.

The first one she gets five years after I been on the ward, a twisted sinewy
dwarf the color of cold asphalt. His mother was raped in Georgia while his
papa stood by tied to the hot iron stove with plow traces, blood streaming
into his shoes. The boy watched from a closet, five years old and squinting his

eye to peep out the crack between the door and the jamb, and he never grew an inch after. Now his eyelids hang loose and thin from his brow like he's got a bat perched on the bridge of his nose. Eyelids like thin gray leather, he lifts them up just a bit whenever a new white man comes on the ward, peeks out from under them and studies the man up and down and nods just once like he's oh yes made positive certain of something he was already sure of. He wanted to carry a sock full of birdshot when he first came on the job, to work the patients into shape, but she told him they didn't do it that way anymore, made him leave the sap at home and taught him her own technique; taught him not to show his hate and to be calm and wait, wait for a little advantage, a little slack, then twist the rope and keep the pressure steady. All the time. That's the way you get them into shape, she taught him.

The other two black boys come two years later, coming to work only about a month apart and both looking so much alike I think she had a replica made of the one who came first. They are tall and sharp and bony and their faces are chipped into expressions that never change, like flint arrowheads. Their eyes come to points. If you brush against their hair it rasps the hide right off you.

All of them black as telephones. The blacker they are, she learned from that long dark row that came before them, the more time they are likely to devote to cleaning and scrubbing and keeping the ward in order. For instance, all three of these boys' uniforms are always spotless as snow. White and cold and stiff as her own.

All three wear starched snow-white pants and white shirts with metal snaps down one side and white shoes polished like ice, and the shoes have red rubber soles silent as mice up and down the hall. They never make any noise when they move. They materialize in different parts of the ward every time a patient figures to check himself in private or whisper some secret to another guy. A patient'll be in a corner all by himself, when all of a sudden here's a squeak and frost forms along his cheek, and he turns in that direction and there's a cold stone mask floating above him against the wall. He just sees the black face. No body. The walls are white as the white suits, polished clean as a refrigerator door, and the black face and hands seem to float against it like a ghost.

Years of training, and all three black boys tune in closer and closer with the Big Nurse's frequency. One by one they are able to disconnect the direct wires and operate on beams. She never gives orders out loud or leaves written instructions that might be found by a visiting wife or schoolteacher. Doesn't need to any more. They are in contact on a high-voltage wave length of hate, and the black boys are out there performing her bidding before she even thinks it.

So after the nurse gets her staff, efficiency locks the ward like a watchman's clock. Everything the guys think and say and do is all worked out months in advance, based on the little notes the nurse makes during the day. This is typed and fed into the machine I hear humming behind the steel door in the rear of the Nurses' Station. A number of Order Daily Cards are returned, punched with a pattern of little square holes. At the beginning of each day the properly dated OD card is inserted in a slot in the steel door and the walls hum up: Lights flash on in the dorm at six-thirty: the Acutes up out of bed quick as the black boys can prod them out, get them to work buffing the floor, emptying ash trays, polishing the scratch marks off the wall where one old fellow shorted out a day ago, went down in an awful twist of smoke and smell of burned rubber. The Wheelers swing dead log legs out on the floor and wait like seated statues for somebody to roll chairs in to them. The Vegetables piss the bed, activating an electric shock and buzzer, rolls them off on the tile where the black boys can hose them down and get them in clean greens. . . .

Six-forty-five the shavers buzz and the Acutes line up in alphabetic order at the mirrors, A, B, C, D. . . . The walking Chronics like me walk in when the Acutes are done, then the Wheelers are wheeled in. The three old guys left, a film of yellow mold on the loose hide under their chins, they get shaved in their lounge chairs in the day room, a leather strap across the forehead to keep them from flopping around under the shaver.

Some mornings—Mondays especially—I hide and try to buck the schedule. Other mornings I figure it's cagier to step right into place between A and C in the alphabet and move the route like everybody else, without lifting my feet—powerful magnets in the floor maneuver personnel through the ward like arcade puppets. . . .

Seven o'clock the mess hall opens and the order of line-up reverses: the Wheelers first, then the Walkers, then the Acutes pick up trays, corn flakes, bacon and eggs, toast—and this morning a canned peach on a piece of green, torn lettuce. Some of the Acutes bring trays to the Wheelers. Most Wheelers are just Chronics with bad legs, they feed themselves, but there's these three of them got no action from the neck down whatsoever, not much from the neck up. These are called Vegetables. The black boys push them in after everybody else is sat down, wheel them against a wall, and bring them identical trays of muddy-looking food with little white diet cards attached to the trays. Mechanical Soft, reads the diet cards for these toothless three: eggs, ham, toast, bacon, all chewed thirty-two times apiece by the stainless-steel machine in the kitchen. I see it purse sectioned lips, like a vacuum-cleaner hose, and spurt a clot of chewed-up ham onto a plate with a barnyard sound.

The black boys stoke the sucking pink mouths of the Vegetables a shade too fast for swallowing, and the Mechanical Soft squeezes out down their little knobs of chins onto the greens. The black boys cuss the Vegetables and ream the mouths bigger with a twisting motion of the spoon, like coring a rotten apple: "This ol' fart Blastic, he's comin' to pieces befo' my very eyes. I can't tell no more if I'm feeding him bacon puree or chunks of his own fuckin' tongue." . . .

Seven-thirty back to the day room. The Big Nurse looks out through her special glass, always polished till you can't tell it's there, and nods at what she sees, reaches up and tears a sheet off her calendar one day closer to the goal. She pushes a button for things to start. I hear the wharrup of a big sheet of tin being shook someplace. Everybody come to order. Acutes: sit on your side of the day room and wait for cards and Monopoly games to be brought out. Chronics: sit on your side and wait for puzzles from the Red Cross box. Ellis: go to your place at the wall, hands up to receive the nails and pee running down your leg. Pete: wag your head like a puppet. Scanlon: work your knobby hands on the table in front of you, constructing a make-believe bomb to blow up a make-believe world. Harding: begin talking, waving your dove hands in the air, then trap them under your armpits because grown men aren't supposed to wave their pretty hands that way. Sefelt: begin moaning about your teeth hurting and your hair falling out. Everybody: breath in . . . and out . . . in perfect order; hearts all beating at the rate the OD cards have ordered. Sound of matched cylinders.

Like a cartoon world, where the figures are flat and outlined in black, jerking through some kind of goofy story that might be real funny if it weren't for the cartoon figures being real guys. . . .

Seven-forty-five the black boys move down the line of Chronics taping catheters on the ones that will hold still for it. Catheters are second-hand condoms the ends clipped off and rubber-banded to tubes that run down pant-legs to a plastic sack marked DISPOSABLE NOT TO BE RE-USED, which it is my job to wash out at the end of each day. The black boys anchor the condom by taping it to the hairs; old Catheter Chronics are hairless as babies from tape removal. . . .

Eight o'clock the walls whirr and hum into full swing. The speaker in the ceiling says, "Medications," using the Big Nurse's voice. We look in the glass case where she sits, but she's nowhere near that microphone; in fact, she's ten feet away from the microphone, tutoring one of the little nurses how to pre-pare a neat drug tray with pills arranged orderly. The Acutes line up at the glass door, A, B, C, D, then the Chronics, then the Wheelers (the Vegetables get theirs later, mixed in a spoon of applesauce). The guys file by and get a capsule in a paper cup—throw it to the back of the throat and get the cup filled with water by the little nurse and wash the capsule down. On rare occasions some fool might ask what he's being required to swallow.

"Wait just a shake, honey; what are these two little red capsules in here with my vitamin?"

I know him. He's a big, griping Acute, already getting the reputation of being a troublemaker.

"It's just medication, Mr. Taber, good for you. Down it goes, now."

"But I mean what *kind* of medication. Christ, I can see that they're pills—"

"Just swallow it all, shall we, Mr. Taber—just for me?" She takes a quick look at the Big Nurse to see how the little flirting technique she is using is accepted, then looks back at the Acute. He still isn't ready to swallow something he don't know what is, not even just for her.

"Miss, I don't like to create trouble. But I don't like to swallow something without knowing what it is, neither. How do I know this isn't one of those funny pills that makes me something I'm not?"

"Don't get upset, Mr. Taber—"

"Upset? All I want to *know,* for the lova Jesus—"

But the Big Nurse has come up quietly, locked her hand on his arm, paralyzes him all the way to the shoulder. "That's all right, Miss Flinn," she says. "If Mr. Taber chooses to act like a child, he may have to be treated as such. We've tried to be kind and considerate with him. Obviously, that's not the answer. Hostility, hostility, that's the thanks we get. You can go, Mr. Taber, if you don't wish to take your medication orally."

"All I wanted to *know,* for the—"

"You can go."

He goes off, grumbling, when she frees his arm, and spends the morning moping around the latrine, wondering about those capsules. I got away once holding one of those same red capsules under my tongue, played like I'd swallowed it, and crushed it open latter in the broom closet. For a tick of time, before it all turned into white dust, I saw it was a miniature electronic element like the ones I helped the Radar Corps work with in the Army, microscopic wires and girds and transistors, this one designed to dissolve on contact with air. . . .

Eight-twenty the cards and puzzles go out. . . .

Eight-twenty-five some Acute mentions he used to watch his sister taking her bath; the three guys at the table with him fall all over each other to see who gets to write it in the log book. . . .

Eight-thirty the ward door opens and two technicians trot in, smelling like grape wine; technicians always move at a fast walk or a trot because they're always leaning so far forward they have to move fast to keep standing. They always lean forward and they always smell like they sterilized their instruments in wine. They pull the lab door to behind them, and I sweep up close and can make out voices over the vicious zzzth-zzzth-zzzth of steel on whetstone.

"What we got already at this ungodly hour of the morning?"

"We got to install an Indwelling Curiosity Cutout in some nosy booger. Hurry-up job, she says, and I'm not even sure we got one of the gizmos in stock."

"We might have to call IBM to rush one out for us; let me check back in Supply—"

"Hey; bring out a bottle of that pure grain while you're back there: it's getting so I can't install the simplest frigging component but what I need a bracer. Well, what the hell, it's better'n garage work. . . ."

Their voices are forced and too quick on the comeback to be real talk—more like cartoon comedy speech. I sweep away before I'm caught eavesdropping.

The two big black boys catch Taber in the latrine and drag him to the mattress room. He gets one a good kick in the shins. He's yelling bloody murder. I'm surprised how helpless he looks when they hold him, like he was wrapped with bands of black iron.

They push him face down on the mattress. One sits on his head, and the other rips his pants open in back and peels the cloth until Taber's peach-colored rear is framed by the ragged lettuce-green. He's smothering curses into the mattress and the black boy sitting on his head saying, "Tha's right, Mistuh Taber, tha's right. . . ." The nurse comes down the hall, smearing Vaseline on a long needle, pulls the door shut so they're out of sight for a second, then comes right back out, wiping the needle on a shred of Taber's pants. She's left the Vaseline jar in the room. Before the black boy can close the door after her I see the one still sitting on Taber's head, dabbing at him with a Kleenex. They're in there a long time before the door opens up again and they come out, carrying him across the hall to the lab. His greens are ripped clear off now and he's wrapped up in a damp sheet. . . .

Nine o'clock young residents wearing leather elbows talk to Acutes for fifty minutes about what they did when they were little boys. The Big Nurse is suspicious of the crew-cut looks of these residents, and that fifty minutes they are on the ward is a tough time for her. While they are around, the machinery goes to fumbling and she is scowling and making notes to check the records of these boys for old traffic violations and the like. . . .

Nine-fifty the residents leave and the machinery hums up smooth again. The nurse watches the day room from her glass case; the scene before her takes on that blue-steel clarity again, that clean orderly movement of a cartoon comedy.

Taber is wheeled out of the lab on a Gurney bed.

"We had to give him another shot when he started coming up during the spine tap," the technician tells her. "What do you say we take him right on over to Building One and buzz him with EST while we're at it—that way not waste the extra Seconal?"

"I think it is an excellent suggestion. Maybe after that take him to the electroencephalograph and check his head—we may find evidence of a need for brain work."

The technicians go trotting off, pushing the man on the Gurney, like cartoon men—or like puppets, mechanical puppets in one of those Punch and Judy acts where it's supposed to be funny to see the puppet beat up by the Devil and swallowed headfirst by a smiling alligator. . . .

Ten o'clock the mail comes up. Sometimes you get the torn envelope. . . .

Ten-thirty Public Relation comes in with a ladies' club following him. He claps his fat hands at the day-room door. "Oh, hello, guys; stiff lip. . . . Look around, girls; isn't it so clean, so bright? This is Miss Ratched. I chose this ward because it's *her* ward. She's, girls, just like a mother. Not that I mean age, but you girls understand. . . ."

Public Relation's shirt collar is so tight it bloats his face up when he laughs, and he's laughing most of the time I don't ever know what at, laughing high and fast like he wishes he could stop but can't do it. And his face bloated up red and round as a balloon with a face painted on it. He got no hair on his face and none on his head to speak of; it looks like he glued some on once but it kept slipping off and getting in his cuffs and his shirt pocket and down his collar. Maybe that's why he keeps his collar so tight, to keep the little pieces of hair out.

Maybe that's why he laughs so much, because he isn't able to keep all the pieces out.

He conducts these tours—serious women in blazer jackets, nodding to him as he points out how much things have improved over the years. He points out the TV, the big leather chairs, the sanitary drinking fountains; then they all go have coffee in the Nurses' Station. Sometimes he'll be by himself and just stand in the middle of the day room and clap his hands (you can *hear* they are wet), clap them two or three times till they stick, then hold them prayerlike together under one of his chins and start spinning. Spin round and around there in the middle of the floor, looking wild and frantic at the TV, the new pictures on the walls, the drinking fountain. And laughing.

What he sees that's so funny he don't ever let us in on, and the only thing I can see funny is him spinning round and around out there like a rubber toy —if you push him over he's weighted on the bottom and straightaway rocks back upright, goes to spinning again. He never, never looks at the men's faces. . . .

Ten-forty, -forty-five, -fifty, patients shuttle in and out to appointments in ET or OT or PT, or in queer little rooms somewhere where the walls are never the same size and the floors aren't level. The machinery sounds about you reach a steady cruising speed.

The ward hums the way I heard a cotton mill hum once when the football team played a high school in California. After a good season one year the boosters in the town were so proud and carried away that they paid to fly us to California to play a championship high-school team down there. When we flew into the town we had to go visit some local industry. Our coach was one for convincing folks that athletics was educational because of the learning afforded by travel, and every trip we took he herded the team around to creameries and beet farms and canneries before the game. In California it was the cotton mill. When we went in the mill most of the team took a look and left to go sit in the bus over stud games on suitcases, but I stayed inside over in a corner out of the way of the Negro girls running up and down the aisles of machines. The mill put me in a kind of dream, all the humming and clicking and rattling of people and machinery, jerking around in a pattern. That's why I stayed when the others left, that, and because it reminded me somehow of the men in the tribe who'd left the village in the last days to do work on the gravel crusher for the dam. The frenzied pattern, the faces hypnotized by routine . . . I wanted to go out with the team, but I couldn't.

It was morning in early winter and I still had on the jacket they'd given us when we took the championship—a red and green jacket with leather sleeves and a football-shaped emblem sewn on the back telling what we'd won—and it was making a lot of the Negro girls stare. I took it off, but they kept staring. I was a whole lot bigger in those days.

One of the girls left her machine and looked back and forth up the aisles to see if the foreman was around, then came over to where I was standing. She asked if we was going to play the high school that night and she told me she had a brother played tailback for them. We talked a piece about football and the like and I noticed how her face looked blurred, like there was a mist between me and her. It was the cotton fluff sifting from the air.

I told her about the fluff. She rolled her eyes and ducked her mouth to laugh in her fist when I told her how it was like looking at her face out on a misty morning duck-hunting. And she said, "Now what in the everlovin' world would you want with me out alone in a duck blind?" I told her she could take care of my gun, and the girls all over the mill went to giggling in their fists. I laughed a little myself, seeing how clever I'd been. We were still talking and laughing when she grabbed both my wrists and dug in. The features of her face snapped into brilliant focus; I saw she was terrified of something.

"Do," she said to me in a whisper, "do take me, big boy. Outa this here mill, outa this town, outa this life. Take me to some ol' duck blind someplace. Someplace *else*. Huh, big boy, huh?"

Her dark, pretty face glittered there in front of me. I stood with my mouth open, trying to think of some way to answer her. We were locked together this way for maybe a couple of seconds; then the sound of the mill jumped a hitch, and something commenced to draw her back away from me. A string somewhere I didn't see hooked on that flowered red skirt and was tugging her back. Her fingernails peeled down my hands and as soon as she broke contact with me her face switched out of focus again, became soft and runny like melting chocolate behind that blowing fog of cotton. She laughed and spun around and gave me a look of her yellow leg when the skirt billowed out. She threw me a wink over her shoulder as she ran back to her machine where a pile of fiber was spilling off the table to the floor; she grabbed it up and ran featherfooted down the aisle of machines to dump the fiber in a hopper; then she was out of sight around the corner.

All those spindles reeling and wheeling and shuttles jumping around and bobbins wringing the air with string, whitewashed walls and steel-gray machines and girls in flowered skirts skipping back and forth, and the whole thing webbed with flowing white lines stringing the factory together—it all stuck with me and every once in a while something on the ward calls it to mind.

Yes. This is what I know. The ward is a factory for the Combine. It's for fixing up mistakes made in the neighborhoods and in the schools and in the churches, the hospital is. When a completed product goes back out into society, all fixed up good as new, *better* than new sometimes, it brings joy to the Big Nurse's heart; something that came in all twisted different is now a functioning, adjusted component, a credit to the whole outfit and a marvel to behold. Watch him sliding across the land with a welded grin, fitting into some nice little neighborhood where they're just now digging trenches along the street to lay pipes for city water. He's happy with it. He's adjusted to surroundings finally. . . .

"Why, I've never seen anything to beat the change in Maxwell Taber since he's got back from that hospital; a little black and blue around the eyes, a little weight lost, and, you know what? he's a *new man*. Gad, modern American science . . ."

And the light is on in his basement window way past midnight every night as the Delayed Reaction Elements the technicians installed lend nimble skills to his fingers as he bends over the doped figure of his wife, his two little girls just four and six, the neighbor he goes bowling with Mondays; he adjusts them like he was adjusted. This is the way they spread it.

When he finally runs down after a pre-set number of years, the town loves him dearly and the paper prints his picture helping the Boy Scouts last year on Graveyard Cleaning Day, and his wife gets a letter from the principal of the high school how Maxwell Wilson Taber was an inspirational figure to the youth of our fine community.

Even the embalmers, usually a pair of penny-pinching tightwads, are swayed. "Yeah, look at him there: old Max Taber, he was a good sort. What do you say we use that expensive thirty-weight at no extra charge to his wife. No, what the dickens, let's make it on the house."

A successful Dismissal like this is a product brings joy to the Big Nurse's heart and speaks good of her craft and the whole industry in general. Everybody's happy with a Dismissal.

But an Admission is a different story. Even the best-behaved Admission is bound to need some work to swing into routine, and, also, you never can tell when just that *certain* one might come in who's free enough to foul things up right and left, really make a hell of a mess and constitute a threat to the whole smoothness of the outfit. And, like I explain, the Big Nurse gets real put out if anything keeps her outfit from running smooth.

STUDS TERKEL

Carmelita Lester

She arrived from the West Indies in 1962. She has been a practical nurse for the past five years. "You study everything about humanity, the human body, all the way through. How to give the patient cares, how to make comfortable . . . Most of the time I work seven days."

We're in a private room at a nursing home for the elderly. "Most of them are upper, above middle class. I only work for private patients. Some may have a stroke, some are maybe confused. Some patients have nothing wrong with them, but relatives just bring them and leave them here."

As she knits, she glances tenderly at the old, old woman lying in the bed. "My baby here has cerebral thrombosis. She is ninety-three years old."[1]

I get in this morning about eight-thirty. I shake her, make sure that she was okay. I took her tray, wipe her face, and give her cereal and a cup of orange juice and an egg. She's unable to chew hard foods. You have to give her liquids through a syringe. She's supposed to get two thousand cc per day. If not, it would get dry and she would get a small rash and things like those.

The first thing in the morning, after breakfast, I sponge her and I give her a back rub. And I keep her clean. She's supposed to be turned every two hours. If we don't turn her every two hours, she will have sores. Even though she's asleep, she's got to be turned.

I give her lunch. The trays come up at twelve thirty. I feed her just the same as what I feed her in the morning. In the evening I go to the kitchen and pick up her tray at four o'clock and I do the same thing again. About five thirty I leave here and go home. She stays here from five thirty until eleven at night as floor care, until the night nurse come.

You have to be very, very used to her to detect it that she's having an attack. I go notify that she's having a convulsion, so the nurse come and give her two grains of sodium amytal in her hips. When she gets the needle it will bring down her blood pressure. Because she has these convulsions, her breathing stops, trying to choke. If there's nobody around, she would stifle.

Some days she's awake. Some days she just sleeps. When she's awake she's very alert. Some people believe she isn't, but she knows what's going on. You will hear her voice say something very simple. Other than that, she doesn't

---

1. Four years before, I visited "her baby" when she was eighty-nine years old. It was a gracefully appointed apartment; she was most hospitable. Bright-eyed, alert, witty, she recounted her experiences during the Great Depression.

say a word. Not since she had that last heavy stroke last year. Before that, she would converse. Now she doesn't converse any more. Oh, she knows what's going on. She's aware. She knows people by the voices. If a man comes in this room, once she hears that voice, I just cannot undress her. (Laughs.)

She knows when I'm not here. If I'm away too long, she gets worried, sick. But she got used to it that I have to go out sometimes. She knows I'll be back, so she's more relaxed now. Oh, sometimes I sit here and get drowsy. I think of the past and the future. Sometime I think when I was a little girl in Cuba and the things I used to do.

If I'm not doing nothing after I get through with her, it's a drag day. I laugh and I keep myself busy doing something. I may make pillows. I sell 'em. Sometimes I'll be writing up my bills. That's my only time I have, here. If I don't feel like doing that, well, I'll make sure she's okay, I'll go down into the street and take a walk.

The work don't leave my mind. I have been so long with her that it became part of me. In my mind it's always working: "How's she getting along?" I worry what happened to her between those hours before the night nurse report. If I go off on a trip, I'll be talking about her. I'll say, "I wonder what happened to my baby." My girl friend will say, "Which baby are you talking about?" I'll say, "My patient." (Laughs.) I went to Las Vegas. I spent a week there. Every night I called. Because if she has these convulsions . . .

My baby, is not everyone can take of her through this illness. Anybody will be sittin' here and she will begin to talk and you don't know it. So you have to be a person that can detect this thing coming along. I called every night to find out how she was doin'. My bill was seventy-eight dollars. (Laughs.) If she's sick, I have to fly back. She stays on my mind, but I don't know why. (Laughs.)

She works through a nurses' registry. "You go where they send you. Maybe you get a little baby." She had worked at a general hospital before. "I used to float around, I worked with geriatric, I worked with pediatric, I worked with teen-agers, I worked with them all. Medical-surgical. I've been with her two years. As long as she's still going." (Laughs.)

In America, people doesn't keep their old people at home. At a certain age they put them away in America. In my country, the old people stay in the home until they die. But here, not like that. It's surprising to me. They put them away. The first thing they think of is a nursing home. Some of these people don't need a nursing home. If they have their own bedroom at home, look at television or listen to the radio or they have themselves busy knitting . . . We all, us foreigners, think about it.

Right now there's a lady here, nothing wrong with her, but they put her away. They don't come to see her. The only time they see her is when she say, "I can't breathe." She wants some attention. And that way she's just aging. When I come here, she was a beautiful woman. She was looking very nice. Now she is going down. If they would come and take her out sometimes . . .

We had one lady here about two years ago, she has two sons. She fell and had a broken hip. They called the eldest son. He said, "Why call on me? Call the little one. She gave all the money to that little one." That was bad. I was right there.

All these people here are not helpless. But just the family get rid of them. There is a lady here, her children took her for a ride one day and push her out of the car. Let her walk and wander. She couldn't find her way home. They come and brought her here. And they try to take away all that she has. They're tryin' to make her sign papers and things like those. There's nothing wrong with her. She can dress herself, comb her hair, take a walk . . . They sign her in here, made the lawyers sign her in. They're just in for the money. She will tell you, "There's nothin' wrong with me."

Things that go on here. I've seen many of these patients, they need help, but they don't have enough help. Sometimes they eat and sometimes they don't. Sometimes there's eight hours' wait. Those that can have private nurse, fine. Those that can't suffer. And this is a high-class place. Where *poor* old people . . . (She shakes her head.)

"The reason I got so interested in this kind of work, I got sick. One evening my strength just went. My legs and everything couldn't hold. For one year I couldn't walk. I had twelve doctors. They couldn't find out what was wrong. I have doctors from all over the United States come to see. Even a professor from Germany. A doctor from South Carolina came, he put it in a book. My main doctor said, 'You have to live with your condition 'cause there's nothing we can do.' I said to him, 'Before I live this way, I'd rather die.' 'Cause I couldn't feed myself, I couldn't do nothin'. This life is not for me.

"They took me home. I started prayin' and prayin' to God and things like those and this. Oral Roberts, I wrote to him several letters. Wrote from my heart. Still I was crippled. Couldn't put a glass of water to my mouth. The strength had been taken away. I prayed hard.

"One night I was in bed and deeply down in my sleep, I heard electricity. Like when you take an electric wire and touch it. It shot through both legs. Ooohhh, it shocked so hard that I woke up. When I woke up; I felt it three times. The next morning I could raise this leg up. I was surprised.

"The next night I felt the same thing. The third night I felt the same thing. So I got up and went to the bathroom. I went back to the doctor and he said, 'That's surprising.' Ooohhh, I can't believe it. There is a miracle. This is very shocking."

What do you think cured you?

"God."

Did Oral Roberts help?

"*Yes.*"

How?

"*By prayin' sincere from his heart.*

"*I was a nurse before, but I wasn't devoted. I saw how they treated people when I was there. Oh, it was pitiful. I couldn't stand it. And from that, I have tender feelings. That changed me. That's when I decided to devote myself.*"

I feel sorry for everybody who cannot help themselves. For that reason I never rest. As soon as I'm off one case I am on another. I have to sometimes say, "Don't call me for a week." I am so tired. Sometimes I have to leave the house and hide away. They keep me busy, busy, busy all the time. People that I take care of years ago are callin' back and askin' for me.

Plenty of nurses don't care. If they get the money, forget it. They talk like that all the time: They say to me, "You still here?" I say, "Yes." "Oh, you still worry about that old woman." I say, "That's why she pays me, to worry about her." Most of the nurses have feelings.

If I had power in this country, first thing I'd do in nursing homes, I would hire someone that pretended to be sick. 'Cause that's the only way you know what's goin' on. I would have government nursing homes. Free care for everybody. Those hospitals that charge too much money and you don't have insurance and they don't accept you, I would change that—overnight.

Things so bad for old people today—if I could afford to buy a few buildings, I would have that to fall on. You got to be independent. So you don't have to run there and there and there in your old age. They don't have enough income. I don't want to be like that.

An elderly person is a return back to babyhood. It give you a feeling how when you were a teen-ager, you're adult, you think you're strong and gay, and you return back to babyhood. The person doesn't know what's happening. But you take care of the person, you can see the difference. It makes you sad, because if you live long enough, you figure you will be the same.

POSTSCRIPT: *A few months after this conversation, her "baby" died.*

ALEKSANDR I. SOLZHENITSYN

Not Cancer at All

The cancer wing was Ward No. 13. Pavel Nikolayevich Rusanov had never been superstitious, had never thought he could be, but something inside him sank when they wrote "Ward 13" on his registration card. They should have had the tact to call it something like "prosthetic" or "intestinal," not "13."

In the whole territory there was no other hospital that could help him now.

"But surely I don't have cancer? Doctor? Surely I don't have cancer?" Pavel Nikolayevich asked hopefully as he gently rubbed the right side of his neck, where the angry swelling seemed to be growing day by day, stretching the unoffending white skin.

"No, no, of course not," Doctor Dontsova reassured him for the tenth time as she continued scribbling the case history in her sprawling handwriting. When she wrote she wore eyeglasses with convex, elliptical lenses; when she stopped writing she took them off. She was no longer young, and she looked pale and very tired, as when she had received him in the outpatient clinic a few days ago. Even when the appointment was simply for a checkup at the outpatient clinic, a person who was directed to the cancer division did not sleep nights. And Dontsova had ordered Pavel Nikolayevich to enter the hospital immediately.

It was not only the illness—unforeseen, unprepared for, descending like a squall two weeks ago upon a happy, carefree Pavel Nikolayevich—that weighed on his spirits now; he was equally depressed at having to enter this hospital as a common ward patient. It was so long since he had been an ordinary ward patient that he could not remember when it had been. He began telephoning—to Yevgeny Semyonovich and Shendyapin Ulmasbasbayev—and they in turn telephoned others to ask whether the hospital had prominent specialists on the staff, whether special arrangements could be made for him, whether they could set up even a small private room, at least temporarily. But the hospital was so crowded that nothing could be done.

The only privileges they managed to obtain for him, through the chief doctor of the entire medical center, were the right to bypass the reception routine and skip the hospital bath in the common tub, and permission to wear his own pajamas instead of the coarse hospital garb.

In the family's pale blue Moskvich, Yura drove his father and mother right up to the portico of Ward 13.

Despite the cold, two women in repulsive cotton twill bathrobes stood in the open on the stone veranda; they were shivering, and their arms hugged their chests, yet they stood there.

Everything about the place, beginning with these slovenly bathrobes, repelled Pavel Nikolayevich: the footworn cement of the veranda, the tarnished
door handles rubbed by patients' hands, and the waiting room. In the waiting
room the floor paint was peeling, the high paneled walls were a dirty olive
color, and the large slatted benches did not provide enough space for all the
patients who had come from far off. Many sat on the floor—Uzbeks in quilted
cotton gowns, old Uzbek women wearing white kerchiefs, young ones wearing
lilac or red or green kerchiefs, and all in boots or galoshes. One Russian fellow lay stretched out on a bench, his coat open, its edges trailing on the
ground. He was emaciated, his belly was swollen, and he cried out in pain.
His wails rang in Pavel Nikolayevich's ears and so pierced him that he felt the
fellow was crying out not about himself but about him.

Pavel Nikolayevich blanched to his lips, stopped, and whispered:

"Kapa! I'll die here. Better not stay. Let's go back."

Kapitolina Matveyevna took his hand firmly and squeezed it.

"Pashenka! Where would we go back to? And then what?"

"Maybe I could still get into a Moscow hospital."

Kapitolina Matveyevna turned and focused on her husband with the whole
of her wide face, made even broader by her trimmed, thick, copper-colored
curls.

"Pashenka! Moscow might take two more weeks, and we might not be able
to arrange it in any case. How can you wait? It is bigger every morning!"

His wife squeezed his wrist to give him courage. In work and public affairs
Pavel Nikolayevich was himself a resolute person; hence in family matters he
liked to rely on his wife to decide the important things—she always made the
right decisions unhesitatingly.

The young fellow on the bench was tearing himself apart, crying out in
pain.

"Perhaps we could get the doctors to treat me at home. We'd pay," Pavel
Nikolayevich said, holding back uncertainly.

"Pasik!" his wife insisted, though she shared her husband's distress. "You
know I'm always the first to call someone in and pay him. But we asked.
These doctors don't go out on calls and they don't accept money. Besides,
they need equipment. It can't be done."

Pavel Nikolayevich himself realized it couldn't be done. He had spoken in
a vain hope.

By agreement with the chief doctor of the oncological division, they were
to be met here at two o'clock. The senior nurse was to have been waiting for
them at the foot of the staircase, which a patient was now cautiously descending on crutches. But of course the nurse was not there, and there was a small
padlock on the door of her supply room.

"You can't depend on anyone!" Kapitolina Matveyevna burst out. "What
do they get paid for?"

Kapitolina Matveyevna, her shoulders covered by a huge collar of two silver-black foxes, strode down the corridor past the sign: "Check Coats Before Entering."

Pavel Nikolayevich remained standing in the waiting room. Fearfully, bending his head slightly to the right, he felt the swelling between collar bone and jaw. It seemed as though it had grown in the half hour since he had looked at himself in the mirror at home as he was wrapping the muffler around his neck. Pavel Nikolayevich was suddenly weak and wanted to sit down. But the benches looked dirty, and he would have had to ask a kerchiefed woman, with a large, grease-stained bundle at her feet, to move. Pavel Nikolayevich was defenseless against his sense of smell, and the stench of the bundle reached him even from this distance.

When will our people learn to travel with neat, clean suitcases? (Come to think of it, considering the tumor, all this didn't matter.)

Tormented by the groans of the young fellow and everything that assailed his eyes and nose, Pavel Nikolayevich leaned against a projection of the wall. A patient entered, carrying a half-liter jar brimming with yellow liquid. He did not conceal the jar, but held it up proudly, as if it were a mug of beer that he had waited in line to buy. He stopped directly in front of Pavel Nikolayevich, almost proffering the jar; he was about to ask something, but he looked at the sealskin hat, turned aside and walked on to the patient on crutches: "Friend, where do I take this, eh?"

The man on crutches pointed to the laboratory door.

Pavel Nikolayevich felt nauseated.

The outer door opened again and a nurse entered. She wore a white gown, nothing warmer; her face was narrow and plain. She immediately noticed Pavel Nikolayevich, realized who he was, and came up to him.

"Please excuse me," she stammered, so breathless from hurrying that her face was as red as her lips. "Please excuse me. I hope you haven't been waiting long. They brought a delivery of medicines, and I had to sign for it."

Pavel Nikolayevich wanted to reply caustically, but he restrained himself. He was glad that at least the waiting was over. Yura entered, carrying the suitcase and the shopping bag filled with food, and walked calmly toward them, forelock dangling over his forehead. He was without coat or hat, just as he had been when he drove.

"This way," said the senior nurse, leading them toward her supply room under the staircase. "I know, Nizamutdin Bakhramovich told me you would bring your own pajamas. But they must be new, never worn before."

"Straight from the store."

"That's the regulation. Otherwise they have to be disinfected, you understand. You can dress in here."

She opened the plywood door and turned on the light. The supply room, with its slanted ceiling, had no windows. On the walls hung many charts marked in colored pencil.

Yura silently brought the suitcase and left, while Pavel Nikolayevich entered to dress. The senior nurse turned impatiently to go on another errand, but at that moment Kapitolina Matveyevna came forward.

"Young lady, where are you rushing to?"

"I have to—"

"What is your name?"

"Mita."

"Strange name. You're not Russian, then?"

"German."

"You kept us waiting."

"Please forgive me. I'm supposed to sign for the medicines and—"

"Now listen, Mita, I want you to know that my husband is a prominent man, a very important official. His name is Pavel Nikolayevich."

"Pavel Nikolayevich, good, I'll remember."

"You understand, he's always been used to being looked after, and now he has this serious illness. Couldn't we arrange to have a day and a night nurse at his bedside?"

Mita's anxious, restless expression became even more troubled. She shook her head.

"Except for the operating room, we have only three nurses on duty during the day to care for sixty patients. And two at night."

"There, you see! A person could be dying here, he could cry for help, and no one would come."

"Why do you say that? We come to everyone who needs help."

"Pavel Nikolayevich isn't 'everyone.' And your nurses change."

"Yes, they take turns in twelve-hour shifts."

"Such impersonal care! My daughter and I would be glad to stay at his bedside if we could. I would bring a nurse at our own expense, but they tell me that is impossible too. Is it?"

"I think it's not allowed. No one has ever done it. There isn't even room for a nurse's chair in the ward."

"My God, I can imagine what the ward is like! I'd better take a look at this ward. How many beds are there?"

"Nine. It's a privilege that he's going right into the ward. New patients are usually assigned beds on the staircase landings or in the corridors."

"Young lady, I insist, won't you please—it would be easier for you to arrange things, you know your people here—arrange with the nurse or the orderly to see that Pavel Nikolayevich doesn't get just routine attention." She had already unsnapped her large black handbag and was taking three fifty-ruble bills from it.

Her son, standing silently nearby with his straight blond forelock, turned away.

Mita put both her hands behind her back.

"No, no. We can't accept—"

"But I'm not giving it to you!" Kapitolina Matveyevna said, thrusting the outspread bills at the nurse. "It's just that I'm paying for the work, since it can't be arranged officially. All I ask of you is to have the kindness, the kindness to pass the money on!"

"No, no!" the nurse said, her voice cold. "We don't do these things."

With a creak of the door, Pavel Nikolayevich emerged from the supply room, dressed in new green-and-brown pajamas and wearing warm bedroom slippers with fur trimming. He had a new raspberry-colored *tyubeteika*—the Central Asian skullcap—on his almost bald head. Without his winter collar and muffler to hide it, the fist-size swelling on the side of his neck seemed particularly menacing. He did not hold his head straight, but to one side.

His son went into the supply room to collect the street clothes and put them in the suitcase. His wife, tucking the money back in her purse, looked at her husband in concern.

"Won't you be cold? We should tave taken your warm bathrobe. I'll bring it. Here's a scarf." She pulled it from her pocket. "Wrap up, don't let it get chilled." In her furs and coat she seemed three times her husband's size. "Now go to the ward and get settled. Put away the food, look around and see what you might need. I'll wait here. Come down and tell me, and I'll bring it all this evening."

She never got rattled, she always thought of everything. She was a real life-comrade. Pavel Nikolayevich looked at her in gratitude and suffering, and then at his son.

"So you're ready to set off, Yura?"

"The train leaves tonight." Yura was always respectful toward his father, but he never exhibited emotion, and now he exhibited none at parting with a father left behind in a hospital. He took everything in a subdued manner.

"So, son. This will be your first big assignment. Start off on the right foot. Take the proper tone. Don't be a weakling! Soft-heartedness will ruin you! Always remember that you are not Yura Rusanov, a private individual; you are the rep–re–sent–a–tive of—the—law, you understand?"

Whether Yura understood or not, Pavel Nikolayevich found it hard to think of more precise words. Mita shifted from foot to foot, impatient to go.

"I'll wait here with Mamma." Yura smiled. "Don't say good-bye yet, Papa. Go on up."

"Are you able to get there by yourself?" Mita asked.

"My God, the man can hardly walk, can't you help him to his bed? Carry his bag!" Kapitolina Matveyevna said.

Overcome by self-pity, Pavel Nikolayevich looked at his wife and son, refused Mita's supporting hand, and, holding the banister, began to climb the stairs. His heart beat fast, not entirely from the effort of climbing. He walked up the stairs as—how to put it?—a condemned man mounts the scaffold to put his head on the block.

The senior nurse, running ahead, dashed upstairs with his bag of food, called out to someone named Maria, and, before Pavel Nikolayevich had mounted the first flight, had already run down the stairs on the other side and out of the ward, showing Kapitolina Matveyevna what kind of care her husband could expect here.

Pavel Nikolayevich slowly ascended to a wide, deep landing such as one finds only in old buildings. On the landing stood two occupied beds. They did not block movement on the staircase, even though each had a bedstand beside it. One of the patients was gravely ill, exhausted, and sucking on an oxygen balloon.

Trying not to stare at his hopeless face, Rusanov turned and walked on, looking upward. He found nothing encouraging at the top of the second flight of stairs. The nurse Maria stood there. No smile, no welcome lit up her dark, icon-like face. Tall, thin, erect, she waited like a soldier, and immediately crossed the upper vestibule, leading the way. Several doors opened off this vestibule, and wherever the doors were ajar he saw beds occupied by patients. In a windowless corner stood the nurse's desk, with its eternally lit desk lamp and instrument stand; on the wall above hung a medicine chest with a frosted-glass door bearing the Red Cross insignia. Beyond this and past several more beds Maria pointed a long, bony finger and said: "Second from the window."

She was already hurrying to leave: an unpleasant feature of a hospital for the general public—no one stops, no one pauses to chat.

The double doors to the ward were kept wide open, yet as he crossed the threshold Pavel Nikolayevich was assailed by a damp, fusty mixture of smells, partly medicinal. With his sensitivity to odors, it was hard to bear.

The beds stood close together. They jutted from the walls, separated only by the width of bedstands, and the aisle down the middle of the room was barely wide enough for two persons.

In this aisle stood a stocky, broad-shouldered patient in rose-striped pajamas. His whole neck was bandaged tightly and thickly almost up to the lobes of his ears. The pressure of the white wrappings prevented him from freely moving his heavy, squat head, with its thick mop of brown hair.

This patient was talking hoarsely to another who listened from a bed. When Rusanov entered, the patient in the aisle turned to him with his entire torso, on which his head seemed tightly fixed and immobile, looked at Rusanov indifferently, and said:

"Here comes another cancer."

Pavel Nikolayevich did not consider it necessary to reply to this familiarity. He felt that the whole room was looking at him, but he did not want to respond by glancing around at these strange faces or even saying hello. He simply gestured to the brown-haired patient to move out of the way. The patient let Pavel Nikolayevich pass and then turned again in the same manner, moving his entire trunk, with the head riveted on top, to face Rusanov.

"Listen, brother, what kind of cancer have you got? Cancer of the what?" he asked in a muffled voice.

This question grated on Pavel Nikolayevich, who had by this time reached his bed. He looked up at the insolent fellow, tried to control his temper (though his shoulders shook), and said with dignity:

"Cancer of the *nothtng*. I don't have cancer."

The brown-haired man snorted and passed judgment for the whole ward to hear:

"Now there's a fool! If he didn't have cancer, why would they put him in here?"

Translated by Rebecca Frank

Topics for Discussion and Writing

1. Interview a registered nurse who works on the staff of a local hospital and is willing to help you gather material for an essay on the topic "Professional Nursing and Lingering Stereotypes." You might ask, for instance, if the nurse's responsibilities and status have changed much since Alcott's 1863 hospital sketch, "A Night." After the interview and some reflection, decide on your thesis; then plan and write the paper for both your class members and your instructor.

2. Alcott's "A Night" and Whitman's "The Wound-Dresser" have much in common thematically, even though their literary forms are different. Do you prefer Alcott's prose sketch to Whitman's poem? Why? Why not? Can Alcott's prose medium achieve some effects that Whitman's poetic medium cannot (and vice versa)? Why? Why not?

3. Keeping in mind Whitman's experiences as a volunteer male nurse in the Civil War, try to determine—perhaps by inquiring at a local hospital school of nursing, at a local community college school of nursing, or at a local university school of nursing—roughly how many men are in training to become registered nurses today. Are there opportunities for men to succeed in this traditionally female-dominated field? Must the word "nurse" always have a woman referent? Look up "nurse" in a college edition dictionary and report on its several meanings.

4. Discuss the doctor-narrator's attitude in "Jean Beicke" toward the nurses he works with. Examine, specifically, the implications of the following passage: "I often kid the girls. Why not? I look at some miserable specimens they've dolled up for me when I make the rounds in the morning and I tell them: Give it an enema, maybe it will get well and grow up into a cheap prostitute or something. The country needs you, brat."

5. Explain the conflict between Miss Ratched and Mr. Taber. Who finally

wins? How is it ironic that Chief Bromden, an inmate, functions as the general narrator for Kesey's novel, of which this selection is a part?

6. Comment on the Big Nurse's remark: " 'You seem to forget, *Miss* Flinn, that this is an institution for the insane.' " Is Miss Ratched at all typical of nurses you have previously encountered in literature?

7. Using *Medicine in Literature* as your primary source, locate and discuss the various nurses and other allied health personnel in literary selections. Can you draw any supportable conclusions about how creative writers usually portray these important people?

8. Write an evaluative character sketch of Carmelita Lester. Try to concentrate on her dominant personality traits and on what motivates her in the interview from Terkel's *Working*.

9. Who is Rusanov's doctor? Describe her. How do you account for the fact that in literature it is almost as surprising to find a woman doctor as it is to find a male nurse?

10. How does Solzhenitsyn's Mita come close to embodying the qualities we look for today in a professional nurse? How well does she seem to function in the admittedly poor hospital conditions?

11. In a thesis-and-support essay, compare and contrast Mita with Carmelita Lester.

Part 6

Medicine and
Its Limitations

Throughout the course of the past five parts of this anthology, we have explored—albeit selectively—what various creative writers have had to say about the topics of medicine and interpersonal relationships, medicine and humor, medicine and mental health, medicine and the scientific impulse, and medicine and the nurse. This last part of *Medicine in Literature* delves into the related themes of death, fate, and the limits of medicine. It concludes the anthology at the same time that it demonstrates how the book's six parts overlap and interconnect.

Thomas Nashe, John Donne, John Keats, and Emily Dickinson are four poets who speak both vividly and intensely about the themes of this closing part. Nashe's "Litany in Time of Plague" asserts the temporariness of life in the face of the 1592 London plague. Money cannot buy health; indeed, "Physic himself must fade." In "Hymn to God My God, in My Sickness," the poet-clergyman Donne reveals the "I" of the poem preparing for death and singing a hymn to God. His several "physicians" are now powerless, for while they can diagnose death by fever, it is man's responsibility to look beyond death to his hoped-for resurrection in the Lord: "Therefore that he may raise the Lord throws down." Keats' "When I have fears that I may cease to be" is a rather angry sonnet in which the poet, who was himself briefly in the medical profession and who was soon to die of consumption, expresses his doubts and fears when he considers what it might be like to die before his poetic and romantic goals are achieved. In Dickinson's "Death is like the insect," we are told that death can kill but that it may also be "decoyed" through drugs and surgery. And yet, if a deadly illness has progressed too "Out of reach of skill," we should fatalistically allow the disease (and therefore death) to have its will.

As we know from reading "The Haunted Quack" and "Rappaccini's Daughter" earlier, a Hawthorne story can usually be counted on to be suspenseful, provocative, and well-crafted. And "Dr. Heidegger's Experiment," a tale of youth versus age, of appearance versus reality, of the magical use of water supposedly from the famous Fountain of Youth in Florida, is no exception. Old Dr. Heidegger assembles "four venerable friends" in his study to try out this special potion on them. Do they grow younger in reality or only in their minds? Hawthorne is ambivalent on the matter. The moral of the story seems to be that we cannot reverse the aging process for long and that we don't become much wiser with age. While "Dr. Heidegger's Experiment" calls to mind the humorous and the scientific themes in two earlier parts, it also points up the limits of medicine that still exist over a hundred years after Hawthorne wrote about the "Water of Youth."

Two relatively modern poets, Robert Bridges and W. H. Auden, handle in quite different ways the death of a person whom medical science cannot save. The child is already dead in Bridges' "On a Dead Child" when the poet-physician begins his lament: "Perfect little body, without fault or stain on thee, / With promise of strength and manhood full and fair!" As the doctor readies the child for burial, he is startled by how lifelike the little one still looks, and he questions whether there is something beyond this world "that rights the disaster of this." On the other hand, Edith Gee is very much alive at the opening of Auden's seriocomic "Miss Gee." This lonely, churchgoing woman has dreams of sexual fantasy, yet prays to be kept " 'a good girl, please.' " Rather suddenly she bicycles down to see the local doctor about " 'a pain inside me.' " He wonders why she didn't come in sooner, for she has cancer, " 'And she's a goner, I fear.' " All too quickly, however, Miss Gee enters a frightening hospital ward and gets dissected (Auden purposely omits any humane description of her intervening death), laughed at, and probed by an instructor and his medical students. It is not hard to realize that Miss Gee's personhood has been sadly ignored by the world around her.

Stoicism plays an important role in both the short story "In Another Country" and the poem "Intimations of Mortality." Set in a Milan hospital, Ernest Hemingway's story sketches the wartime friendship between an American fighting for the Italians and an Italian major who unexpectedly loses his wife due to pneumonia. The futility of war, the inevitability of suffering, and the limits of medical cures are the central themes. Especially interesting is Hemingway's description of "the machines" that the men are hooked up to and that are supposed to help in therapy with their wounded limbs. Do such contraptions cure men or just help them pass the time? Does the answer make any difference? The subtitle of Phyllis McGinley's poem "Intimations of Mortality," which reads "On being told by the dentist that 'this will be over soon,' " triggers some perceptive reflections in the patient-poet on the shortness of life, the transitory nature of good and bad events, and the necessity of fate in human affairs. But while stoic acceptance is stressed, the patient is, in a sense, in control of the situation during the dental work because she sees more deeply into the nature of reality than do other people.

And finally, as a closing selection there is "The Curse of Eve" by doctor-writer Arthur Conan Doyle. This excellent story makes the perfect conclusion for *Medicine in Literature*, for it clearly brings together the book's six thematic parts. Doyle presents not only a husband and wife about to become parents for the first time, but also an exceptionally illuminating portrait of two doctors. The attentive reader of this tale of medicine and life in turn-of-the-century London will discover (1) developing interpersonal relationships; (2) several light or humorous passages; (3) the growing psychological awareness and insight of the protagonist, Robert Johnson; (4) uses for medical science as the crisis nears; (5) the presence of the nursing role in Mrs. Peyton; and (6) how at last "the great cat Fate" takes over where medicine leaves off. In short, the Doyle selection recapitulates the six main themes with which we have been concerned. Significantly, "The Curse of Eve" finishes on an essentially optimistic note: "The night had been long and dark but the day was the sweeter and the purer in consequence. London was waking up."

THOMAS NASHE

Litany in Time of Plague

Adieu, farewell earth's bliss,
This world uncertain is:
Fond are life's lustful joys,
Death proves them all but toys,
None from his darts can fly.
I am sick, I must die.
        Lord, have mercy on us!

Rich men, trust not in wealth,
Gold cannot buy you health;
Physic himself must fade,
All things to end are made.
The plague full swift goes by.
I am sick, I must die.
        Lord, have mercy on us!

Beauty is but a flower
Which wrinkles will devour;
Brightness falls from the air,
Queens have died young and fair,
Dust hath closed Helen's eye.
I am sick, I must die.
        Lord, have mercy on us!

Strength stoops unto the grave,
Worms feed on Hector brave,
Swords may not fight with fate,
Earth still holds ope her gate.
Come! come! the bells do cry.
I am sick, I must die.
        Lord, have mercy on us!

Wit with his wantonness
Tasteth death's bitterness;
Hell's executioner
Hath no ears for to hear
What vain art can reply.
I am sick, I must die.
        Lord, have mercy on us!

Haste, therefore, each degree,
To welcome destiny.
Heaven is our heritage,
Earth but a player's stage;
Mount we unto the sky.
I am sick, I must die.
        Lord, have mercy on us!

JOHN DONNE

Hymn to God My God, in My Sickness

Since I am coming to that holy room,
    Where, with thy choir of saints for evermore,
I shall be made thy music; as I come
    I tune the instrument here at the door,
    And what I must do then, think now before.

Whilst my physicians by their love are grown
    Cosmographers, and I their map, who lie
Flat on this bed, that by them may be shown
    That this is my south-west discovery
    Per fretum febris, by these strains to die,

I joy, that in these straits, I see my west;
   For, though their currents yield return to none,
What shall my west hurt me? As west and east
   In all flat maps (and I am one) are one,
   So death doth touch the resurrection.

Is the Pacific Sea my home? Or are
   The eastern riches? Is Jerusalem?
Anyan, and Magellan, and Gibraltar,
   All straits, and none but straits, are ways to them,
   Whether where Japhet dwelt, or Cham, or Shem.

We think that Paradise and Calvary,
   Christ's cross, and Adam's tree, stood in one place;
Look Lord, and find both Adams met in me;
   As the first Adam's sweat surrounds my face,
   May the last Adam's blood my soul embrace.

So, in his purple wrapped receive me Lord,
   By these his thorns give me his other crown;
And as to others' souls I preached thy word,
   Be this my text, my sermon to mine own,
   Therefore that he may raise the Lord throws down.

JOHN KEATS

When I have fears that I may cease to be

When I have fears that I may cease to be
   Before my pen has gleaned my teeming brain,
Before high-pilèd books, in charact'ry,
   Hold like rich garners the full-ripened grain;
When I behold, upon the night's starred face,
   Huge cloudy symbols of a high romance,
And think that I may never live to trace
   Their shadows, with the magic hand of chance;
And when I feel, fair creature of an hour,
   That I shall never look upon thee more,

Never have relish in the faery power
　　Of unreflecting love!—then on the shore
Of the wide world I stand alone, and think
Till Love and Fame to nothingness do sink.

EMILY DICKINSON

Death is like the insect

Death is like the insect
Menacing the tree,
Competent to kill it,
But decoyed may be.

Bait it with the balsam,
Seek it with the saw,
Baffle, if it cost you
Everything you are.

Then, if it have burrowed
Out of reach of skill—
Wring the tree and leave it,
'Tis the vermin's will.

NATHANIEL HAWTHORNE

Dr. Heidegger's Experiment

That very singular man, old Dr. Heidegger, once invited four venerable friends to meet him in his study. There were three white-bearded gentlemen, Mr. Medbourne, Colonel Killigrew, and Mr. Gascoigne, and a withered gentle-woman, whose name was the Widow Wycherly. They were all melancholy old creatures, who had been unfortunate in life, and whose greatest misfortune it was that they were not long ago in their graves. Mr. Medbourne, in the vigor of his age, had been a prosperous merchant, but had lost his all by a frantic speculation, and was now little better than a mendicant. Colonel Killigrew

had wasted his best years, and his health and substance, in the pursuit of
sinful pleasures, which had given birth to a brood of pains, such as the gout,
and divers other torments of soul and body. Mr. Gascoigne was a ruined
politician, a man of evil fame, or at least had been so till time had buried
him from the knowledge of the present generation, and made him obscure
instead of infamous. As for the Widow Wycherly, tradition tells us that she
was a great beauty in her day; but, for a long while past, she had lived in deep
seclusion, on account of certain scandalous stories which had prejudiced the
gentry of the town against her. It is a circumstance worth mentioning that each
of these three old gentlemen, Mr. Medbourne, Colonel Killigrew, and Mr.
Gascoigne, were early lovers of the Widow Wycherly, and had once been on the
point of cutting each other's throats for her sake. And, before proceeding
further, I will merely hint that Dr. Heidegger and all his four guests were
sometimes thought to be a little beside themselves,—as is not unfrequently the
case with old people, when worried either by present troubles or woful
recollections.

"My dear old friends," said Dr. Heidegger, motioning them to be seated,
"I am desirous of your assistance in one of those little experiments with which
I amuse myself here in my study."

If all stories were true, Dr. Heidegger's study must have been a very curious
place. It was a dim, old-fashioned chamber, festooned with cobwebs, and be-
sprinkled with antique dust. Around the walls stood several oaken bookcases,
the lower shelves of which were filled with rows of gigantic folios and black-
letter quartos, and the upper with little parchment-covered duodecimos. Over
the central bookcase was a bronze bust of Hippocrates, with which, according
to some authorities, Dr. Heidegger was accustomed to hold consultations in
all difficult cases of his practice. In the obscurest corner of the room stood a
tall and narrow oaken closet, with its door ajar, within which doubtfully appeared a skeleton. Between two of the bookcases hung a looking-glass, presenting its high and dusty plate within a tarnished gilt frame. Among many
wonderful stories related of this mirror, it was fabled that the spirits of all
the doctor's deceased patients dwelt within its verge, and would stare him
in the face whenever he looked thitherward. The opposite side of the chamber
was ornamented with the full-length portrait of a young lady, arrayed in the
faded magnificence of silk, satin, and brocade, and with a visage as faded as
her dress. Above half a century ago, Dr. Heidegger had been on the point of
marriage with this young lady; but, being affected with some slight disorder,
she had swallowed one of her lover's prescriptions, and died on the bridal evening. The greatest curiosity of the study remains to be mentioned; it was a
ponderous folio volume, bound in black leather, with massive silver clasps.
There were no letters on the back, and nobody could tell the title of the
book. But it was well known to be a book of magic; and once, when a
chambermaid had lifted it, merely to brush away the dust, the skeleton had
rattled in its closet, the picture of the young lady had stepped one foot upon

the floor, and several ghastly faces had peeped forth from the mirror; while
the brazen head of Hippocrates frowned, and said,—"Forbear!"

Such was Dr. Heidegger's study. On the summer afternoon of our tale a
small round table, as black as ebony, stood in the centre of the room, sustaining a cut-glass vase of beautiful form and elaborate workmanship. The sunshine came through the window, between the heavy festoons of two faded
damask curtains, and fell directly across this vase; so that a mild splendor was
reflected from it on the ashen visages of the five old people who sat around.
Four champagne glasses were also on the table.

"My dear old friends," repeated Dr. Heidegger, "may I reckon on your aid
in performing an exceedingly curious experiment?"

Now Dr. Heidegger was a very strange old gentleman, whose eccentricity
had become the nucleus for a thousand fantastic stories. Some of these fables,
to my shame be it spoken, might possibly be traced back to my own veracious
self; and if any passages of the present tale should startle the reader's faith, I
must be content to bear the stigma of a fiction monger.

When the doctor's four guests heard him talk of his proposed experiment,
they anticipated nothing more wonderful than the murder of a mouse in an
air pump, or the examination of a cobweb by the microscope, or some similar
nonsense, with which he was constantly in the habit of pestering his intimates.
But without waiting for a reply, Dr. Heidegger hobbled across the chamber,
and returned with the same ponderous folio, bound in black leather, which
common report affirmed to be a book of magic. Undoing the silver clasps, he
opened the volume, and took from among its black-letter pages a rose, or what
was once a rose, though now the green leaves and crimson petals had assumed
one brownish hue and the ancient flower seemed ready to crumble to dust in
the doctor's hands.

"This rose," said Dr. Heidegger, with a sigh, "this same withered and
crumbling flower, blossomed five and fifty years ago. It was given me by
Sylvia Ward, whose portrait hangs yonder; and I meant to wear it in my
bosom at our wedding. Five and fifty years it has been treasured between the
leaves of this old volume. Now, would you deem it possible that this rose of
half a century could ever bloom again?"

"Nonsense!" said the Widow Wycherly, with a peevish toss of her head.
"You might as well ask whether an old woman's wrinkled face could ever
bloom again."

"See!" answered Dr. Heidegger.

He uncovered the vase, and threw the faded rose into the water which it
contained. At first, it lay lightly on the surface of the fluid, appearing to imbibe none of its moisture. Soon, however, a singular change began to be visible. The crushed and dried petals stirred, and assumed a deepening tinge of
crimson, as if the flower were reviving from a deathlike slumber; the slender
stalk and twigs of foliage became green; and there was the rose of half a
century, looking as fresh as when Sylvia Ward had first given it to her lover.

It was scarcely full blown; for some of its delicate red leaves curled modestly around its moist bosom, within which two or three dewdrops were sparkling.

"That is certainly a very pretty deception," said the doctor's friends; carelessly, however, for they had witnessed greater miracles at a conjurer's show; "pray how was it effected?"

"Did you ever hear of the 'Fountain of Youth?'" asked Dr. Heidegger, "which Ponce De Leon, the Spanish adventurer, went in search of two or three centuries ago?"

"But did Ponce De Leon ever find it?" said the Widow Wycherly.

"No," answered Dr. Heidegger, "for he never sought it in the right place. The famous Fountain of Youth, if I am rightly informed, is situated in the southern part of the Floridian peninsula, not far from Lake Macaco. Its source is overshadowed by several gigantic magnolias, which, though numberless centuries old, have been kept as fresh as violets by the virtues of this wonderful water. An acquaintance of mine, knowing my curiosity in such matters, has sent me what you see in the vase."

"Ahem!" said Colonel Killigrew, who believed not a word of the doctor's story; "and what may be the effect of this fluid on the human frame?"

"You shall judge for yourself, my dear colonel," replied Dr. Heidegger; "and all of you, my respected friends, are welcome to so much of this admirable fluid as may restore to you the bloom of youth. For my own part, having had much trouble in growing old, I am in no hurry to grow young again. With your permission, therefore, I will merely watch the progress of the experiment."

While he spoke, Dr. Heidegger had been filling the four champagne glasses with the water of the Fountain of Youth. It was apparently impregnated with an effervescent gas, for little bubbles were continually ascending from the depths of the glasses, and bursting in silvery spray at the surface. As the liquor diffused a pleasant perfume, the old people doubted not that it possessed cordial and comfortable properties; and though utter sceptics as to its rejuvenescent power, they were inclined to swallow it at once. But Dr. Heidegger besought them to stay a moment.

"Before you drink, my respectable old friends," said he, "it would be well that, with the experience of a lifetime to direct you, you should draw up a few general rules for your guidance, in passing a second time through the perils of youth. Think what a sin and shame it would be, if, with your peculiar advantages, you should not become patterns of virtue and wisdom to all the young people of the age!"

The doctor's four venerable friends made him no answer, except by a feeble and tremulous laugh; so very ridiculous was the idea that, knowing how closely repentance treads behind the steps of error, they should ever go astray again.

"Drink, then," said the doctor, bowing: "I rejoice that I have so well selected the subjects of my experiment."

With palsied hands, they raised the glasses to their lips. The liquor, if it really possessed such virtues as Dr. Heidegger imputed to it, could not have been bestowed on four human beings who needed it more wofully. They looked as if they had never known what youth or pleasure was, but had been the offspring of Nature's dotage, and always the gray, decrepit, sapless, miserable creatures, who now sat stooping round the doctor's table, without life enough in their souls or bodies to be animated even by the prospect of growing young again. They drank off the water, and replaced their glasses on the table.

Assuredly there was an almost immediate improvement in the aspect of the party, not unlike what might have been produced by a glass of generous wine, together with a sudden glow of cheerful sunshine brightening over all their visages at once. There was a healthful suffusion on their cheeks, instead of the ashen hue that had made them look so corpse-like. They gazed at one another, and fancied that some magic power had really begun to smooth away the deep and sad inscriptions which Father Time had been so long engraving on their brows. The Widow Wycherly adjusted her cap, for she felt almost like a woman again.

"Give us more of this wondrous water!" cried they, eagerly. "We are younger—but we are still too old! Quick—give us more!"

"Patience, patience!" quoth Dr. Heidegger, who sat watching the experiment with philosophic coolness. "You have been a long time growing old. Surely, you might be content to grow young in half an hour! But the water is at your service."

Again he filled their glasses with the liquor of youth, enough of which still remained in the vase to turn half the old people in the city to the age of their own grandchildren. While the bubbles were yet sparkling on the brim, the doctor's four guests snatched their glasses from the table, and swallowed the contents at a single gulp. Was it delusion? even while the draught was passing down their throats, it seemed to have wrought a change on their whole systems. Their eyes grew clear and bright; a dark shade deepened among their silvery locks, they sat around the table, three gentlemen of middle age, and a woman, hardly beyond her buxom prime.

"My dear widow, you are charming!" cried Colonel Killigrew, whose eyes had been fixed upon her face, while the shadows of age were flitting from it like darkness from the crimson daybreak.

The fair widow knew, of old, that Colonel Killigrew's compliments were not always measured by sober truth; so she started up and ran to the mirror, still dreading that the ugly visage of an old woman would meet her gaze. Meanwhile, the three gentlemen behaved in such a manner as proved that the water of the Fountain of Youth possessed some intoxicating qualities; unless, indeed, their exhilaration of spirits were merely a lightsome dizziness caused by the sudden removal of the weight of years. Mr. Gascoigne's mind seemed to run on political topics, but whether relating to the past, present, or future, could not easily be determined, since the same ideas and phrases have been in vogue these fifty years. Now he rattled forth full-throated sentences about patriotism, national glory, and the people's right; now he muttered some perilous stuff or other, in a sly and doubtful whisper, so cautiously that even his own conscience could scarcely catch the secret; and now, again, he spoke in measured accents, and a deeply deferential tone, as if a royal ear were listening to his well-turned periods. Colonel Killigrew all this time had been trolling forth a jolly bottle song, and ringing his glass in symphony with the chorus, while his eyes wandered toward the buxom figure of the Widow Wycherly. On the other side of the table, Mr. Medbourne was involved in a calculation of dollars and cents, with which was strangely intermingled a project for supplying the East Indies with ice, by harnessing a team of whales to the polar icebergs.

As for the Widow Wycherly, she stood before the mirror courtesying and simpering to her own image, and greeting it as the friend whom she loved better than all the world beside. She thrust her face close to the glass, to see whether some long-remembered wrinkle or crow's foot had indeed vanished. She examined whether the snow had so entirely melted from her hair that the venerable cap could be safely thrown aside. At last, turning briskly away, she came with a sort of dancing step to the table.

"My dear old doctor," cried she, "pray favor me with another glass!"

"Certainly, my dear madam, certainly!" replied the complaisant doctor; "see! I have already filled the glasses."

There, in fact, stood the four glasses, brimful of this wonderful water, the delicate spray of which, as it effervesced from the surface, resembled the tremulous glitter of diamonds. It was now so nearly sunset that the chamber had grown duskier than ever; but a mild and moonlike splendor gleamed from within the vase, and rested alike on the four guests and on the doctor's venerable figure. He sat in a highbacked, elaborately-carved, oaken arm-chair, with a gray dignity of aspect that might have well befitted that very Father Time, whose power had never been disputed, save by this fortunate company. Even while quaffing the third draught of the Fountain of Youth, they were almost awed by the expression of his mysterious visage.

But, the next moment, the exhilarating gush of young life shot through their veins. They were now in the happy prime of youth. Age, with its miserable train of cares and sorrows and diseases, was remembered only as the trouble of a dream, from which they had joyously awoke. The fresh gloss of the soul, so early lost, and without which the world's successive scenes had been but a gallery of faded pictures, again threw its enchantment over all their prospects. They felt like new-created beings in a new-created universe.

"We are young! We are young!" they cried exultingly.

Youth, like the extremity of age, had effaced the strongly-marked characteristics of middle life, and mutually assimilated them all. They were a group of merry youngsters, almost maddened with the exuberant frolicsomeness of

their years. The most singular effect of their gayety was an impulse to mock
the infirmity and decrepitude of which they had so lately been the victims.
They laughed loudly at their old-fashioned attire, the wide-skirted coats and
flapped waistcoats of the young men, and the ancient cap and gown of the
blooming girl. One limped across the floor like a gouty grandfather; one set a
pair of spectacles astride of his nose, and pretended to pore over the black-
letter pages of the book of magic; a third seated himself in an arm-chair, and
strove to imitate the venerable dignity of Dr. Heidegger. Then all shouted
mirthfully, and leaped about the room. The Widow Wycherly—if so fresh a
damsel could be called a widow—tripped up to the doctor's chair, with a
mischievous merriment in her rosy face.

"Doctor, you dear old soul," cried she, "get up and dance with me!" And
then the four young people laughed louder than ever, to think what a queer
figure the poor old doctor would cut.

"Pray excuse me," answered the doctor quietly. "I am old and rheumatic,
and my dancing days were over long ago. But either of these gay young gentlemen will be glad of so pretty a partner."

"Dance with me, Clara!" cried Colonel Killigrew.

"No, no, I will be her partner!" shouted Mr. Gascoigne.

"She promised me her hand, fifty years ago!" exclaimed Mr. Medbourne.

They all gathered round her. One caught both her hands in his passionate
grasp—another threw his arm about her waist—the third buried his hand
among the glossy curls that clustered beneath the widow's cap. Blushing,
panting, struggling, chiding, laughing, her warm breath fanning each of their
faces by turns, she strove to disengage herself, yet still remained in their
triple embrace. Never was there a livelier picture of youthful rivalship, with
bewitching beauty for the prize. Yet, by a strange deception, owing to the
duskiness of the chamber, and the antique dresses which they still wore, the
tall mirror is said to have reflected the figures of the three old, gray, withered
grandsires, ridiculously contending for the skinny ugliness of a shrivelled
grandam.

But they were young: their burning passions proved them so. Inflamed to
madness by the coquetry of the girl-widow, who neither granted nor quite
withheld her favors, the three rivals began to interchange threatening glances.
Still keeping hold of the fair prize, they grappled fiercely at one another's
throats. As they struggled to and fro, the table was overturned, and the vase
dashed into a thousand fragments. The precious Water of Youth flowed in a
bright stream across the floor, moistening the wings of a butterfly, which,
grown old in the decline of summer, had alighted there to die. The insect
fluttered lightly through the chamber, and settled on the snowy head of Dr.
Heidegger.

"Come, come, gentlemen!—come, Madam Wycherly," exclaimed the doctor, "I really must protest against this riot."

They stood still and shivered; for it seemed as if gray Time were calling them back from their sunny youth, far down into the chill and darksome vale of years. They looked at old Dr. Heidegger, who sat in his carved arm-chair, holding the rose of half a century, which he had rescued from among the fragments of the shattered vase. At the motion of his hand, the four rioters resumed their seats; the more readily, because their violent exertions had wearied them, youthful though they were.

"My poor Sylvia's rose!" ejaculated Dr. Heidegger, holding it in the light of the sunset clouds; "it appears to be fading again."

And so it was. Even while the party were looking at it, the flower continued to shrivel up, till it became as dry and fragile as when the doctor had first thrown it into the vase. He shook off the few drops of moisture which clung to its petals.

"I love it as well thus as in its dewy freshness," observed he, pressing the withered rose to his withered lips. While he spoke, the butterfly fluttered down from the doctor's snowy head, and fell upon the floor.

His guests shivered again. A strange chillness, whether of the body or spirit they could not tell, was creeping gradually over them all. They gazed at one another, and fancied that each fleeting moment snatched away a charm, and left a deepening furrow where none had been before. Was it an illusion? Had the changes of a lifetime been crowded into so brief a space, and were they now four aged people, sitting with their old friend, Dr. Heidegger?

"Are we grown old again, so soon?" cried they, dolefully.

In truth they had. The Water of Youth possessed merely a virtue more transient than that of wine. The delirium which it created had effervesced away. Yes! they were old again. With a shuddering impulse, that showed her a woman still, the widow clasped her skinny hands before her face, and wished that the coffin lid were over it, since it could be no longer beautiful.

"Yes, friends, ye are old again," said Dr. Heidegger, "and lo! the Water of Youth is all lavished on the ground. Well—I bemoan it not; for if the fountain gushed at my very doorstep, I would not stoop to bathe my lips in it—no, though its delirium were for years instead of moments. Such is the lesson ye have taught me!"

But the doctor's four friends had taught no such lesson to themselves. They resolved forthwith to make a pilgrimage to Florida, and quaff at morning, noon, and night, from the Fountain of Youth.

ROBERT BRIDGES

On a Dead Child

Perfect little body, without fault or stain on thee,
   With promise of strength and manhood full and fair!
       Though cold and stark and bare,
The bloom and the charm of life doth awhile remain on thee.

Thy mother's treasure wert thou;—alas! no longer
   To visit her heart with wondrous joy; to be
       Thy father's pride;—ah, he
Must gather his faith together, and his strength make
       stronger.

To me, as I move thee now in the last duty,
   Dost thou with a turn or gesture anon respond;
       Startling my fancy fond
With a chance attitude of the head, a freak of beauty.

Thy hand clasps, as 'twas wont, my finger, and holds it:
   But the grasp is the clasp of Death, heartbreaking and stiff;
       Yet feels to my hand as if
'Twas still thy will, thy pleasure and trust that enfolds it.

So I lay thee there, thy sunken eyelids closing,—
   Go lie thou there in thy coffin, thy last little bed!—
       Propping thy wise, sad head,
Thy firm, pale hands across thy chest disposing.

So quiet! doth the change content thee?—Death, whither
       hath he taken thee?
   To a world, do I think, that rights the disaster of this?
       The vision of which I miss,
Who weep for the body, and wish but to warm thee and
       awaken thee?

Ah! little at best can all our hopes avail us
   To lift this sorrow, or cheer us, when in the dark,
       Unwilling, alone we embark,
And the things we have seen and have known and have
       heard of, fail us.

W. H. AUDEN

Miss Gee

Let me tell you a little story
   About Miss Edith Gee;
She lived in Clevedon Terrace
   At Number 83.

She'd a slight squint in her left eye,
   Her lips they were thin and small,
She had narrow sloping shoulders
   And she had no bust at all.

She'd a velvet hat with trimmings,
   And a dark grey serge costume;
She lived in Clevedon Terrace
   In a small bed-sitting room.

She'd a purple mac for wet days,
   A green umbrella too to take,
She'd a bicycle with shopping basket
   And a harsh back-pedal brake.

The Church of Saint Aloysius
   Was not so very far;
She did a lot of knitting,
   Knitting for that Church Bazaar.

Miss Gee looked up at the starlight
   And said, "Does anyone care
That I live in Clevedon Terrace
   On one hundred pounds a year?"

She dreamed a dream one evening
   That she was the Queen of France
And the Vicar of Saint Aloysius
   Asked Her Majesty to dance.

But a storm blew down the palace,
   She was biking through a field of corn,

And a bull with the face of the Vicar
   Was charging with lowered horn.

She could feel his hot breath behind her,
   He was going to overtake;
And the bicycle went slower and slower
   Because of that back-pedal brake.

Summer made the trees a picture,
   Winter made them a wreck;
She bicycled to the evening service
   With her clothes buttoned up to her neck.

She passed by the loving couples,
   She turned her head away;
She passed by the loving couples
   And they didn't ask her to stay.

Miss Gee sat down in the side-aisle,
   She heard the organ play;
And the choir it sang so sweetly
   At the ending of the day.

Miss Gee knelt down in the side-aisle,
   She knelt down on her knees;
"Lead me not into temptation
   But make me a good girl, please."

The days and nights went by her
   Like waves round a Cornish wreck;
She bicycled down to the doctor
   With her clothes buttoned up to her neck.

She bicycled down to the doctor,
   And rang the surgery bell;
"O, doctor, I've a pain inside me,
   And I don't feel very well."

Doctor Thomas looked her over,
   And then he looked some more;
Walked over to his wash-basin,
   Said, "Why didn't you come before?"

Doctor Thomas sat over his dinner,
    Though his wife was waiting to ring,
Rolling his bread into pellets;
    Said, "Cancer's a funny thing.

"Nobody knows what the cause is,
    Though some pretend they do;
It's like some hidden assassin
    Waiting to strike at you.

"Childless women get it,
    And men when they retire;
It's as if there had to be some outlet
    For their foiled creative fire."

His wife she rang for the servant,
    Said, "Don't be so morbid, dear";
He said: "I saw Miss Gee this evening
    And she's a goner, I fear."

They took Miss Gee to the hospital,
    She lay there a total wreck,
Lay in the ward for women
    With the bedclothes right up to her neck.

They laid her on the table,
    The students began to laugh;
And Mr. Rose the surgeon
    He cut Miss Gee in half.

Mr. Rose he turned to his students,
    Said, "Gentlemen, if you please,
We seldom see a sarcoma
    As far advanced as this."

They took her off the table,
    They wheeled away Miss Gee
Down to another department
    Where they study Anatomy.

They hung her from the ceiling,
    Yes, they hung up Miss Gee;
And a couple of Oxford Groupers
    Carefully dissected her knee.

ERNEST HEMINGWAY

In Another Country

In the fall the war was always there, but we did not go to it any more. It was cold in the fall in Milan and the dark came very early. Then the electric lights came on, and it was pleasant along the streets looking in the windows. There was much game hanging outside the shops, and the snow powdered in the fur of the foxes and the wind blew their tails. The deer hung stiff and heavy and empty, and small birds blew in the wind and the wind turned their feathers. It was a cold fall and the wind came down from the mountains.

We were all at the hospital every afternoon, and there were different ways of walking across the town through the dusk to the hospital. Two of the ways were alongside canals, but they were long. Always, though, you crossed a bridge across a canal to enter the hospital. There was a choice of three bridges. On one of them a woman sold roasted chestnuts. It was warm, standing in front of her charcoal fire, and the chestnuts were warm afterward in your pocket. The hospital was very old and very beautiful, and you entered through a gate and walked across a courtyard and out a gate on the other side. There were usually funerals starting from the courtyard. Beyond the old hospital were the new brick pavilions, and there we met every afternoon and were all very polite and interested in what was the matter, and sat in the machines that were to make so much difference.

The doctor came up to the machine where I was sitting and said: "What did you like best to do before the war? Did you practise a sport?"

I said: "Yes, football."

"Good," he said. "You will be able to play football again better than ever."

My knee did not bend and the leg dropped straight from the knee to the ankle without a calf, and the machine was to bend the knee and make it move as in riding a tricycle. But it did not bend yet, and instead the machine lurched when it came to the bending part. The doctor said: "That will pass. You are a fortunate young man. You will play football again like a champion."

In the next machine was a major who had a little hand like a baby's. He winked at me when the doctor examined his hand, which was between two leather straps that bounced up and down and flapped the stiff fingers, and said: "And will I too play football, captain-doctor?" He had been a very great fencer, and before the war the greatest fencer in Italy.

The doctor went to his office in a back room and brought a photograph which showed a hand that had been withered almost as small as the major's, before it had taken a machine course, and after was a little larger. The major held the photograph with his good hand and looked at it very carefully. "A wound?" he asked.

"An industrial accident," the doctor said.

"Very interesting, very interesting," the major said, and handed it back to the doctor.

"You have confidence?"

"No," said the major.

There were three boys who came each day who were about the same age I was. They were all three from Milan, and one of them was to be a lawyer, and one was to be a painter, and one had intended to be a soldier, and after we were finished with the machines, sometimes we walked back together to the Café Cova, which was next door to the Scala. We walked the short way through the communist quarter because we were four together. The people hated us because we were officers, and from a wine-shop some one would call out, "A basso gli ufficiali!" as we passed. Another boy who walked with us sometimes and made us five wore a black silk handkerchief across his face because he had no nose then and his face was to be rebuilt. He had gone out to the front from the military academy and been wounded within an hour after he had gone into the front line for the first time. They rebuilt his face, but he came from a very old family and they could never get the nose exactly right. He went to South America and worked in a bank. But this was a long time ago, and then we did not any of us know how long it was going to be afterward. We only knew then that there was always the war, but that we were not going to it any more.

We all had the same medals, except the boy with the black silk bandage across his face, and he had not been at the front long enough to get any medals. The tall boy with a very pale face who was to be a lawyer had been a lieutenant of Arditi and had three medals of the sort we each had only one of. He had lived a very long time with death and was a little detached. We were all a little detached, and there was nothing that held us together except that we met every afternoon at the hospital. Although, as we walked to the Cova through the tough part of town, walking in the dark, with light and singing coming out of the wine-shops, and sometimes having to walk into the street when the men and women would crowd together on the sidewalk so that we would have had to jostle them to get by, we felt held together by there being something that had happened that they, the people who disliked us, did not understand.

We ourselves all understood the Cova, where it was rich and warm and not too brightly lighted, and noisy and smoky at certain hours, and there were always girls at the tables and the illustrated papers on a rack on the wall. The girls at the Cova were very patriotic, and I found that the most patriotic people in Italy were the café girls—and I believe they are still patriotic.

The boys at first were very polite about my medals and asked me what I had done to get them. I showed them the papers, which were written in very beautiful language and full of *fratellanza* and *abnegazione,* but which really said, with the adjectives removed, that I had been given the medals because I was an American. After that their manner changed a little toward me, although I was their friend against outsiders. I was a friend, but I was never really one of them after they had read the citations, because it had been different with them and they had done very different things to get their medals. I had been wounded, it was true; but we all knew that being wounded, after all, was really an accident. I was never ashamed of the ribbons, though, and sometimes, after the cocktail hour, I would imagine myself having done all the things they had done to get their medals; but walking home at night through the empty streets with the cold wind and all the shops closed, trying to keep near the street lights, I knew that I would never have done such things, and I was very much afraid to die, and often lay in bed at night by myself, afraid to die and wondering how I would be when I went back to the front again.

The three with the medals were like hunting-hawks; and I was not a hawk, although I might seem a hawk to those who had never hunted; they, the three, knew better and so we drifted apart. But I stayed good friends with the boy who had been wounded his first day at the front, because he would never know now how he would have turned out; so he could never be accepted either, and I liked him because I thought perhaps he would not have turned out to be a hawk either.

The major, who had been the great fencer, did not believe in bravery, and spent much time while we sat in the machines correcting my grammar. He had complimented me on how I spoke Italian, and we talked together very easily. One day I had said that Italian seemed such an easy language to me that I could not take a great interest in it; everything was so easy to say. "Ah, yes," the major said. "Why, then, do you not take up the use of grammar?" So we took up the use of grammar, and soon Italian was such a difficult language that I was afraid to talk to him until I had the grammar straight in my mind.

The major came very regularly to the hospital. I do not think he ever missed a day, although I am sure he did not believe in the machines. There was a time when none of us believed in the machines, and one day the major said it was all nonsense. The machines were new then and it was we who were to prove them. It was an idiotic idea, he said, "a theory, like another." I had not learned my grammar, and he said I was a stupid impossible disgrace, and he was a fool to have bothered with me. He was a small man and he sat straight up in his chair with his right hand thrust into the machine and looked straight ahead at the wall while the straps thumped up and down with his fingers in them.

"What will you do when the war is over if it is over?" he asked me. "Speak grammatically!"

"I will go to the States."

"Are you married?"

"No, but I hope to be."

"The more of a fool you are," he said. He seemed very angry. "A man must not marry."

"Why, Signor Maggiore?"

"Don't call me 'Signor Maggiore.'"

"Why must not a man marry?"

"He cannot marry. He cannot marry," he said angrily. "If he is to lose everything, he should not place himself in a position to lose that. He should not place himself in a position to lose. He should find things he cannot lose."

He spoke very angrily and bitterly, and looked straight ahead while he talked.

"But why should he necessarily lose it?"

"He'll lose it," the major said. He was looking at the wall. Then he looked down at the machine and jerked his little hand out from between the straps and slapped it hard against his thigh. "He'll lose it," he almost shouted. "Don't argue with me!" Then he called to the attendant who ran the machines. "Come and turn this damned thing off."

He went back into the other room for the light treatment and the massage. Then I heard him ask the doctor if he might use his telephone and he shut the door. When he came back into the room, I was sitting in another machine. He was wearing his cape and had his cap on, and he came directly toward my machine and put his arm on my shoulder.

"I am so sorry," he said, and patted me on the shoulder with his good hand. "I would not be rude. My wife has just died. You must forgive me."

"Oh—" I said, feeling sick for him. "I am so sorry."

He stood there biting his lower lip. "It is very difficult," he said. "I cannot resign myself."

He looked straight past me and out through the window. Then he began to cry. "I am utterly unable to resign myself," he said and choked. And then crying, his head up looking at nothing, carrying himself straight and soldierly, with tears on both his cheeks and biting his lips, he walked past the machines and out the door.

The doctor told me that the major's wife, who was very young and whom he had not married until he was definitely invalided out of the war, had died of pneumonia. She had been sick only a few days. No one expected her to die. The major did not come to the hospital for three days. Then he came back at the usual hour, wearing a black band on the sleeve of his uniform. When he came back, there were large framed photographs around the wall, of all sorts of wounds before and after they had been cured by the machines. In front of the machine the major used were three photographs of hands like his that were completely restored. I do not know where the doctor got them. I always understood we were the first to use the machines. The photographs did not make much difference to the major because he only looked out of the window.

PHYLLIS McGINLEY

Intimations of Mortality

On being told by the dentist that "this will be over soon"

Indeed, it will soon be over, I shall be done
    With the querulous drill, the forceps, the clove-smelling
       cotton.
I can go forth into fresher air, into sun,
    This narrow anguish forgotten.

In twenty minutes or forty or half an hour,
    I shall be easy, and proud of my hard-got gold.
But your apple of comfort is eaten by worms, and sour.
    Your consolation is cold.

This will not last, and the day will be pleasant after.
    I'll dine tonight with a witty and favorite friend.
No doubt tomorrow I shall rinse my mouth with laughter.
    And also that will end.

The handful of time that I am charily granted
    Will likewise pass, to oblivion duly apprenticed.
Summer will blossom and autumn be faintly enchanted.
    Then time for the grave, or the dentist.

Because you are shrewd, my man, and your hand is clever,
    You must not believe your words have a charm to spell
       me.
There was never a half of an hour that lasted forever.
    Be quiet. You need not tell me.

SIR ARTHUR CONAN DOYLE

The Curse of Eve

Robert Johnson was an essentially commonplace man, with no feature to
distinguish him from a million others. He was pale of face, ordinary in looks,
neutral in opinions, thirty years of age, and a married man. By trade he was
a gentleman's outfitter in the New North Road, and the competition of business squeezed out of him the little character that was left. In his hope of
conciliating customers he had become cringing and pliable, until working
ever in the same routine from day to day he seemed to have sunk into a soul-
less machine rather than a man. No great question had ever stirred him. At
the end of this smug century, self-contained in his own narrow circle, it
seemed impossible that any of the mighty, primitive passions of mankind
could ever reach him. Yet birth, and lust, and illness, and death are change-
less things, and when one of these harsh facts springs out upon a man at
some sudden turn of the path of life, it dashes off for the moment his mask
of civilisation and gives a glimpse of the stranger and stronger face below.

Johnson's wife was a quiet little woman, with brown hair and gentle ways.
His affection for her was the one positive trait in his character. Together
they would lay out the shop window every Monday morning, the spotless
shirts in their green cardboard boxes below, the neckties above hung in
rows over the brass rails, the cheap studs glistening from the white cards at
either side, while in the background were the rows of cloth caps and the bank
of boxes in which the more valuable hats were screened from the sunlight.
She kept the books and sent out the bills. No one but she knew the joys and
sorrows which crept into his small life. She had shared his exultation when
the gentleman who was going to India had bought ten dozen shirts and an
incredible number of collars, and she had been stricken as he when, after
the goods had gone, the bill was returned from the hotel address with the
intimation that no such person had lodged there. For five years they had
worked, building up the business, thrown together all the more closely because their marriage had been a childless one. Now, however, there were
signs that a change was at hand, and that speedily. She was unable to come
downstairs, and her mother, Mrs. Peyton, came over from Camberwell to
nurse her and to welcome her grandchild.

Little qualms of anxiety came over Johnson as his wife's time approached.
However, after all, it was a natural process. Other men's wives went through it
unharmed, and why should not his? He was himself one of a family of fourteen, and yet his mother was alive and hearty. It was quite the exception

for anything to go wrong. And yet in spite of his reasonings the remembrance of his wife's condition was always like a sombre background to all his other thoughts.

Doctor Miles of Bridport Place, the best man in the neighbourhood, was retained five months in advance, and, as time stole on, many little packets of absurdly small white garments with frill work and ribbons began to arrive among the big consignments of male necessities. And then one evening, as Johnson was ticketing the scarves in the shop, he heard a bustle upstairs, and Mrs. Peyton came running down to say that Lucy was bad and that she thought the doctor ought to be there without delay.

It was not Robert Johnson's nature to hurry. He was prim and staid and liked to do things in an orderly fashion. It was a quarter of a mile from the corner of the New North Road where his shop stood to the doctor's house in Bridport Place. There were no cabs in sight, so he set off on foot, leaving the lad to mind the shop. At Bridport Place he was told that the doctor had just gone to Harman Street to attend a man in a fit. Johnson started off for Harman Street, losing a little of his primness as he became more anxious. Two full cabs but no empty ones passed him on the way. At Harman Street he learned that the doctor had gone on to a case of measles, fortunately he had left the address—69 Dunstan Road, at the other side of the Regent's Canal. Johnson's primness had vanished now as he thought of the women waiting at home, and he began to run as hard as he could down the Kingsland Road. Some way along he sprang into a cab which stood by the curb and drove to Dunstan Road. The doctor had just left, and Robert Johnson felt inclined to sit down upon the steps in despair.

Fortunately he had not sent the cab away, and he was soon back in Bridport Place. Doctor Miles had not returned yet, but they were expecting him every instant. Johnson waited, drumming his fingers on his knees, in a high, dim-lit room, the air of which was charged with a faint, sickly smell of ether. The furniture was massive, and the books in the shelves were sombre, and a squat black clock ticked mournfully on the mantelpiece. It told him that it was half-past seven, and that he had been gone an hour and a quarter. Whatever would the women think of him! Every time that a distant door slammed he sprang from his chair in a quiver of eagerness. His ears strained to catch the deep notes of the doctor's voice. And then, suddenly, with a gush of joy he heard a quick step outside, and the sharp click of the key in the lock. In an instant he was out in the hall, before the doctor's foot was over the threshold.

"If you please, doctor, I've come for you," he cried; "the wife was taken bad at six o'clock."

He hardly knew what he expected the doctor to do. Something very energetic, certainly—to seize some drugs, perhaps, and rush excitedly with him through the gaslit streets. Instead of that Doctor Miles threw his umbrella into the rack, jerked off his hat with a somewhat peevish gesture, and pushed Johnson back into the room.

"Let's see! You *did* engage me, didn't you?" he asked in no very cordial voice.

"Oh, yes, doctor, last November. Johnson, the outfitter, you know, in the New North Road."

"Yes, yes. It's a bit overdue," said the doctor, glancing at a list of names in a note-book with a very shiny cover. "Well, how is she?"

"I don't——"

"Ah, of course, it's your first. You'll know more about it next time."

"Mrs. Peyton said it was time you were there, sir."

"My dear sir, there can be no very pressing hurry in a first case. We shall have an all-night affair, I fancy. You can't get an engine to go without coals, Mr. Johnson, and I have had nothing but a light lunch."

"We could have something cooked for you—something hot and a cup of tea."

"Thank you, but I fancy my dinner is actually on the table. I can do no good in the earlier stages. Go home and say that I'm coming, and I will be round immediately afterwards."

A sort of horror filled Robert Johnson as he gazed at this man who could think about his dinner at such a moment. He had not imagination enough to realise that the experience which seemed so appallingly important to him, was the merest everyday matter of business to the medical man who could not have lived for a year had he not, amid the rush of work, remembered what was due to his own health. To Johnson he seemed little better than a monster. His thoughts were bitter as he sped back to his shop.

"You've taken your time," said his mother-in-law reproachfully, looking down the stairs as he entered.

"I couldn't help it!" he gasped. "Is it over?"

"Over! She's got to be worse, poor dear, before she can be better. Where's Doctor Miles?"

"He's coming after he's had dinner."

The old woman was about to make some reply, when, from the half-opened door behind, a high, whinnying voice cried out for her. She ran back and closed the door, while Johnson, sick at heart, turned into the shop. There he sent the lad home and busied himself frantically in putting up shutters and turning out boxes. When all was closed and finished he seated himself in the parlour behind the shop. But he could not sit still. He rose incessantly to walk a few paces and then fall back into a chair once more. Suddenly the clatter of china fell upon his ear, and he saw the maid pass the door with a cup on a tray and a smoking teapot.

"Who is that for, Jane?" he asked.

"For the mistress, Mr. Johnson. She says she would fancy it."

There was immeasurable consolation to him in that homely cup of tea. It wasn't so very bad after all if his wife could think of such things. So light-hearted was he that he asked for a cup also. He had just finished it when the doctor arrived, with a small black-leather bag in his hand.

"Well, how is she?" he asked genially.

"Oh, she's very much better," said Johnson, with enthusiasm.

"Dear me, that's bad!" said the doctor. "Perhaps it will do if I look in on my morning round?"

"No, no," cried Johnson, clutching at his thick frieze overcoat. "We are so glad that you have come. And, doctor, please come down soon and let me know what you think about it."

The doctor passed upstairs, his firm, heavy steps resounding through the house. Johnson could hear his boots creaking as he walked about the floor above him, and the sound was a consolation to him. It was crisp and decided, the tread of a man who had plenty of self-confidence. Presently, still straining his ears to catch what was going on, he heard the scraping of a chair as it was drawn along the floor, and a moment later he heard the door fly open, and some one came rushing downstairs. Johnson sprang up with his hair bristling, thinking that some dreadful thing had occurred, but it was only his mother-in-law, incoherent with excitement and searching for scissors and some tape. She vanished again and Jane passed up the stairs with a pile of newly-aired linen. Then, after an interval of silence, Johnson heard the heavy, creaking tread and the doctor came down into the parlour.

"That's better," said he, pausing with his hand upon the door. "You look pale, Mr. Johnson."

"Oh no, sir, not at all," he answered deprecatingly, mopping his brow with his handkerchief.

"There is no immediate cause for alarm," said Doctor Miles. "The case is not all that we could wish it. Still we will hope for the best."

"Is there danger, sir?" gasped Johnson.

"Well, there is always danger, of course. It is not altogether a favourable case, but still it might be much worse. I have given her a draught. I saw as I passed that they have been doing a little building opposite to you. It's an improving quarter. The rents go higher and higher. You have a lease of your own little place, eh?"

"Yes, sir, yes!" cried Johnson, whose ears were straining for every sound from above, and who felt none the less that it was very soothing that the doctor should be able to chat so easily at such a time. "That's to say no, sir, I am a yearly tenant."

"Ah, I should get a lease if I were you. There's Marshall, the watchmaker, down the street, I attended his wife twice and saw him through the typhoid when they took up the drains in Prince Street. I assure you his landlord sprung his rent nearly forty a year and he had to pay or clear out."

"Did his wife get through it, doctor?"

"Oh yes, she did very well. Hullo! Hullo!"

He slanted his ear to the ceiling with a questioning face, and then darted swiftly from the room.

It was March and the evenings were chill, so Jane had lit the fire, but the wind drove the smoke downwards and the air was full of its acrid taint. Johnson felt chilled to the bone, though rather by his apprehensions than by the weather. He crouched over the fire with his thin white hands held out to the blaze. At ten o'clock Jane brought in the joint of cold meat and laid his place for supper, but he could not bring himself to touch it. He drank a glass of the beer, however, and felt the better for it. The tension of his nerves seemed to have reacted upon his hearing, and he was able to follow the most trivial things in the room above. Once, when the beer was still heartening him, he nerved himself to creep on tiptoe up the stair and to listen to what was going on. The bedroom door was half an inch open, and through the slit he could catch a glimpse of the clean-shaven face of the doctor, looking wearier and more anxious than before. Then he rushed downstairs like a lunatic, and running to the door he tried to distract his thoughts by watching what was going on in the street. The shops were all shut, and some rollicking boon companions came shouting along from the public-house. He stayed at the door until the stragglers had thinned down, and then came back to his seat by the fire. In his dim brain he was asking himself questions which had never intruded themselves before. Where was the justice of it? What had his sweet, innocent little wife done that she should be used so? Why was Nature so cruel? He was frightened at his own thoughts, and yet wondered that they had never occurred to him before.

As the early morning drew in, Johnson, sick at heart and shivering in every limb, sat with his great-coat huddled round him, staring at the grey ashes and waiting hopelessly for some relief. His face was white and clammy, and his nerves had been numbed into a half-conscious state by the long monotony of misery. But suddenly all his feelings leapt into keen life again as he heard the bedroom door open and the doctor's steps upon the stair. Robert Johnson was precise and unemotional in everyday life, but he almost shrieked now as he rushed forward to know if it were over.

One glance at the stern, drawn face which met him showed that it was no pleasant news which had sent the doctor downstairs. His appearance had altered as much as Johnson's during the last few hours. His hair was on end, his face flushed, his forehead dotted with beads of perspiration. There was a peculiar fierceness in his eye, and about the lines of his mouth, a fighting look as befitted a man who for hours on end had been striving with the hungriest of foes for the most precious of prizes. But there was a sadness too, as though his grim opponent had been overmastering him. He sat down and leaned his head upon his hand like a man who is fagged out.

"I thought it my duty to see you, Mr. Johnson, and to tell you that it is a very nasty case. Your wife's heart is not strong, and she has some symptoms which I do not like. What I wanted to say is that if you would like to have a second opinion I shall be very glad to meet any one whom you might suggest."

Johnson was so dazed by his want of sleep and the evil news that he could hardly grasp the doctor's meaning. The other, seeing him hesitate, thought that he was considering the expense.

"Smith or Hawley would come for two guineas," said he. "But I think Pritchard of the City Road is the best man."

"Oh yes, bring the best man," cried Johnson.

"Pritchard would want three guineas. He is a senior man, you see."

"I'd give him all I have if he would pull her through. Shall I run for him?"

"Yes. Go to my house first and ask for the green baize bag. The assistant will give it to you. Tell him I want the A.C.E. mixture. Her heart is too weak for chloroform. Then go for Pritchard and bring him back with you."

It was heavenly for Johnson to have something to do and to feel that he was of some use to his wife. He ran swiftly to Bridport Place, his footfalls clattering through the silent streets, and the big dark policemen turning their yellow funnels of light on him as he passed. Two tugs at the night-bell brought down a sleepy, half-clad assistant, who handed him a stoppered glass bottle and a cloth bag which contained something which clinked when you moved it. Johnson thrust the bottle into his pocket, seized the green bag, and pressing his hat firmly down ran as hard as he could set foot to ground until he was in the City Road and saw the name of Pritchard engraved in white upon a red ground. He bounded in triumph up the three steps which led to the door, and as he did so there was a crash behind him. His precious bottle was in fragments upon the pavement.

For a moment he felt as if it were his wife's body that was lying there. But the run had freshened his wits and he saw that the mischief might be repaired. He pulled vigorously at the night-bell.

"Well, what's the matter?" asked a gruff voice at his elbow. He started back and looked up at the windows, but there was no sign of life. He was approaching the bell again with the intention of pulling it, when a perfect roar burst from the wall.

"I can't stand shivering here all night," cried the voice. "Say who you are and what you want or I shut the tube."

Then for the first time Johnson saw that the end of a speaking tube hung out of the wall just above the bell. He shouted up it—

"I want you to come with me to meet Doctor Miles at a confinement at once."

"How far?" shrieked the irascible voice.

"The New North Road, Hoxton."

"My consultation fee is three guineas, payable at the time."

"All right," shouted Johnson. "You are to bring a bottle of A.C.E. mixture with you."

"All right! Wait a bit!"

Five minutes later an elderly, hard-faced man with grizzled hair flung open the door. As he emerged a voice from somewhere in the shadows cried—

"Mind you take your cravat, John," and he impatiently growled something over his shoulder in reply.

The consultant was a man who had been hardened by a life of ceaseless labour, and who had been driven, as so many others have been, by the needs of his own increasing family to set the commercial before the philanthropic side of his profession. Yet beneath his rough crust he was a man with a kindly heart.

"We don't want to break a record," said he, pulling up and panting after attempting to keep up with Johnson for five minutes. "I would go quicker if I could, my dear sir, and I quite sympathise with your anxiety, but really I can't manage it."

So Johnson, on fire with impatience, had to slow down until they reached the New North Road, when he ran ahead and had the door open for the doctor when he came. He heard the two meet outside the bedroom, and caught scraps of their conversation. "Sorry to knock you up—nasty case—decent people." Then it sank into a mumble and the door closed behind them.

Johnson sat up in his chair now, listening keenly, for he knew that a crisis must be at hand. He heard the two doctors moving about, and was able to distinguish the step of Pritchard, which had a drag in it, from the clean, crisp sound of the other's footfall. There was silence for a few minutes and then a curious drunken, mumbling sing-song voice came quavering up, very unlike anything which he had heard hitherto. All the same time a sweetish, insidious scent, imperceptible perhaps to any nerves less strained than his, crept down the stairs and penetrated into the room. The voice dwindled into a mere drone and finally sank away into silence, and Johnson gave a long sigh of relief for he knew that the drug had done its work and that, come what might, there should be no more pain for the sufferer.

But soon the silence became even more trying to him than the cries had been. He had no clue now as to what was going on, and his mind swarmed with horrible possibilities. He rose and went to the bottom of the stairs again. He heard the clink of metal against metal, and the subdued murmur of the doctors' voices. Then he heard Mrs. Peyton say something, in a tone as of fear or expostulation, and again the doctors murmured together. For twenty minutes he stood there leaning against the wall, listening to the occasional rumbles of talk without being able to catch a word of it. And then of a sudden there rose out of the silence the strangest little piping cry, and Mrs. Peyton screamed out in her delight and the man ran into the parlour and flung himself down upon the horse-hair sofa, drumming his heels on it in his ecstasy.

But often the great cat Fate lets us go, only to clutch us again in a fiercer grip. As minute after minute passed and still no sound came from above save those thin, glutinous cries, Johnson cooled from his frenzy of joy, and lay breathless with his ears straining. They were moving slowly about. They were talking in subdued tones. Still minute after minute passing, and no word from the voice for which he listened. His nerves were dulled by his night of trouble, and he waited in limp wretchedness upon his sofa. There he still sat when the doctors came down to him—a bedraggled, miserable figure with his face grimy and his hair unkempt from his long vigil. He rose as they entered, bracing himself against the mantelpiece.

"Is she dead?" he asked.

"Doing well," answered the doctor.

And at the words that little conventional spirit which had never known until that night the capacity for fierce agony which lay within it, learned for the second time that there were springs of joy also which it had never tapped before. His impulse was to fall upon his knees, but he was shy before the doctors.

"Can I go up?"

"In a few minutes."

"I'm sure, doctor. I'm very—I'm very——" he grew inarticulate. "Here are your three ginueas, Doctor Pritchard. I wish they were three hundred."

"So do I," said the senior man, and they laughed as they shook hands.

Johnson opened the shop door for them and heard their talk as they stood for an instant outside.

"Looked nasty at one time."

"Very glad to have your help."

"Delighted, I'm sure. Won't you step round and have a cup of coffee?"

"No, thanks. I'm expecting another case."

The firm step and the dragging one passed away to the right and the left. Johnson turned from the door still with that turmoil of joy in his heart. He seemed to be making a new start in life. He felt that he was a stronger and a deeper man. Perhaps all this suffering had an object then. It might prove to be a blessing both to his wife and to him. The very thought was one which he would have been incapable of conceiving twelve hours before. He was full of new emotions. If there had been a harrowing, there had been a planting too.

"Can I come up?" he cried, and then, without waiting for an answer, he took the steps three at a time.

Mrs. Peyton was standing by a soapy bath with a bundle in her hands. From under the curve of a brown shawl there looked out at him the strangest little red face with crumpled features, moist, loose lips, and eyelids which quivered like a rabbit's nostrils. The weak neck had let the head topple over, and it rested upon the shoulder.

"Kiss it, Robert!" cried the grandmother. "Kiss your son!"

But he felt a resentment to the little, red, blinking creature. He could not forgive it yet for that long night of misery. He caught sight of a white face in the bed and he ran towards it with such love and pity as his speech could find no words for.

"Thank God it is over! Lucy, dear, it was dreadful!"

"But I'm so happy now. I never was so happy in my life."

Her eyes were fixed upon the brown bundle.

"You mustn't talk," said Mrs. Peyton.

"But don't leave me," whispered his wife.

So he sat in silence with his hand in hers. The lamp was burning dim and the first cold light of dawn was breaking through the window. The night had been long and dark but the day was the sweeter and the purer in consequence. London was waking up. The roar began to rise from the street. Lives had come and lives had gone, but the great machine was still working out its dim and tragic destiny.

Topics for Discussion and Writing

1. Nashe's "Litany in Time of Plague" is but one short poem on a topic that has interested creative writers throughout the ages, from classical to modern times. Read your library's copy of *The Plague* (1947) by Albert Camus. Report to the class on this medical novel's themes and characters. Try to persuade the class to read *The Plague* sometime in the near future. Be concrete and specific in your report.

2. How exactly is the physician limited in the Nashe and Donne poems? Where do both poets turn for hope or salvation?

3. Explicate the last two and one-half lines of Keats' sonnet. How do they serve to summarize this rather bitter poem?

4. Explain the gardener-tree versus physician-patient analogy in "Death is like the insect." Does Dickinson seem to be advocating a kind of euthanasia at the end of her short poem?

5. Write one well-developed and very specific paragraph discussing the "lesson" that Dr. Heidegger finally claims his four old friends have taught him.

6. Contrast Bridges' treatment of the child in "On a Dead Child" with Auden's treatment of Edith Gee in "Miss Gee." How does the tone of the first poem differ from that of the second?

7. What is the significance of Miss Gee's bicycling "down to the doctor / With her clothes buttoned up to her neck"? And why does Auden tell that she "Lay in the ward for women / With the bedclothes right up to her neck"?

8. Can you detect any instances of irony in the story "In Another Country"? How do these contribute to Hemingway's theme? What, in fact, is the theme or central message here?

9. Write a brief continuation of Hemingway's story. Pick up where the last sentence—"The photographs did not make much difference to the major because he only looked out of the window"—leaves off. Be prepared to share your fictional continuation with the class.

10. Write an argument paper in which you defend why *your* continuation of "In Another Country" is appropriate. Be sure to attach your brief continuation (see topic 9 above) to your essay.

11. Why in McGinley's "Intimations of Mortality" is the dentist's "apple of comfort . . . eaten by worms, and sour"? And why is his consolation "cold"?

12. In order to review the general topic of medicine in literature, trace the various resonances of this anthology's six major thematic areas throughout Doyle's "The Curse of Eve."

A Selected Bibliography

GETTING STARTED: GENERAL REFERENCE WORKS

Ehrenreich, Barbara, and English, Deirdre. *Witches, Midwives, and Nurses.* Old Westbury, N.Y.: Feminist Press, 1972.

Gibson, William Carleton. *Creative Minds in Medicine: Scientific, Humanistic, and Cultural Contributions by Physicians.* Springfield, Ill.: Charles C. Thomas, 1963.

Hoffman, Frederick. *The Mortal No: Death and the Modern Imagination.* Princeton, N.J.: Princeton University Press, 1964.

Hughes, Muriel Joy. *Women Healers in Medieval Life and Literature.* New York: King's Crown Press, 1943.

Majno, Guido. *The Healing Hand: Man and Wound in the Ancient World.* Cambridge, Mass.: Harvard University Press, 1975.

Osborne, Nancy F. *The Doctor in the French Literature of the Sixteenth Century.* New York: King's Crown Press, 1946.

Riedman, Sarah R. *Masters of the Scalpel: The Story of Surgery.* New York: Rand McNally, 1962.

Selzer, Richard. *Mortal Lessons: Notes on the Art of Surgery.* New York: Simon & Schuster, 1976.

Sigerist, Henry E. *Civilization and Disease.* Chicago: University of Chicago Press, 1965.

Silvette, Herbert. *The Doctor on the Stage: Medicine and Medical Men in Seventeenth-Century England,* edited by Francelia Butler. Knoxville: University of Tennessee Press, 1967.

Stone, Alan A., and Stone, Sue Smart. *The Abnormal Personality Through Literature.* Englewood Cliffs, N.J.: Prentice-Hall, 1966.

Thomas, Clayton L., ed. *Taber's Cyclopedic Medical Dictionary.* 12th rev. ed. Philadelphia: F. A. Davis, 1973.

Trautmann, Joanne, and Pollard, Carol. *Literature and Medicine: Topics, Titles & Notes.* Philadelphia: Society for Health and Human Values, 1975.

Ussery, Huling E. *Chaucer's Physician: Medicine and Literature in Fourteenth-Century England.* New Orleans: Tulane Studies in English, 1971.

Young, Francis Brett. "The Doctor in Literature." In *Essays by Divers Hands: Transactions of the Royal Society of Literature of the United Kingdom,* edited by Hugh Walpole. London: Oxford University Press, 1936.

PART ONE: MEDICINE AND INTERPERSONAL RELATIONSHIPS

Aldridge, Ira. *The Black Doctor.* In *Black Theater, U.S.A.*, edited by James V. Hatch and Ted Shine. New York: Free Press, 1974.

Chekhov, Anton. "An Attack of Nerves." In *The Portable Chekhov*, edited by Avrahm Yarmolinsky. New York: Viking Press, 1965.

Cronin, A. J. *The Citadel.* Boston: Little, Brown, 1937.

Maugham, W. Somerset. "Sanatorium." In *The Complete Short Stories of W. Somerset Maugham: Vol. 2, The World Over.* Garden City, N.Y.: Doubleday, 1952.

Norris, Frank. *McTeague.* New York: New American Library, 1964.

Oates, Joyce Carol. *Wonderland.* Greenwich, Conn.: Fawcett, 1971.

Schnitzler, Arthur. *La Ronde.* In *Drama in the Modern World: Plays and Essays, Alternate Edition*, edited by Samuel A. Weiss. Lexington, Mass.: D. C. Heath, 1974.

Selzer, Richard. *Rituals of Surgery.* New York: Harper's Magazine Press, 1974.

Sexton, Anne. "The Abortion." In *All My Pretty Ones.* Boston: Houghton Mifflin, 1962.

Sheed, Wilfred. *People Will Always Be Kind.* New York: Farrar, Straus & Giroux, 1973.

PART TWO: MEDICINE AND HUMOR

Fielding, Henry. *An Old Man Taught Wisdom or, The Virgin Unmasked; A Farce.* In *The Complete Works of Henry Fielding, Esq.: Plays and Poems, Vol 10.* New York: Barnes & Noble, 1967.

Holmes, Oliver Wendell. "Rip Van Winkle, M.D." In *The Complete Poetical Works of Oliver Wendell Holmes*, edited by Horace E. Scudder. Boston: Houghton Mifflin, 1923.

Hope, A. D. "The Bed." In *Collected Poems: 1930–1970.* Sydney, Australia: Angus & Robertson, 1972.

Jonson, Ben. *The Alchemist.* In *Stuart Plays*, edited by Arthur H. Nethercot. New York: Holt, Rinehart & Winston, 1971.

———. *Volpone, or The Fox.* In *Stuart Plays*, edited by Arthur H. Nethercot. New York: Holt, Rinehart & Winston, 1971.

Molière. *The Imaginary Invalid.* In *The Misanthrope and Other Plays*, translated by Donald M. Frame. New York: New American Library, 1968.

Nichols, Peter. *Joe Egg.* New York: Grove Press, 1967.

Poe, Edgar Allan. "The Man That Was Used Up." In *Introduction to Poe*, edited by E. W. Carlson. Glenview, Ill.: Scott, Foresman, 1967.

Roth, Philip. *Portnoy's Complaint.* New York: Random House, 1969.

Shapiro, Karl. "Drug Store." In *Selected Poems.* New York: Random House, 1969.

PART THREE: MEDICINE AND MENTAL HEALTH

Crabbe, George. "Sir Eustace Grey." In *The Poetical Works of George Crabbe*, edited by A. J. Carlyle and R. M. Carlyle. London: Oxford University Press, 1932.

Freud, Sigmund. *An Outline of Psychoanalysis*. Translated by James Strachey. New York: W. W. Norton, 1963.

Gide, Andre. *The Immoralist*. Translated by Richard Howard. New York: Bantam Books, 1970.

Green, Hannah. *I Never Promised You a Rose Garden*. New York: New American Library, 1964.

Ibsen, Henrik. *Ghosts*. In *Ghosts and Three Other Plays*, translated by Michael Meyer. Garden City, N.Y.: Anchor Books, 1966.

Oates, Joyce Carol. "In the Region of Ice." In *The Wheel of Love and Other Stories*. New York: Vanguard Press, 1970.

O'Connor, Flannery. "The Lame Shall Enter First." In *Everything That Rises Must Converge*. New York: Farrar, Straus & Giroux, 1965.

Plath, Sylvia. *The Bell Jar*. New York: Bantam Books, 1971.

Sexton, Anne. *To Bedlam and Part Way Back*. Boston: Houghton Mifflin, 1960.

Strindberg, August. *The Father*. In *The Father and A Dream Play*, translated by Valborg Anderson. New York: Appleton-Century-Crofts, 1964.

PART FOUR: MEDICINE AND THE SCIENTIFIC IMPULSE

Doyle, Sir Arthur Conan. "A Medical Document." In *The Man from Archangel and Other Tales of Adventure*. Freeport, N.Y.: Books for Libraries, 1969.

Huxley, Aldous. *Brave New World*. New York: Bantam Books, 1958.

Ibsen, Henrik. *An Enemy of the People*. In *Ghosts and Three Other Plays*, translated by Michael Meyer. Garden City, N.Y.: Anchor Books, 1966.

Lewis, Sinclair. *Arrowsmith*. New York: New American Library, 1961.

More, Thomas. *Utopia*. Translated by H. V. S. Ogden. New York: Appleton-Century-Crofts, 1949.

Neihardt, John G. "The Powers of the Bison and the Elk." In *Black Elk Speaks*. New York: Pocket Books, 1972.

Pasternak, Boris. *Doctor Zhivago*. New York: New American Library, 1960.

Poe, Edgar Allan. "Sonnet—To Science." In *Introduction to Poe*, edited by E. W. Carlson. Glenview, Ill.: Scott, Foresman, 1967.

Shaw, Bernard. "Preface on Doctors" and *The Doctor's Dilemma*. In *Complete Plays with Prefaces. Vol. 1*. New York: Dodd, Mead, 1962.

Williams, William Carlos. "A Night in June." In *The Farmers' Daughters: The Collected Stories of William Carlos Williams*. Norfolk, Conn.: New Directions, 1961.

PART FIVE: MEDICINE AND THE NURSE

Aiken, Conrad. "Mr. Arcularis." In *The Collected Short Stories of Conrad Aiken.* Cleveland: World, 1960.

Alcott, Louisa May. *Hospital Sketches.* Edited by Bessie Z. Jones. Cambridge, Mass.: Harvard University Press, 1960.

Boyle, Kay. "The White Horses of Vienna." In *The White Horses of Vienna and Other Stories.* New York: Harcourt, Brace, 1936.

Burgess, Anthony. *The Doctor Is Sick.* New York: W. W. Norton, 1960.

Choromanski, Michal. *Jealousy and Medicine.* Translated by Eileen Arthurton-Barker. Norfolk, Conn.: New Directions, 1964.

Kesey, Ken. *One Flew Over the Cuckoo's Nest.* New York: New American Library, 1962.

Lessing, Doris. *A Proper Marriage.* New York: Simon & Schuster, 1964.

Porter, Katherine Anne. "Pale Horse, Pale Rider." In *Pale Horse, Pale Rider.* New York: Harcourt, Brace, 1937.

Roth, Philip. *The Breast.* New York: Holt, Rinehart & Winston, 1972.

Solzhenitsyn, Aleksandr I. *The Cancer Ward.* Translated by Rebecca Frank. New York: Dell, 1968.

PART SIX: MEDICINE AND ITS LIMITATIONS

Camus, Albert. *The Plague.* Translated by Stuart Gilbert. New York: Modern Library, 1948.

Defoe, Daniel. *A Journal of the Plague Year.* New York: New American Library, 1960.

Hemingway, Ernest. *A Farewell to Arms.* New York: Scribner's, 1929.

Johnson, Samuel. "On the Death of Dr. Robert Levet." In *Rasselas, Poems, and Selected Prose,* edited by Bertrand H. Bronson. New York: Holt, Rinehart & Winston, 1958.

Kafka, Franz. *The Metamorphosis.* Translated by Stanley Corngold. New York: Bantam Books, 1972.

Keats, John. "To Charles Brown, 30 November 1820." In *The Letters of John Keats: 1814–1821. vol. 2,* edited by Hyder Edward Rollins. Cambridge, Mass.: Harvard University Press, 1958.

Lawrence, D. H. "The Ship of Death." In *Selected Poems.* New York: Viking Press, 1959.

Marlowe, Christopher. *Tamburlaine the Great: Part Two.* In *The Complete Plays of Christopher Marlowe,* edited by Irving Ribner. New York: Odyssey Press, 1963.

Orwell, George. "How the Poor Die." In *The Orwell Reader.* New York: Harcourt, Brace, 1956.

Tolstoy, Leo. "The Death of Ivan Ilych." In *The Narrative Sensibility: An Introduction to Fiction,* edited by Reloy Garcia and Lloyd Hubenka. New York: David McKay, 1976.